ANESTHETIC TOXICITY

ANESTHETIC TOXICITY

Editors

Susan A. Rice, Ph.D., D.A.B.T.
Susan A. Rice and Associates, Inc.
Sunnyvale, California and
Department of Anesthesia
Stanford University School of Medicine
Stanford, California

Kevin J. Fish, M.Sc., M.B., Ch.B., F.R.C.A., F.R.C.P.(C)
Department of Anesthesia
Stanford University School of Medicine
Stanford, California and
Department of Anesthesia
Veterans Affairs Medical Center
Palo Alto, California

RAVEN PRESS 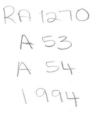 **NEW YORK**

Raven Press, Ltd., 1185 Avenue of the Americas, New York, New York 10036

Made in the United States of America

Library of Congress Cataloging-in-Publication Data

Anesthetic toxicity / editors, Susan A. Rice and Kevin J. Fish.
      p.   cm.
    Includes bibliographical references and index.
    ISBN 0-7817-0202-X
    1. Anesthetics—Toxicology.   I. Rice, Susan A.   II. Fish, Kevin J.
    [DNLM: 1. Anesthetics—toxicity.   QV 81 A579 1994]
  RA1270.A53A54   1994
  617.9′6—dc20
  DNLM/DLC
  for Library of Congress   93-39550

9 8 7 6 5 4 3 2 1

Contents

Contributors

C. Murray Ardies, Ph.D.   *Center for Exercise Science and Cardiovascular Research, Northeastern Illinois University, 5500 N. St. Louis Avenue, Chicago, Illinois 60625*

Max T. Baker, Ph.D.   *Department of Anesthesia, University of Iowa, Iowa City, Iowa 52242*

Kristie L. Ebi, Ph.D., M.P.H.   *EMF Health Studies Program, Environment Division, Electric Power Research Institute, 3412 Hillview Avenue, Palo Alto, California 94304*

Hal S. Feldman, D.Sc.   *Department of Anesthesia Research Laboratories, Brigham and Women's Hospital, Harvard Medical School, 75 Francis Street, Boston, Massachusetts 02115*

Kevin J. Fish, M.Sc., M.B., Ch.B., F.R.C.A., F.R.C.P.(C)   *Department of Anesthesia, Stanford University School of Medicine, Stanford, California 94305, and Department of Anesthesia, Veterans Affairs Medical Center, 3801 Miranda Avenue, Palo Alto, California 94304*

Brian P. Kavanagh, M.B., M.R.C.P.(I), F.R.C.P.(C)   *Intensive Care Medicine, Stanford University School of Medicine, Stanford, California 94305*

Donald D. Koblin, Ph.D., M.D.   *Anesthesiology Service, Veterans Administration Medical Center, 4150 Clement Street, San Francisco, California 94121*

Marilyn Green Larach, M.D., F.A.A.P.   *The North American Malignant Hyperthermia Registry, Departments of Anesthesia and Pediatrics, Pennsylvania State University College of Medicine, P.O. Box 850, Hershey, Pennsylvania 17033*

Victor S. Lukas, Jr., D.V.M., D.A.C.L.A.M.   *Syntex Discovery Research, Institute of Pathology, Toxicology, and Metabolism, Department of Laboratory Animal Resources, 3401 Hillview Avenue, Palo Alto, California 94304*

Girish C. Moudgil, M.B., B.S., M.Sc., F.F.A.R.C.S., F.R.C.P.(C)   *Department of Anesthesiology, Tulane University Medical School, 1430 Tulane Avenue, New Orleans, Louisiana 70112*

Ronald G. Pearl, M.D., Ph.D.   *Department of Anesthesia, Stanford University School of Medicine, Stanford, California 94305*

Susan A. Rice, Ph.D., D.A.B.T.   *Susan A. Rice and Associates, Inc., 448 Cumulus Avenue, Sunnyvale, California 94087, and Department of Anesthesia, Stanford University School of Medicine, Stanford, California 94305*

Russell A. Van Dyke, Ph.D.   *Department of Anesthesiology, Henry Ford Hospital, 2799 W. Grand Boulevard, Detroit, Michigan 48202*

Lucy Waskell, M.D., Ph.D. *Department of Anesthesia, University of California, San Francisco, California 94143, and Anesthesiology Service, Veterans Administration Medical Center, 4150 Clement Street, San Francisco, California 94121*

Margaret Wood, M.D. *Departments of Anesthesiology and Pharmacology, Vanderbilt University School of Medicine, Nashville, Tennessee 37232-2125*

Acknowledgment

Somewhat to our surprise, we had very little difficulty recruiting the authors for this book. It was with some trepidation that we approached them because we understood how busy they were and we knew how much work we were asking them to undertake. They have our heartfelt thanks for the enthusiastic way they agreed to contribute to this book and we thank them all for their thoughtful contributions.

Preface

In recent years, we have seen an explosion in the number of scientific articles written on the toxicity of anesthetics. This topic is being explored by researchers in many disciplines including biochemistry, genetics, and immunology. The results of their research have been published in journals and books not normally associated with anesthesia. The purpose of this book is to provide a single-source summary of the current knowledge of toxicity of the anesthetic agents. To be as inclusive as possible, we have defined toxicity in its broadest sense to mean an adverse effect, whether that effect is the result of pharmacologic, toxicologic, physiologic, or other mechanism.

The authors have been chosen to reflect the diversity in current research. Our instructions to the individual authors were to provide a concise review of their field of expertise that includes the historical development of the subject, the current state of knowledge, and the possible future direction of research. This book was inspired in part by the now classic 1977 book *Metabolism of Volatile Anesthetics—Implications for Toxicity,* authored by Ellis Cohen and Russell Van Dyke. Since that time, there has not been another book that has dealt exclusively with the toxicity of anesthetics.

This book is of interest to anyone who is using anesthetic agents to anesthetize humans or animals for clinical care or research. It should also be read by anyone who is examining anesthetic effects on whole organ or tissue preparations or studying *in vitro* anesthetic metabolism. For the clinician who wishes to become acquainted with the toxicity of anesthetics on a more than superficial level, this book will be a major resource. There are some very thought-provoking and important immunologic aspects of anesthetic administration in this book that should be considered by the clinician administering anesthetic agents for prolonged periods of time to patients in intensive care. The book will help the clinician planning clinical trials to avoid some important confounding anesthetic factors affecting drug metabolism. For the laboratory researcher planning studies involving anesthesia, whether related to anesthetic drugs or not, there is a wealth of information within these pages to assist in choosing the correct animal and anesthetic technique. As editors, we have learned new and interesting facts about clinical anesthesia and research on anesthetic toxicity. Having been educated during the preparation of this book about the digestive habits of rabbits, we are thankful that in our own studies, we have avoided studying rabbits thus far!

The initial chapters provide a background to enhance an appreciation and understanding of the factors that impact toxicity and the ways in which the adverse effects of the anesthetics can be investigated. The subsequent chapters present and summarize anesthetic toxicity, some of which will be familiar, such as nephrotoxicity and hepatotoxicity. Other chapters offer new insights into the anesthetics and their interactions, such as the immunologic effects of anesthesia and the impact of pharmacogenetics.

In summary, we believe that there is so much new information available and new ways that old information is being interpreted, in light of recent developments in the basic sciences, that the information in this book is essential to practitioners in all the above-mentioned areas.

Susan A. Rice
Kevin J. Fish

ANESTHETIC TOXICITY

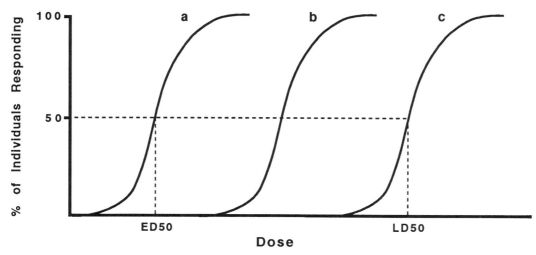

FIG. 1. Three dose–response curves are shown. The percent of individuals responding is shown on the abscissa and the log dose on the ordinate. Curve "a" represents the pharmacologic effect (e.g., depressed blood pressure), curve "b" represents a specific toxic effect (e.g., cardiac arrhythmias), and curve "c" represents lethality.

dose and the number of doses used to define the dose–response relationship. Thus, the LOEL or LOAEL may not, in fact, be the lowest dose at which a specific pharmacologic or other effect may occur. Other measures or terms, therefore, are helpful to represent doses at which there is no observed effect (NOEL) and the level at which there is no observed adverse effect (NOAEL). Note that for each compound there can be only one LOEL, LOAEL, NOEL, and NOAEL, even though there may be several different pharmacologic and toxicologic effects.

One can think of dose–response curves in terms of either acute or chronic effects. From the pharmacologic perspective, we tend to think of the acute effects of the anesthetic agents. From the toxicologic perspective, both the acute and chronic effects are equally important. In the case of the anesthetic gases, generally the former is important for the patient, and the latter is important for the occupationally exposed health care worker.

There is some debate about whether a threshold dose exists below which there is no effect. One could argue that effects at the molecular level are significant, and, therefore, there is no dose at which there is not an effect. This debate has proved most controversial in the arena of carcinogenicity, where exposure to a single molecule of a carcinogen represents a finite risk. This interpretation generates discussion for a number of reasons, among which is the fact that the body has the ability to repair itself if there is not some genetic defect to prevent that repair. The process of natural cell death and replacement by new cells (turnover) is another mechanism for recovery. Thus, injury at one point in time does not necessarily mean that function is significantly affected or that recovery is precluded.

GENERAL MECHANISMS OF TOXICITY

Tissue injury can result from the direct and indirect actions of a drug or its metabolites when their intracellular concentrations surpass the threshold for toxicity. The adverse effect is dependent on the concentration of the drug or metabolite, the interactions of the drug or metabolite with its receptors, the reserve capacity of the affected system, the turnover of affected cellular components (e.g., enzymes, membranes, and substrates), and the regenerative capacity of any repair mechanisms.

Enzymatic or structural systems maintaining cellular integrity (e.g., mitochondrial energy production and membrane ion transport) may be inhibited or modified, intracellular substrates may be depleted, or unwanted pharmacologic actions may result from excess drug or metabolite in a target cell or organelle (e.g., renal tubular cell damage from inorganic fluoride).

Drug metabolism inadvertently may be the first step in the pathogenesis of anesthetic toxicity. During phase I metabolism, a reactive intermediate may be produced from drugs that are not themselves reactive (see chapter by Waskell). These intermediates initiate toxicity by covalently binding with cellular macromolecules (e.g., enzymes and nucleic acids) to form adducts or to initiate aberrant, free-radical chain reactions.

Adducts of tissue macromolecules may initiate toxicity by altering the function of cellular components, such as the endoplasmic reticulum or mitochondria. Covalent binding also may deplete the cell of endogenous compounds necessary for normal cell function. For example, intracellular sulfhydryl-containing compounds, such as glutathione, act as natural cellular antioxidants and thus help maintain cellular homeostasis. When the cell is depleted of glutathione, it is susceptible to the oxidant effects of normal cellular metabolism and those resulting from drug-induced, uncontrolled, free-radical chain reactions. Normally, glutathione conjugates the free radicals and thus interrupts potentially destructive chain reactions. In the absence of glutathione or other natural antioxidants, destructive reactions continue and cell death can ensue.

Toxicity encompasses a spectrum of potential adverse effects ranging in severity from minimal physiologic disturbance (e.g., tachycardia) to death. Toxicity also can be manifest as an idiosyncratic reaction or an anaphylactic reaction where there may be extreme sensitivity even to a low dose. Toxicity can be immediate or delayed in expression, reversible or irreversible in effect, and localized or systemic in specificity.

Drug overdose results in a form of toxicity manifest as an excess of pharmacologic activity. In the case of the anesthetics, excessive pharmacologic activity results in excessive respiratory or cardiovascular depression or both. Drugs also may have toxic effects that are unrelated to their pharmacologic effects. In their mildest form, these unrelated effects are referred to as side effects; an example is chlorpheniramine-induced sedation. For the anesthetics, suppression of adrenal corticosteroid secretion by etomidate may be considered a side effect. In their most severe form, the unwanted effects that cause injury are identified as toxic effects; an example of this is halothane-induced arrhythmias. These effects are observed with the parent compound, but unwanted toxic effects may also be experienced with a drug's metabolite. One example of this is the induction of methemoglobinemia by *o*-toluidine, a metabolite of the local anesthetic agent prilocaine. Another example is the nephrotoxicity associated with inorganic fluoride produced from metabolism of methoxyflurane and other fluorine-containing volatile anesthetic agents. The toxic effects of metabolites may be unrelated to the pharmacologic or toxic effects directly attributable to the parent compound.

DETERMINANTS OF TOXICITY

Factors that determine and influence toxicity include species, age, gender, genetics, metabolism, dose, route of administration, duration of administration, and health status. Interactions of a drug or metabolite with other drugs and nutritional deficiencies or excesses are also significant determinants of toxicity. Aspects of species and health status are discussed by Lukas. Genetics in relation to drug disposition, metabolism, and action is discussed by Wood. Drug metabolism and its influences are discussed by Waskell. Several toxicology textbooks are listed in the references (2–4).

Toxicity of the anesthetics is dependent on the amount of the anesthetic absorbed and the amount of active toxic agent (parent drug or metabolite) that reaches the site of toxic action. Pharmacokinetics (toxicokinetics) can be used to describe the rates of distribution of the drug to the sites of pharmacologic (toxicologic) effect. It is equally important to understand the factors that influence the metabolism of the parent drug to any active pharmacologic or toxicologic metabolites. Pharmacodynamics (toxicodynamics) describe the effects of interaction of the active agent with the target site.

Measurement of the plasma or serum concentration of a drug or its metabolite is a surrogate for measurement at the site of action. In many cases, the correlation among the dose administered, the concentration in the plasma, and the concentration at the target site is sufficiently good to permit extrapolation from one to the other. This direct relationship between the plasma concentration and the effect seems to work best when predicting pharmacologic effects and less well when predicting some toxic effects. When the relationship is not good it is presumably because the appropriate surrogate, or biomarker, has not been identified (see chapter by Ardies).

TOXICITY AND EXPOSURE

Two very different exposure scenarios present very different patterns of potential anesthetic toxicity. The patient population receiving anesthesia for surgery is represented by the acute, high-dose exposure scenario. The occupational population exposed to waste anesthetic gases is represented by the chronic, low-dose exposure scenario. This latter group is exposed to very low concentrations for hours at a time over months and years of clinical practice. There is some crossover between the patient and the occupational groups because some patients are exposed to relatively high concentrations of anesthetics for pain control or sedation in the intensive care unit for days or weeks, and some occupationally exposed workers are inadvertently exposed to high anesthetic concentrations as a result of certain work practices or occupational accidents.

These two different exposure patterns require different ways of investigating potential toxicity. The patient population is monitored individually for signs of acute toxicity by observation of physiologic perturbations, such as hyperthermia or cardiac arrhythmias. In this setting, toxicity, such as malignant hyperthermia or halothane hepatitis, can occur even when the anesthetic is administered at the usual concentration for the usual duration. For patients, biomarkers, such as temperature, might alert the clinician to toxic effects.

The occupational population, on the other hand, is not closely monitored, and, therefore, the techniques used to identify toxicity and to show an association between exposure and an adverse health outcome are different. The latter case is one in which epidemiologic approaches, coupled with laboratory research, become indispensable. The basics of epidemiology are covered in the chapter by Ebi.

OCCUPATIONAL EXPOSURE

Over the years, numerous studies have measured the ambient air environment of human and veterinary operating rooms and dental operatories to quantify concentrations of the waste anesthetic gases. This information could be used to estimate the daily and yearly exposure of occupationally exposed health care personnel. The problems of quantifying exposure for use in epidemiologic studies is formidable (see chapter by Ebi).

The advent and use of scavenging systems has decreased significantly the ambient concentration of anesthetic gas and vapor, probably by several orders of magnitude. Although the rationale for many governmental regulatory actions and recommendations is questionable, many countries have adopted exposure limits or guidelines. The early history of anesthetic health assessments and the involvement of the U.S. regulatory agencies in setting guidelines has been discussed by Mazze (5). In the United States and other countries, exposures still occur above the NIOSH recommended concentrations of 2 ppm for the halogenated agents and 25 ppm for nitrous oxide (N_2O). With the new scavenging systems, these excursions are generally the result of equipment malfunctions, anesthetic spills, and a few anesthetic techniques (e.g., mask induction).

Many studies regarding anesthetic concentrations in operating rooms and dental operatories have been published over the years. A study recently performed at seven different hospitals in Canada by Sass-Kortsak et al. (6) exemplifies the concentrations of waste anesthetic gases that currently are measured in many institutions. Anesthesiologists and OR nurses (circulating and scrub) wore personal detectors for N_2O and for halogenated vapors (halothane, isoflurane, and enflurane). The N_2O concentrations ranged from 3.1 to 13.1 ppm for geometric means and from 4.6 to 53.6 ppm for arithmetic means. For these exposure estimates, the total amount of exposure to three halogenated agents currently in use (i.e., halothane, isoflurane, and enflurane) was summed to arrive at one value referred to as the sum of halogenated anesthetic agents (SHAA). This SHAA was expressed in $\mu mol/m^3$ (halothane = 197 g/ mole; isoflurane = 184 g/mole;

enflurane = 184 g/mole). The SHAA geometric means ranged from 3.2 to 24.2 $\mu mol/m^3$, and the arithmetic means ranged from 13.4 to 127.9 $\mu mol/m^3$. Considering the individual samples taken in this study, 27% of all measurements of anesthetists' time-weighted average N_2O exposures were in excess of the 25-ppm standard; 14% of nurses' exposures were in excess. For purposes of comparison, 2 ppm of halothane is equivalent to 81 $\mu mol/m^3$. A total of 15% of samples taken on anesthetists and 8% of nurses exceeded this value. The authors determined that the age of the anesthetic equipment was a significant factor in determining the degree of exposure to the anesthetics. Equipment more than 10 years old was associated with significantly higher ambient anesthetic concentrations.

TOPICS NOT ADDRESSED

Various topics have not been included in this book because either there is not sufficient evidence for toxicity, the toxicity is self-evident, or there is no new significant information. There are two general areas that are well researched where there are few, if any, recent publications (i.e., mutagenicity, carcinogenicity). Findings from tests for genetic and related effects and from studies of DNA damage, chromosomal effects, and mutation in humans and for carcinogenicity in humans and experimental animals were summarized and updated by the 1986–1987 IARC Working Group (7). Overall, this group evaluated carcinogenicity for humans for 628 agents. Individual volatile anesthetics have either no adequate data or insufficient data for classification as a carcinogen in experimental animals. As a class, the volatile anesthetics in humans have inadequate evidence for carcinogenicity and are classified in class 3. Mutagenicity is of concern also for its relationship to teratogenicity (see chapter by Rice). Anaphylaxis is another topic that is only mentioned in passing in this book. The interested reader is referred to a recent publication by Levy (8).

SUMMARY

Earlier anesthetics, such as chloroform, had a high incidence of hepatic necrosis and other adverse effects. The consistent strategy for designing newer anesthetics has been the development of safer anesthetics. The study of anesthetic toxicity has greatly advanced the understanding of the mechanisms of toxicity and has helped in the prediction of what molecular configurations would be the most resistant to metabolism and the production of toxicity. With a better understanding of metabolic pathways and mechanisms of toxicity, the significance of the metabolic products, the design of metabolically resistant drugs, and the use of pharmacologic interventions, such as dantrolene, anesthesia has become safer for the surgical patient. Occupational exposure to N_2O and the volatile agents is a continuing problem.

For this book, we have defined toxicity in its broadest sense to mean an adverse effect whether that effect is the result of a pharmacologic, toxicologic, or, in some cases,

physiologic mechanism. We believe that summarizing the available information about anesthetic toxicity from many sources and diverse fields into one book will be both useful and of great interest to clinicians and researchers.

REFERENCES

1. Klaassen C D, Eaton D L. Principles of toxicology. In: Amdur M O, Doull J, Klaassen C D, eds. *Casarett and Doull's toxicology—The basic science of poisons,* 4th ed. Elmsford, NY: Pergamon Press, 1991:12–49.
2. Amdur M O, Doull J, Klaassen C D, eds. *Casarett and Doull's toxicology—The basic science of poisons.* 4th ed. Elmsford, NY: Pergamon Press, 1991.
3. Hayes W A, ed. *Principles and methods of toxicology,* 2nd ed. New York: Raven Press, 1989.
4. Ottoboni M A. *The dose makes the poison,* 2nd ed. New York: Van Nostrand Reinhold, 1991.
5. Mazze R I. Waste anesthetic gases and the regulatory agencies. *Anesthesiology* 1980;52:248–256.
6. Sass-Kortsak A M, Purdham J T, Bozek P R, Murphy J H. Exposure of hospital operating room personnel to potentially harmful environmental agents. *Am Ind Hyg Assoc J* 1992;53:203–209.
7. IARC. *IARC monographs on the evaluation of carcinogenic risks to humans, overall evaluations of carcinogenicity; an updating of IARC monographs.* Suppl 7, Vol 1–42, Lyon, 1987:38–57.
8. Levy J H. *Anaphylactic reactions in anesthesia and intensive care,* 3rd ed. Boston: Butterworths, 1992.

Anesthetic Toxicity, edited by
Susan A. Rice and Kevin J. Fish.
Raven Press, Ltd., New York © 1994.

2

Animal Use in Toxicity Evaluation

Victor S. Lukas, Jr.

*Syntex Discovery Research, Institute of Pathology, Toxicology, and Metabolism,
Department of Laboratory Animal Resources, Palo Alto, California 94304*

The use of laboratory animals is critical to the study of anesthetic toxicity. A carefully designed and executed animal study avoids confounders that typically plague human clinical and epidemiologic studies: concurrent drug administration and differences in age, weight, diet, physical condition, and ethnic background. If an adequate sample size is assigned to the treatment and control groups, animal studies can provide greater power to detect statistically significant differences in the resulting data. In addition, due to the relatively short life span of rodents, certain animal studies, such as research into carcinogenicity and teratogenicity, take less time than similar studies conducted in humans, thus allowing research to progress more rapidly. Finally, animal testing can provide a level of confidence in the safety of a new drug before advancing to human clinical studies. Researchers must remember that there are no perfect animal models. Animal testing only approximates, not duplicates, the results of human studies performed under similar conditions. It is critical, therefore, to base selection of the most appropriate animal model on a variety of criteria.

This chapter discusses selecting an animal model, practical animal health and husbandry information (which potentially affects the outcome of laboratory studies), technical information for researchers who perform surgery, other routine research procedures, such as sample collection, animal identification, and dosing, and interactions of drugs, species-specific drug toxicities, and potential research complications of certain drugs.

ANIMAL MODEL SELECTION

The primary goal in selecting an animal model for biomedical research is to increase the capability of predicting human responses under similar conditions. Unfortunately for the investigator, there are no perfect animal models, nor is there any one animal species that best approximates human physiology. In fact, in certain situations, valuable information may be generated by comparing responses in animal species known to have anatomic or physiologic differences from humans. It is critical for the investigator to define clearly the goals of his or her research and to select the most appropriate animal model based on sound scientific judgment. Selecting the incorrect animal model will waste valuable human and animal resources and may result in erroneous conclusions.

The ideal animal model accurately reproduces the human condition under study and is available in adequate numbers to investigators at other institutions. Animals should be large enough to allow investigators to obtain multiple samples, if required, and most animal facilities should be able to provide the necessary husbandry for them.

The animals should be handled easily and survive long enough to be usable.

The importance of appropriate animal model selection was emphasized by a study that compared toxic lesions produced by 20 pharmaceutical agents in seven animal species and humans (1). The primary toxicity for each of the 20 agents was reported, i.e., nephrotoxicity for acetaminophen, uterine tumors for bromocriptine, ulcerogenesis for indomethacin. An average of four animal species was used to compare each agent. Data in humans were available for 14 of the 20 agents. Of the 14 agents studied, lesions developed from 5. The rat, mouse, and monkey accurately predicted the absence or presence of toxic lesions in humans in 71%, 73%, and 83% of the comparison, respectively. Accurate predictions of human toxicity based on the other species' responses were considerably less: dogs (45%), rabbits (50%), guinea pigs (20%), and hamsters (33%). The ability to predict the presence of toxic lesions in humans was best with rats (80%) and worse in the other species (40% or less). Although the number of pharmaceutical agents and the number of comparisons were limited, this study demonstrated the importance of proper species selection and the potential pitfalls of relying on a single species in the absence of reliable scientific information.

Metabolic Disposition

The metabolic disposition of the pharmaceutical agents is often the basis of species similarities and differences in reactions to the agents. The sources of species differences in metabolic disposition include the amount of compound absorbed by the different routes of administration, the processes of distribution, biotransformation, and excretion, and the interaction of the compound or its metabolites with the target receptors.

Differential biotransformation of compounds may be the most important source of species differences (2). Species variation in biotransformation may be due to a species-specific presence or absence of a particular metabolic reaction or to variations in the ratio of metabolic reactions. For example, dogs are deficient in acetylations and cats in glucuronidations. An example of a metabolic reaction that is limited to humans and some nonhuman primates is N1-glucuronidation of sulfadimethoxine and other methoxysulfonamides (3). Laboratory animals may metabolize drugs more quickly than humans because their livers are larger relative to their body weight, or the concentration of liver enzymes, such as cytochrome P450, may be much greater (4).

Differential plasma protein binding may contribute to species differences because the concentration of free, unbound drug circulating in blood affects the potential toxicity of compounds. A comparison of the plasma protein binding of five drugs in five animal species and humans suggests that binding is highest in human serum, lowest in mouse serum, and variable in other species (2). Thus, for a given compound, the concentration of free or unbound drug may be greater in animals than in humans, and, therefore, the potential toxic effects may be greater.

Another significant source of variation among species is the excretion rate of compounds. For example, rats and dogs generally are more efficient in biliary excretion than mice, which are more efficient than guinea pigs, monkeys, and humans. For compounds that are excreted in the bile, absorbed in the intestine, and returned to the liver by the portal system, the potential for toxicity is greatly increased in species with efficient biliary excretion. To further emphasize species-specific anatomic and physiologic differences, selected examples follow.

Mice

Mice have a relatively large surface area for their weight that results in profound physiologic changes in response to ambient temperature fluctuations. When acclimated to cold temperatures, mice can triple their metabolic rate to generate heat. In response to increased environmental temperatures, the mouse's body temperature may increase several degrees. Mice cannot sweat or pant to lose heat, but their metabolic rate decreases and vascularization to the ears increases to improve heat loss.

The renal glomeruli are about the size of glomeruli in rats, but there are 4.8 times as many. The mouse can concentrate urine up to 4300 mOsm/L, more than the maximum concentration of humans. A large amount of protein is excreted in mouse urine.

Mice are spontaneous ovulators. Pheromones and the social environment affect the estrous cycle. Estrus is suppressed when females are housed in large groups (Whitten effect), but suppression is counteracted by pheromones from male mice. Pheromones from a strange male mouse may prevent pregnancy in recently bred females (Bruce effect). Pheromones released from mice under different circumstances, such as stress, may affect the behavior of other mice in the same room. Gestation is 19 to 21 days. Estrus occurs in mice about 14 to 24 hours after parturition. However, fertile matings occur less frequently than with a normal estrus.

Rats

Rats are used in a wide variety of research applications, more than any other animal. The rat digestive system has some unusual anatomic features. The stomach is divided into the forestomach (nonglandular) and the corpus (glandular) by a limiting ridge. The esophagus enters the stomach in a fold of the limiting ridge, which prevents rats from vomiting. The rat is unique among laboratory animals in that it has no gallbladder. The bile ducts from the four lobes of the liver form the common bile duct that enters the duodenum.

Most rat strains are docile and easily trained to a variety of sensory stimuli for behavioral research. Most of their activity and feeding occurs at night or early morning. Rats are coprophagic like other rodents and rabbits, which may increase the amount of a drug absorbed if the drug is excreted in the feces. Rats are less prone to fight than mice, and males can be safely housed together. They also adapt to single caging better than mice.

Hamsters

The Syrian (golden) hamster, *Mesocricetus auratus,* is used more commonly in research than is the Chinese, American, European, or Siberian hamster. The Syrian hamster's natural environment is the desert, where it avoids the heat by living nocturnally in deep tunnels. This animal is useful in research because it has a short life cycle, is resistant to most pathogenic agents of rats and mice, and has several unique anatomic and physiologic characteristics.

Hamsters have cheek pouches that lack intact lymphatic drainage. Foreign tissues transplanted into the walls of the cheek pouches do not generally experience immunologic rejection. Their immune system differs from other species in that skin allograft rejection occurs less frequently than with other rodents, although hamsters are more susceptible to certain viruses, such as tumor viruses.

Other unique characteristics include the ability to hibernate when exposed to cold temperatures, a high level of resistance to irradiation, and ingesta fermentation in the nonglandular forestomach. The conductive airways of the respiratory tract have relatively few glandular structures, and the pulmonary vascular bed is similar to that of humans.

Guinea Pigs

Guinea pigs are rodents that are more closely related to chinchillas and porcupines than to rats. They differ from other laboratory rodents because they have no tail, one pair of mammae, and four digits on the forefeet and three on the hindfeet. The most common outbred stocks are Dunkan-Hartley and Hartley. The two most common inbred strains are designated strains 2 and 13. Guinea pigs are used to study antigen-induced immediate respiratory anaphylaxis (5). Fatal bronchoconstriction may result when a sensitizied guinea pig is exposed to an antigen by i.v. injection or inhalation. They also are a common model for delayed hypersensitivity reactions (6).

Unique aspects of guinea pig reproduction include a long estrous cycle (15 to 17 days) and gestation period (59 to 72 days) and the birth of precocious young. Neonates are born fully haired, with teeth and open eyes and ears. They are capable of walking almost immediately after birth and will consume solid feed within several days, although not typically weaned until 15 to 28 days of age.

Guinea pigs and nonhuman primates are the only two common laboratory animal species that require vitamin C in their diet. Guinea pigs are strict herbivores and may not accept unfamiliar feeds. They also typically reject overly bitter, salty, sweet, or chemically pure diets. They tend to spill and foul their food and water bowls and inject ingesta into water bottle sipper tubes. Due to these characteristics, providing accurate amounts of medication in their feed or water is challenging.

Guinea pigs are very social and usually move, sleep, and eat in groups. When startled, a group behaves uniquely by either freezing or frantically scattering in all directions. This reaction may complicate behavioral research.

Rabbits

Rabbits are lagomorphs, not rodents. The two most common breeds used in research are the New Zealand White and the smaller Dutch Belted rabbits. One reason rabbits may not be popular for anesthesia research is because of their small mouth and larynx, which makes tracheal intubation difficult. Rabbits readily develop reflex laryngospasm during intubation and inhalation of volatile anesthetics.

The rabbit gastrointestinal tract has several unique characteristics. Like rats, rabbits cannot vomit. They have a very large cecum that has a capacity of approximately 10 times that of the stomach. Once or twice daily, elimination of hard fecal pellets is replaced by cecotrophs or soft pellets. Cecotrophs are consumed directly from the anus and are rich in B vitamins and minerals. Because this behavior cannot be prevented, the amount of a drug absorbed from the digestive tract may be increased if it is excreted in the feces.

The genitourinary system also has characteristics not present in other laboratory species. The creatinine clearance is identical to the inulin clearance such that creatinine clearance may be used to measure glomerular filtration rate (GFR). Unlike other mammals, tubules of the rabbit kidney can be conveniently dissected with intact basement membrane, allowing close study of the entire nephron. Rabbits do not have regular estrous cycles but ovulate spontaneously 10 to 13 hours postcoitus, like cats and ferrets. Rabbits are popular in teratology studies because they breed readily, have a relatively short gestation (29 to 35 days), and have large litters (4 to 10) and large fetuses.

Nonhuman Primates

Nonhuman primates consist of a diverse group of approximately 200 species. Of these, only a few species, such as the rhesus and cynomolgus macaques, are used regularly in research. Nonhuman primates are not used more frequently because they generally are not available in large numbers, many species are endangered, they are expensive, most are difficult or dangerous to handle because they are wild, and they have the potential to transmit dangerous zoonotic diseases, such as fatal herpes B encephalitis.

Nonhuman primate species are divided into four groups: prosimians, New World and Old World monkeys, and apes. Prosimians are evolutionarily the most primitive. Prosimians, such as lemurs and galagos, are generally small animals that resemble squirrels or small foxes. They are used infrequently. New World monkeys originate in Central or South America. These monkeys are either no longer available for research or available in limited numbers. The two species used most frequently in research are the common marmoset *(Callithrix jacchus jacchus)* and the squirrel monkey *(Saimiri sciureus)*. Marmosets weigh approximately 0.5 kg and generally give birth to twins. The squirrel monkeys weigh 0.5 to 1 kg and are used in atherosclerosis research.

Old World monkeys originate in Africa and Asia. Two of these are the most common nonhuman primate species used in research, the rhesus *(Macaca mulatta)* and the cynomolgus or crab-eating macaque *(Macaca fascicularis)*. Old World monkeys have the following general characteristics: nonprehensile tails, cheek pouches, and calluses on the ischium, called ischial pads or callosities. Adults weigh approximately 3 to 7 kg. Baboons are available for research but are not commonly used, in part due to their large size, 10 to 25 kg. Captive-bred macaques and baboons typically are more expensive to purchase than feral animals, but they have the advantage generally of being exposed to fewer diseases and have known birth dates.

Apes range in size from the gibbon, 4 to 8 kg, to gorillas, 150 kg or more. Chimpanzees are apes that are used most commonly in research for the study of such diseases as hepatitis B and AIDS. They are available only in very small numbers.

Further information on specific animal models may be found in references 7–14.

ANIMAL HEALTH

Infectious Diseases

Scientifically valid research data are obtained from laboratory animal studies in part by insuring that animals are procured and maintained in a healthy state. Presence of a disease, whether overt or subclinical, can, at best, cast doubts on the conclusions drawn from a study. At worst, disease can result in unnecessary animal mortality, an inability to prove a true hypothesis, or proof of an erroneous hypothesis. Ignorance or disregard of the adverse effects of animal diseases may negate months or years of potentially valuable research.

Rodent Diseases

The list of research complications from infectious diseases varies considerably and is dependent on many factors. General examples of research complications in mice and rats and the respective list of causative agents are provided in Table 1.

As a group, the rodent pathogens that most commonly have an adverse impact on anesthesia research are agents that infect the respiratory system. Examples include Sendai virus, pneumonia virus of mice, K virus, sialodacryoadenitis virus, *Mycoplasma pulmonis,* and *Streptococcus pneumoniae.* Generally, these agents also are among the most common contaminants of laboratory animal facilities because once introduced into a facility, they typically spread from room to room via the air. To further complicate control of a disease outbreak, these agents usually produce subclinical infection rather than overt disease, thereby increasing the potential to produce unrecognized research complications.

Sendai virus is one of the most common rodent colony contaminants that may significantly interfere with research through a variety of mechanisms. Sendai virus is one of the most contagious infections of mice,

TABLE 1. *Potential research complications due to rodent pathogens*

Altered immune response	Contamination of cell cultures
Ectromelia virus	Kilham rat virus
Encephalitozoon cuniculi	Lymphocytic choriomeningitis virus[a]
Eperythrozoon coccoides	Minute virus of mice
Giardia muris[a]	*Mycoplasma arthritidis*
Haemobartonella muris	*Mycoplasma pulmonis*
Kilham rat virus	Polyoma virus
Lactic dehydrogenase-elevating virus	Reovirus-3
Lymphocytic choriomeningitis virus[a]	Contamination of transplantable tumors and altered
Minute virus of mice	host response
Mouse cytomegalovirus	*Encephalitozoon cuniculi*
Mouse hepatitis virus	*Haemobartonella muris*
Mouse thymic virus	H-1 virus
Mycoplasma pulmonis	Kilham rat virus
Myobia musculi	Lactic dehydrogenase-elevating virus
Myocoptes musculinus	Lymphocytic choriomeningitis virus[a]
Salmonella enteritidis	Minute virus of mice
Sendai virus	*Mycoplasma arthritidis*
Spironucleus muris	*Mycoplasma neurolyticum*
Syphacia sp.	*Mycoplasma pulmonis*
Altered physiologic, pharmacologic, or toxicologic	Polyoma virus
response	Reovirus-3
Bacillus piliformis	Sendai virus
Haemobartonella muris	Inapparent infection exacerbated by experimental
Kilham rat virus	immunosuppression
Lactic dehydrogenase-elevating virus	*Bacillus piliformis*
Mouse hepatitis virus	*Corynebacterium kutscheri*
Mycoplasma pulmonis	Ectromelia virus
Salmonella enteritidis[a]	*Eperythrozoon coccoides*
Streptococcus pneumoniae[a]	*Giardia muris*[a]
Carcinogenesis or spontaneous neoplasia	*Haemobartonella muris*
Citrobacter freundii (biotype 4280)	Kilham rat virus
H-1 virus	Mouse hepatitis virus
Lactic dehydrogenase-elevating virus	*Mycoplasma pulmonis*
Lymphocytic choriomeningitis virus	*Pneumocystis carinii*
Mouse mammary tumor virus	*Pseudomonas aeruginosa*
Mycoplasma pulmonis	*Salmonella enteritidis*[a]
Polyoma virus	*Spironucleus muris*
Sendai virus	

Adapted from National Academy of Sciences. *Infectious diseases of mice and rats.* Washington, DC: National Academy Press, 1991.

[a]Rodent pathogens that can infect humans.

rats, hamsters, and guinea pigs. It is an RNA virus in the genus *Paramyxovirus,* species, *parainfluenza 1.* The virus spreads rapidly by direct contact and airborne transmission. Viral replication occurs in the respiratory tract, and natural transmission lasts 1 to 2 weeks postinfection. As serum antibody levels begin to increase at 7 to 9 days postinfection, viral titers in the lungs decline until the virus is eliminated from the host.

In rats, natural infection with Sendai virus usually does not produce clinical signs.

In breeding colonies, a reduction in litter size and growth rate of pups may be observed (15). Experimentally infected pregnant rats experience prolonged gestation, fetal resorptions, retarded embryonic development, and increased neonatal mortality (16,17).

Clinical signs produced by natural infection in mice vary depending on preexisting immunity and the mouse strain. In a previously infected breeding colony, newborn mice are protected by maternal antibodies until 4 to 8 weeks of age. When maternal antibodies decline, infection occurs, typically with minimal clinical signs. Although adults do not carry the virus, the virus is maintained in the colony by a continuous supply of susceptible young mice. In adult mice not previously infected, exposure to Sendai virus typically results in 100% morbidity, with mortality ranging from 0 to 100%, depending on the mouse strain involved. The most susceptible strains include 129/Rej, 129/J, Nude (Swiss), DBA/1J, C3H/Bi, and DBA/2J (18). Clinical signs in these strains may include rapid weight loss, dyspnea, crusting of the eyes, chattering teeth, a hunched posture, a ruffled haircoat, and death. Athymic or immunosuppressed mice typically develop severe clinical signs. Resistant strains usually have asymptomatic infections.

The initial lesions produced by Sendai virus are inflammatory edema of bronchial lamina propria, alveolar ducts, alveoli, and perivascular spaces. Subsequent changes may include necrosis and exfoliation of bronchial and alveolar epithelium and lymphoid infiltration of alveolar septae, epibronchial, and perivascular spaces. By 9 days after the initial infection, regeneration of airway epithelium begins, as evidenced by epithelial hyperplasia, squamous metaplasia, and syncytial giant cell formation. Considerable resolution occurs by 21 days. However, some inflammatory lesions may persist for a year.

Sendai virus infection in mice has been reported to produce profound immunologic effects, including altered pulmonary macrophage function (19,20), persistent B and T cell deficiencies (21–23), transient increase in splenic IgM and IgG plaque-forming cell responses to sheep red blood cells (24), *in vitro* inhibition of lymphocyte mitogenesis (25,26), increased natural killer cell-mediated cytotoxicity (27), altered isograft rejection (28), increased or decreased neoplastic response to respiratory carcinogens (29–33), and delayed wound healing (34).

Diagnosis of Sendai virus infection is best accomplished by demonstration of antibody seroconversion with an enzyme-linked immunosorbant assay (ELISA). Infection control may be achieved by several different methods. The most effective method is prompt elimination of the infected colony to prevent the virus from spreading to other rodent rooms in the facility. Another option is to quarantine the colony for 6 to 8 weeks, remove young and pregnant animals, and keep out susceptible animals until the virus has been naturally eliminated. Other choices include vaccination and cesarean derivation.

Rabbit Diseases

Among the diseases of rabbits, pasteurellosis caused by *Pasteurella multocida* is the most common and has a great potential to interfere with research. The clinical forms of the disease are rhinitis (snuffles), pneumonia, otitis media and interna, conjunctivitis, abscesses, vulvovaginitis, pyometra, balanoposthitis, orchitis, and septicemia. The number and severity of the clinical forms manifested vary considerably. Clinical signs may respond to antibiotic therapy, although recurrence is not uncommon. Prevention of the disease is achieved by procuring rabbits from *Pasteurella*-free sources and isolating them from sources of contamination in the animal facility. Other diseases that affect rabbits are Tyzzer's disease, caused by *Bacillus piliformis,* enterotoxemia, treponematosis, hepatic and intestinal coccidiosis, and ear mites.

Dog Diseases

In dogs acquired from animal shelters or random sources, a variety of diseases may cause illness or interfere with research. The most important of these are typically respiratory infections, enteric infections, and parasitic infestations. Dogs with respiratory disease may exhibit mucopurulent nasal discharge, conjunctivitis, dry or productive cough, dyspnea, depression, and anorexia. Severe cases may progress to fatal bronchopneumonia even with appropriate therapy. Etiologic agents include canine distemper virus, canine parainfluenza virus, canine adenovirus type 2, *Streptococcus zooepidemicus,* and *Bordetella bronchiseptica.* Fatal infections are most commonly caused by distemper virus. Respiratory disease is best prevented by acquiring only healthy dogs and implementing effective quarantine and immunization programs.

Disease Prevention

The first step in ensuring the availability of healthy animals for research is purchasing them disease-free from vendors and transporting them to the animal research facility in a manner that eliminates the potential for contamination. Without control of these two factors, maintaining an animal facility free of significant disease is difficult, if not impossible.

When establishing a disease-free animal facility, an approved animal vendor list should be developed that ensures a supply of the different species, breeds, and strains of animals typically purchased by the institution. In general, the fewer vendors on the list, the less the chance for introducing pathogens into the facility. Selection of approved vendors depends on such criteria as adequate availability, vendor-supplied health information, health of the animals after arrival, vendor screening information provided by the veterinary staff, and availability of reliable transportation.

To evaluate the health status of an animal vendor, information should be gathered from several sources. Vendor-supplied health records are useful but may not be comprehensive because the vendor may not test routinely for certain subclinical diseases. Vendor screening performed by the research institution's veterinary staff may be

comprehensive, but typically only 5 to 10 rodents or rabbits are tested. Also, screening is usually infrequent, one to four times a year, with long intervals between tests. Regular monitoring of animals after arrival can be effective, but once a contamination is discovered, it is likely that other animal rooms are contaminated, and controlling the outbreak will be difficult.

Rodents occasionally are contaminated during transport by common commercial carriers when contact with infected laboratory or feral rodents can occur. Airborne transmission of pathogens may occur when shipping crates containing healthy rodents are placed next to crates of infected rodents or when feral rodents come in close proximity to the shipping crates. To inhibit transmission of pathogens, filter paper may be placed over the breathing holes in the shipping crates. This precaution is helpful, but it cannot completely prevent viral particles from entering the crates. It is best if the animals are trucked directly from the vendor's facility to the animal research facility. This precludes contact with animals from other vendors as well as feral animals and also minimizes shipping stress.

When rodents arrive at a research facility, they must be examined to ensure that they are healthy, and they must be allowed to acclimate to their new environment for 1 to 3 days. A quarantine may be necessary to better evaluate their health status. If the potential for contamination during shipment is significant, rodents should be quarantined for up to 3 weeks to allow development of detectable antibody levels. If there is no such contamination potential, quarantine may be unnecessary.

For larger animals, such as dogs, cats, swine, and nonhuman primates, quarantine is necessary and typically lasts 1 to 4 weeks for all species except nonhuman primates. Nonhuman primates usually are tested for tuberculosis several times at 2-week intervals, which necessitates a 4- to 6-week quarantine. The length of quarantine generally depends on the health of the animals and may be extended if a health problem develops.

In addition to performing physical examinations and observing for signs of illness, it is beneficial to perform a complete blood count (CBC) and to evaluate clinical chemistry parameters, such as serum glucose, protein, blood urea nitrogen (BUN), and alanine aminotransferase (ALT). Vaccinations may be given to dogs for rabies, distemper, hepatitis, parainfluenza, *Bordetella,* parvovirus, and leptospirosis. A test for dirofilariasis (heartworms) is warranted especially for random-source dogs. Cats should be vaccinated for rabies, panleukopenia, rhinotracheitis, and calcivirus. Depending on the source, cats may need to be tested or vaccinated for feline leukemia virus. Swine from dependable breeders typically are vaccinated when they are young and do not require additional boosters in a research facility. Nonhuman primates typically are not vaccinated, except occasionally with a human measles vaccine. They should be tested serologically for herpes B virus, hepatitis A virus, and the simian retroviruses and cultured for enteric pathogens. All of these species should be checked for internal and external parasites and appropriately treated if positive. Additional testing or treatments may be performed during quarantine as necessary depending on specific health problems or to meet the special needs of research protocols.

After animals are released from quarantine, long-term animals must be examined routinely to verify the absence of infectious and noninfectious diseases. In general, dogs, cats, and swine should be examined at least annually. Blood for a CBC and serum chemistries should be collected, a physical examination performed, teeth checked and cleaned, and vaccinations provided as necessary. Nonhuman primates require the same procedures, except vaccinations. Tuberculin skin tests generally are given two to four times annually.

Rodent colonies are monitored by routinely testing a representative sample of animals from each rodent room for serum antibody titers against specific rodent pathogens. The tested rodents are referred to as "sentinels." Usually 6 to 12 sentinels are placed in each room by veterinary services personnel specifically for health monitoring. Sentinels are housed identically to the study animals. The frequency of testing, number of animals tested, testing methodology, and the choice of tests included in the testing regimen vary considerably among institutions. Each monitoring program must be tailored to the needs and resources of the institution. One effective sentinel health monitoring program is described in Table 2.

Testing for serum antibody titers against viruses and *Mycoplasma* is best performed with an ELISA or an indirect fluorescent antibody (IFA) test. The test may be performed by an in-house or a commercial laboratory. Pinworms are easily detected by obtaining an impression of the perianal region with cellophane tape and microscopically examining the tape for pinworm ova.

Transplantable tissues and tumors represent another potential source of contamination of animals that has been unrecognized by most institutions until recently. Such pathogens as lymphocytic choriomeningitis virus (LCMV) and minute virus of mice (MVM) survive in tissue cultures and frozen tissues. Tissues purchased from commercial suppliers usually are not guaranteed to be free of these viruses. To ensure the absence of pathogens, tissue samples should be sent to a commercial laboratory for mouse antibody production (MAP) or rat antibody production (RAP) testing.

Genetic Quality

In addition to animal health, two other fundamental factors have the potential to significantly affect research data generated by animal studies. These factors are genetic

TABLE 2. *Sample rodent sentinel health monitoring program*

Monthly screening profile
  Eight sentinel mice in each mouse room are tested for
    Sendai virus
    Mouse hepatitis virus (MHV)
    Minute virus of mice (MVM)
    Syphacia sp. (pinworms)
  Eight sentinel rats in each rat room are tested for
    Sendai virus
    Sialodacryoadenitis virus (SDAV)/rat coronavirus (RCV)
    Kilham rat virus (KRV)
    Pinworms
Quarterly screening profile
  Eight hamsters and guinea pigs in each hamster and guinea pig room are tested for
    Sendai virus
    Simian virus 5 (SV-5)
    Pneumonia virus of mice (PVM)
    Reovirus-3 (Reo-3)
    Lymphocytic choriomeningitis virus (LCMV)
    Encephalitozoon cuniculi
  If *Pasteurella*-free rabbits are purchased, 4 rabbits in each rabbit room are cultured for intranasal *Pasteurella* and *Bordetella* spp.
Comprehensive profile (performed every third month)
  Eight sentinel mice in each mouse room are tested for the agents in the mouse monthly screening profile plus the following
    PVM
    Reo-3
    LCMV
    Ectromelia virus
    Mouse encephalomyelitis virus (MEV)
    Epizootic diarrhea of infant mice (EDIM)
    Mycoplasma pulmonis
    Mouse adenovirus (MAD)
    Polyoma virus
    Mouse cytomegalovirus (MCMV)
    Mouse thymic virus (MTV)
  Eight sentinel rats in each room are tested for the agents in the rat monthly screening profile plus the following
    PVM
    Reo-3
    LCMV
    Mycoplasma pulmonis
    H-1 virus
    MAD

authenticity of laboratory rodents and the environment in which the animals are maintained. Although these factors typically are not under the researcher's direct control, familiarity with these subjects will provide additional assurances that optimal conditions exist to perform the intended studies.

Genetic variations that are not visually or easily detectable may occur in rodent breeding colonies. Genetic changes may occur that affect biologic characteristics, such as life span, physiologic function, behavior, metabolism, immune function, response to drugs, and susceptibility to infections, transplanted tumors, and spontaneous tumors (35).

Rodent genetic changes may occur due to human error or natural causes. Genetic contamination is the result of inadvertently allowing a different rodent strain to mix with a breeding colony. If both strains have the same phenotype, intermixing of the strains could proceed for a number of generations if adequate genetic testing is not performed. Causes of genetic contamination include improper breeding practices, poor colony management, inadequate record keeping, and lack of personnel training.

Examples of natural causes of genetic changes are genetic drift, mutation, and residual heterozygosity. Inbred rodent strains are produced by allowing only brother–sister matings for 20 or more consecutive generations. Inbred mice are, therefore, essentially genetically identical to other mice of the same strain and sex, unless a genetic change occurs. Random-bred stocks, by contrast, are genetically heterogeneous and are produced by systems that minimize inbreeding. Substrains are produced by separating an inbred colony into two colonies and separately breeding the colonies for 20 or more generations. Differences in the colonies may occur due to genetic drift. Researchers always should use the exact nomenclature when writing reports because using similar but genetically different animals could produce different results. For example, C57BL/6J mice are distinct from C57BL/10J mice.

Most commercial producers of inbred laboratory rodents conduct routine genetic monitoring. Their laboratory reports usually are available on request. Additional questions to pose to breeders include the number of animals tested, frequency, and methods used. Researchers who believe that genetic variation may have affected their studies are encouraged to contact the breeder.

In-house rodent breeding colonies are typically of greater concern because breeding practices and engineering controls may be less controlled than in commercial breeding operations. In addition to maintaining the strictest colony management practices possible, a number of different genetic monitoring methods are available (Table 3). To ensure genetic quality, breeders should use several methods to test animals on a regular basis. The specifics of each program should be tailored to the needs of the researcher and the risk for genetic contamination to occur. An example of a genetic monitoring program for an average, relatively small inbred breeding colony is to test 10 animals annually by monitoring biochemical markers and by performing skin grafts with several pairs of animals, then observing for rejection.

Environmental Factors

In addition to animal health and genetic quality, the third fundamental factor that affects research is the environment in which the animals are maintained. Minor fluctuations in such parameters as ventilation or lighting due to temporary power outages,

TABLE 3. *Genetic monitoring methods*

Monitoring immunogenetic markers
  Skin grafting
  Mixed lymphocyte reactions
  Lymphoid tissue transplantation
  Tumor transplantation
  Serologic methods
Monitoring biochemical markers
  Isoenzyme electrophoretic patterns
Monitoring osteomorphic characteristics
  Mandible analysis
Monitoring coat color
  Test matings between strains with known
    recessive coat color genes
Monitoring chromosomal bands
  Chromosome banding techniques

for example, may affect physiologic responses. These complicating environmental factors can be divided into physical and chemical categories (36).

Acceptable standards for the physical factors that affect laboratory animals are readily available (37). Starting with the animal's immediate environment, cage design affects animals in several ways. Design and construction materials influence ventilation, light, sound, temperature, and humidity. The difference between the environment inside a rodent filter-top plastic cage and that inside a suspended stainless steel wire-bottomed cage is tremendous. Inside the filter-top cage, ventilation is greatly reduced, and as a result, temperature, humidity, and ammonia levels are elevated. The number of animals housed per cage also is important. Housing some species individually may be less stressful than housing several animals per cage. Overcrowding may affect behavior (38) and may compromise the immune system and affect metabolism (39). For example, the interaction of room temperature and group housing may influence study data. The LD_{50} for amphetamine at 27°C was about tenfold less for single-housed mice than for mice in groups of 10 (40). The acceptable room temperature range for mice is 18°C to 26°C (37).

Light intensity and duration are important factors in biologic responses. Light influences the reproductive system by indirectly stimulating the release of gonadotropic and adrenocorticotropic hormones (41). Photoperiod influences enzyme activity, drug metabolism, and drug toxicity. For example, the sleep times in rats treated with pentobarbital were significantly changed if the rats were exposed to different light cycles (42). Placement of cages is important. The light intensity on the top shelf of a rodent cage rack may be 80 times more intense than at the bottom shelf of the rack (41). Light levels of 75 to 100 footcandles have been shown to cause irreversible retinal damage in albino mice and rats. Levels of 30 footcandles appear to be safe. To minimize the compounding effect of such factors, researchers should randomize the position of individual cages on a rack and the position of racks within a room.

Continuous noise above 85 db can have deleterious effects, such as eosinopenia and increased adrenal weights in rats (43,44), reduced fertility in rodents (45), and increased blood pressure in nonhuman primates (46). The DBA/2 mouse is prone to audiogenic seizures (47). Personnel working in animal research facilities should attempt to minimize noise when performing their daily functions. Radios should not be allowed. Noisy animals, such as dogs, should not be housed next to rodent rooms or procedure rooms where studies such as behavioral research are performed.

Unintentional exposure of research animals to chemical contaminants may occur by many routes and may include detergents, disinfectants, acids, herbicides, pesticides, heavy metals, fumes, and mycotoxins. Effects vary widely depending on the animal species exposed, the nature of the chemical, the amount absorbed, the duration, and the route of exposure. Examples of effects include direct cell injury or necrosis, immunostimulation or suppression, teratogenesis, mutagenesis, or carcinogenesis, and enzyme induction or inhibition. Specific examples of chemical exposures are provided later.

Contamination of air generally produces subtle effects on animals that may not be detected quickly because all animals within a room or building are equally exposed. Exterior fumes may originate from a vehicle that is left idling close to the building, paints, insecticides, pesticides, or other airborne pollutants. Various chemicals are intentionally used inside animal research facilities, but they must be selected carefully and used properly to avoid interference with research. Room deodorizers should never be used because they release volatile hydrocarbons that may induce or inhibit hepatic microsomal enzymes (48). Many cleaning agents and disinfectants contain compounds with similar effects (49). Occasional or routine use of pesticides and insecticides is common in animal research facilities. Such chemicals as carbamates or organophosphates can depress hepatic microsomal enzymes, irritate skin, and affect the central nervous and hematopoietic systems. These chemicals should not be used in occupied animal rooms. Other methods of controlling insects and vermin, such as applying traps and sealing cracks and crevices in walls, are safe and effective. Researchers should always be informed before any unusual chemical is used in an animal facility, even if it is not used inside animal rooms.

The generally accepted guideline for ventilation is 10 to 15 room air changes per hour without recirculation from other rooms (37). Inadequate design or maintenance of a ventilation system or animal overcrowding may result in increased carbon dioxide or ammonia levels. Ammonia is produced by the action of urease-positive bacteria on urine and feces. Extended exposure of rats to 25 to 250 ppm of ammonia increases the prevalence of lung lesions of murine mycoplasmosis (50) and may enhance respiratory irritation of other environmental pollutants or alter their deposition in the lungs (51).

The quality of animal drinking water depends on the source of water, the geographical area (i.e., industrial or agricultural), municipal treatment methods, and the plumbing system used to deliver the water. The quality of delivered water may vary from month to month for such reasons as water companies obtaining water from several sources or the runoff from agricultural areas containing varying amounts of herbicides. The majority of identifiable synthetic organic contaminants in water usually are the trihalomethanes, formed by the interaction of chlorine or bromine with methane from natural organic sources. They are found in all drinking water that has been treated with chlorine (48). Environmental carcinogens may act synergistically with other test compounds to increase the incidence of neoplasia during a long-term study.

Inorganic elements, such as cadmium, barium, selenium, arsenic, lead, and nitrates, may contaminate drinking water (52). Microbial contamination may occur in a building's plumbing system, animal room water distribution system, cage rack water system, or in water bottles and sipper tubes. Routine flushing may be necessary to properly maintain these systems. Monitoring of drinking water for chemical and microbial contamination and radioactivity in certain parts of the country should be performed one to four times annually, depending on the type of research performed. If relatively pure water cannot be provided consistently, purification systems, such as chlorination or reverse-osmosis systems, should be installed.

Contamination of grain for animal feed may occur from the use of agricultural chemicals or during the formulation or storage of the feed. Feed contaminants include chlorinated hydrocarbons, organophosphates, polychlorinated biphenyls, heavy metals (i.e., lead, mercury, cadmium, arsenic, and selenium), aflatoxins, nitrates, nitrosamines, and estrogenic compounds (53,54). Chronic exposure to low levels of these chemicals may produce a wide variety of toxic lesions. For example, exposure to dietary cadmium or lead or both has produced morphologic and biochemical changes in cardiac tissues, alterations of the cardiac conduction system, accelerated aortic plaque formation, and hypertension (55,56), alterations of myocardial ATP concentration (55), decreased resistance to infectious agents (57), reduced antibody formation and delayed-type hypersensitivity (58), and reduced embryo implantation, delayed fetal growth, and teratogenesis (59,60).

Excesses or deficiencies in the quantity of nutrients, vitamins, minerals, or energy may affect experimental results. The effects are extremely variable, such as altering drug-metabolizing systems or predisposing to the effects of carcinogens (53).

Excessive caloric intake may adversely affect longevity of rodents on long-term studies.

Fortunately, contamination or improper formulation of laboratory animal diets is a rare event today due to improved manufacture and quality control techniques. However, for certain long-term studies and studies intended to meet the requirements of the Food and Drug Administration's Good Laboratory Practices, specific assurances must be provided. The most common and cost-effective method is to purchase feed that is certified by the manufacturer not to exceed maximum concentrations of key contaminants. Samples from every manufacturing lot are analyzed for heavy metals, aflatoxins, chlorinated hydrocarbons, organophosphates, and specified nutrients. The manufacturer typically will store samples at 0°F for 1 year. Documentation of certification is provided with each feed bag.

Care must be taken to avoid exposure of animals to chemical fumes when they are brought into laboratories. Animal bedding material must be selected that eliminates potential sources of contamination. Bedding derived from cedar and pine trees contain aromatic hydrocarbons that can induce the biosynthesis of hepatic microsomal enzymes (48,61).

Euthanasia

For the purpose of this chapter, euthanasia can be defined as the procedure of killing laboratory animals rapidly and painlessly. The single best source of useful information is the Report of the AVMA Panel on Euthanasia (62). Selecting the most appropriate method is an important decision based on numerous factors, including (a) freedom from pain, fright, struggling, vocalization, or other signs of distress, (b) safe for personnel, (c) in accordance with institutional policies and applicable laws, (d) easy to perform correctly, (e) rapid effect, (f) appropriate for the age, species, health, and number of animals, (g) aesthetically acceptable, (h) reliable and reproducible, (i) irreversible, (j) nonpolluting to the environment, (k) minimal drug abuse potential, (l) economical, and (m) must not interfere with the study or with postmortem evaluation (63).

Sodium pentobarbital injected at a concentration approximately three times the anesthetic dose is probably the most common chemical method to euthanatize laboratory animals. It is typically injected i.v. in rabbits and larger animals and i.p. in rodents. It generally meets the required criteria, but it causes congestion of alveolar capillaries, congestive splenomegaly, and interference with hepatic microsomal enzymes and leaves tissue residues. Carbon dioxide inhalation, used commonly for rodents, does not leave tissue residues but causes focal alveolar hemorrhage, perivascular edema of lungs, and other changes associated with hypoxemia.

Physical methods, such as decapitation of rodents and small rabbits and cervical dislocation of rodents less than 200 g and rabbits less than 1 kg, are effective. The AVMA recommends that these techniques should be used only when scientifically justified because electrical brain activity persists for 13 to 14 seconds after the procedures are performed. It remains unclear if pain is perceived during that interval.

ANESTHESIA AND SURGERY

Management of Anesthesia

Factors that must be considered when selecting an anesthetic protocol include (a) the experimental protocol, (b) the species, (c) the animal's age and physical state, (d) the technical expertise of the personnel, and (e) the anesthetic equipment available. This section provides basic information on the most common anesthetic agents and other factors to consider that may affect research outcome. Additional references

provide further details on the current techniques and agents used in laboratory animals (63–65).

Although the basic principles of anesthesia are the same for animals and humans, many distinct differences exist, such as species-specific anesthetic toxicities and effective dosages. Researchers should not extrapolate information on the use of an agent from one species to another. Animals should be fasted before they are anesthetized to prevent regurgitation and aspiration of gastric contents. Twelve hours is sufficient for most animals, but 2 to 4 hours is preferred for very small mammals with high metabolic rates. Rodents are predominantly nocturnal and consume most of their feed at night. Water should not be withheld. When removing animals from cages or pens, animals should always be handled gently and calmly. Excitation will disturb their circulatory and metabolic status. Attempting to induce anesthesia in a struggling animal will present physical problems and enhance the likelihood of an abnormal physiologic response.

Anticholinergic drugs, such as atropine, are useful in preventing bradycardia due to parasympathetic stimulation of the cardiopulmonary system and reducing bronchial secretions that may occlude small pulmonary airways. Atropine commonly is injected subcutaneously (s.c.) before general anesthesia, and repeat doses may be given as bradycardia develops. Rabbits are unique in that approximately one third have an atropinesterase that inactivates atropine. If atropinesterase is present, larger doses of atropine must be administered on a more frequent basis to maintain an effect.

A presurgical physical examination of animals, such as carnivores, swine, and nonhuman primates, should be performed to ensure that they are in good health. CBC, serum glucose, protein, BUN, and ALT should be measured. Rodents should be observed for obvious signs of illness, such as weight loss or a ruffled hair coat, before they are anesthetized. The anesthesiologist should be familiar with the animal's normal physical characteristics, such as cardiac and respiratory rates, mucous membrane color, and appearance of the eyes, to ensure recognition of abnormal signs during anesthesia.

Animals of the same species generally respond predicably to an anesthetic agent. However, individual variation in the depth of response at a given dose is to be expected. For this reason, initial dosing of injectable anesthetics should be provided at the lower end of the dose range, and supplemental doses should be given as needed. As soon as the agent is administered, monitoring of the animal should begin (Table 4). Not all observations are practical for all species, but a minimum of three to six different observations, such as temperature, pulse, and respiration, should be included in a routine anesthesia-monitoring procedure. The objective is to maintain a con-

stant level of anesthesia in a patient with good vital signs and with no response to surgical stimulation. Every effort should be made to maintain circulation, respiration, and body temperature within normal physiologic limits. Intravenous fluids, such as lactated Ringer's solution, can be administered at a volume of 5% to 10% of the animal's body weight. Fluids can be injected by the s.c. or i.p. route in rodents. Respiration in large animals and rabbits is aided by the use of an endotracheal tube that ensures that the airway remains patent. In the event of respiratory arrest, positive pressure ventilation can be provided quickly. Hypothermia is a significant problem with all anesthetized animals and is particularly critical for small or immature animals. It may be prevented or counteracted by placing the patient on a temperature-controlled warming blanket, using a heat lamp (exercise caution to prevent burns), keeping the animal dry and covered, and administering warm parenteral fluids.

TABLE 4. *Observations for routine monitoring of anesthetized animals*

Cardiovascular system
  Heart rate and rhythm
  Mucous membrane color
  Capillary refill time
  Arterial pulse and pressure
  Electrocardiogram
Respiratory system
  Respiratory rate
  Depth of breathing
  Character of breathing
  Blood gases
Muscle tone
  Jaw or limb tone
  Movement of limbs
Eye
  Position of eye (presence or absence of
    movement)
  Size of pupil
  Responsiveness of pupil to light
  Palpebral reflex
  Corneal reflex
  Lacrimation
Miscellaneous
  Response to pain
  Body temperature
  Swallowing
  Coughing
  Phonation
  Salivation

Tranquilizers

Tranquilizers are useful for producing a physiologic calming of animals to facilitate handling. Most do not produce analgesia. On painful stimulation, arousal may occur, and thus, animals may bite even if they are tranquilized. Most tranquilizers when used alone or in combination with anesthetics cause some cardiovascular and respiratory depression and hypotension. Tranquilizers are desirable when used with anesthetics because they allow lower anesthetic dosages, extend anesthetic duration, and provide a smooth induction and recovery. Some provide an antiemetic effect (i.e., acepromazine) and facilitate muscle relaxation. The commonly used tranquilizers are the phenothiazines (e.g., chlorpromazine, acepromazine, and promazine), butyrophenones (e.g., droperidol), and benzodiazepines (e.g., diazepam).

The most commonly used tranquilizer in

laboratory animals is an alpha-$_2$-adrenergic agonist, xylazine. This drug acts as a CNS depressant that produces analgesia in addition to muscle relaxation. It potentiates anesthetics and is used commonly in combination with ketamine in rodents and rabbits. Xylazine often produces hypotension. Ruminants require a dosage one-tenth or less than carnivores, whereas even a high dose has little to no effect in swine.

Neuromuscular Blocking Agents

The neuromuscular blocking agents (e.g., D-tubocurarine, gallamine, succinylcholine, and decamethonium) must not be used for anesthesia, analgesia, euthanasia, or restraint in any procedure that causes pain. These agents produce motor paralysis but not sedation or analgesia. They may be used with general anesthetics and positive ventilation when additional muscle relaxation is required.

Neuroleptanalgesics

Neuroleptanalgesia is a state of sedation with analgesia produced by the combination of a tranquilizer and an analgesic. A commonly used product is a butyrophenone/narcotic analgesic combination, droperidol/fentanyl. It is useful to sedate dogs for minor surgeries and rabbits for blood collection from the ear vein or artery. The narcotic portion can be reversed with an antagonist (naloxone). Undesirable effects include respiratory depression during prolonged procedures and overdosage of the tranquilizer portion during redosing. It is a DEA schedule II controlled substance. Neuroleptanalgesia is contraindicated in cows, sheep, cats, and guinea pigs.

Dissociative Anesthetics

The most commonly used drug in this class is ketamine, a phencyclidine deriva-

tive. It produces a state of chemical restraint and anesthesia that is characterized by muscle rigidity and an apparent dissociation of the mind from the environment. It is rapidly metabolized to demethylated ketamine via the hepatic P450 microsomal enzymes. It is generally safe in most species and does not significantly depress the cardiovascular or respiratory systems or change hepatic or renal function. The undesirable effects of ketamine include marginal analgesia, increased salivary secretion (prevented with atropine), and persistent swallowing reflex. The eyes remain open, which results in corneal drying if an ophthalmic ointment is not applied, there is muscle rigidity that can be reduced with diazepam, and there can be convulsions, disorientation, and excitement during recovery.

Another available product is a dissociative anesthetic/tranquilizer combination, tiletamine/zolazepam, which provides effective anesthesia for up to 25 minutes. It can be used for minor but not abdominal surgery. It is safe for most laboratory species except for the rabbit, in which this combination may produce nephrotoxicity. As with ketamine, eyes remain open and there is copious salivation.

Barbiturates

The barbiturates are grouped according to duration of action: (a) ultrashort, 5 to 15 minutes (e.g., methohexital), (b) short, 10 to 45 minutes (e.g., thiamyl sodium and thiopental sodium), (c) intermediate, 1 to 3 hours (e.g., pentobarbital sodium), and (d) long, 8 to 24 hours (e.g., phenobarbital and inactin).

The barbiturates provide smooth, rapid induction following i.v. injection in most species and are easily administered i.p. in rodents. When injecting i.v., the safest method to induce anesthesia is to inject one-half the calculated dose, wait 30 to 60 seconds, and titrate to the desired surgical plane. Barbiturates produce numerous undesirable effects, such as cardiovascular and respiratory depression, high mortality with i.p. injection in rodents, local tissue necrosis from perivascular injection (minimized with concentrations of 1% to 2%), prolonged recovery with pentobarbital (especially with cats), transient apnea after i.v. injection, and excitation with intermediate doses. They are either DEA schedule II or III controlled substances.

Other Injectable Anesthetic Agents

These agents are used rarely but may be appropriate for specialized, nonsurvival procedures. Alpha-chloralose provides 8 to 10 hours of stable, light anesthesia with minimal cardiovascular depression. It should not be used alone for painful procedures. It requires heating to dissolve in an aqueous medium and then cooling to body temperature before i.v. injection.

Urethane provides 8 to 10 hours of surgical anesthesia for rodents, with minimal cardiovascular and respiratory depression. It should be avoided when possible because it is carcinogenic and cytotoxic. If used, it should only be handled by trained personnel.

Tribromoethanol produces surgical anesthesia in rodents, with moderate respiratory and cardiovascular depression. Second doses are associated with high mortality. It is recommended for use only in nonsurvival procedures because it may produce peritoneal adhesions and ileus. A recent report suggests that these problems are caused by decomposition products in stock solutions. With proper storage in the dark at 4°C, it may be a safe and effective surgical anesthetic in mice (66).

Chloral hydrate produces 1 to 2 hours of light anesthesia, with minimal effects on the cardiovascular system and on baroreceptor reflexes. It produces poor analgesia, and the higher doses required for surgery produce severe respiratory depression.

Volatile Anesthetics

Diethyl ether is relatively safe for use in rodents because it does not significantly affect blood pressure, it vaporizes in a jar, and it provides good analgesia and muscle relaxation. Because it is highly flammable and explosive, it must be stored in a vented fume hood and used only in fume hoods designed for such agents. Diethyl ether should not be used in guinea pigs because it is irritating to mucous membranes, it causes increased bronchial and salivary secretions, and it may induce laryngospasm.

Methoxyflurane has a low vaporization pressure that provides safe anesthesia for rodents when using the open-drop or jar technique. It provides excellent muscle relaxation and analgesia, which persist into the recovery period. The undesirable effects include prolonged time to change depth of anesthesia and nephrotoxicity (especially in Fischer rats) due to elevated blood fluoride concentrations from hepatic metabolism of methoxyflurane.

Halothane requires a calibrated, precision vaporizer because it has a high saturated vapor pressure. It cannot be used with an open-drop or jar technique because high, lethal concentrations are quickly achieved. When properly administered, it provides rapid control, induction, and recovery. It produces cardiovascular depression, sensitizes the myocardium to catecholamines, and may cause arrhythmias. Halothane has a marked effect on hepatic microsomal cytochrome P450, which may significantly affect metabolism of other drugs, even in the postanesthetic period. Halothane may produce liver dysfunction after prolonged or repeated use. Malignant hyperthermia may be induced in certain breeds of swine (Landrace, Poland-China, and Pietrain) and Greyhound dogs.

Isoflurane is metabolized less than methoxyflurane or halothane and produces minimal interference in drug metabolism and toxicology studies. Similar to halothane, it has a high vaporization pressure that requires a calibrated, precision vaporizer. Isoflurane produces less cardiovascular depression than halothane.

Nitrous oxide can be used as a 50 : 50 or 60 : 40 mixture with oxygen to reduce the concentration of other anesthetic agents that have more marked side effects. It has low anesthetic and analgesic potency and cannot be used alone to produce anesthesia.

Carbon dioxide provides light anesthesia in rodents for approximately 1 to 2 minutes when combined with oxygen. A 60 : 40 CO_2/O_2 mixture appears safest. It is useful because small blood samples may be obtained rapidly by the periorbital route without leaving drug residues in tissues.

Analgesics

Anesthesia or analgesia must be provided to animals that have the potential to experience pain. The Institutional Animal Care and Use Committee (IACUC) at each research institution is legally required to review and approve protocols involving animals. The IACUC may approve withholding the use of anesthetics or analgesics only after reviewing a valid scientific justification detailing why the agents could interfere with the outcome of the study. In most cases, it is obvious which procedures will result in pain. However, other procedures require interpretation of signs displayed by the animal that could indicate perception of pain. In general, assume that procedures that cause pain in humans also cause pain in animals.

Several classes of analgesics are available for use in animals. The most common agents historically are the opioid agonists (e.g., morphine, meperidine, codeine, fentanyl, and propoxyphene). In general, they produce potent hypnotic and analgesic effects. A codeine/acetaminophen elixir may be conveniently mixed with water and offered to rodents, rabbits, and nonhuman primates in water bottles. Undesirable side effects include stimulation of the canine gastrointestinal tract by morphine, depression of the cardiovascular and respiratory systems, short duration of action (2 to 4 hours for morphine), excitation in cats, mice, and farm animals, and stimulation of histamine release, which can produce peripheral vasodilation and hypotension. They are DEA schedule II controlled substances.

Another class of analgesics is the opioid partial agonists (e.g., pentazocine, butorphanol, and buprenorphine). These agents have several advantages over the opioid agonists. They produce mild sedation, may reduce heart rate and blood pressure, generally have fewer side effects, are effective in all laboratory animal species, and are DEA schedule IV or V controlled substances. Buprenorphine has the additional advantage of being a potent analgesic and having a long duration of action (6 to 12 hours).

The final class of analgesics is the nonsteroidal anti-inflammatory drugs (e.g., aspirin, acetaminophen, phenylbutazone, and ibuprofen). These agents have antipyretic, anti-inflammatory, and mild analgesic properties. Their potential side effects are development of hemolytic anemia, hypothermia, and hepatocellular necrosis in cats and gastric irritation and ulceration.

Specific recommendations on the selection and use of anesthetics and analgesics may be provided by the research institution's attending veterinarian.

Surgery

Surgical procedures typically require the highest technical expertise and have the most potential to cause pain or distress in animals. For these reasons, personnel must be given adequate training in surgical and aseptic techniques before they are allowed to perform surgery without supervision.

Major survival surgery on larger animals, such as rabbits, dogs, and nonhuman primates, must be performed in an aseptic surgical room intended for that purpose. Major survival surgery is defined as a surgical intervention that penetrates a body cavity or has the potential for producing a permanent handicap in an animal that is expected to recover (37). Minor survival surgeries, such as skin suturing or peripheral blood vessel cannulation in the larger species, or any nonsurvival surgeries may be performed in a procedure room or laboratory. Survival surgeries in rodents do not require a dedicated aseptic surgical room, but the area should be free of clutter, easily cleaned and disinfected, and isolated from the general movement of personnel.

Regardless of the animal species involved in surgery, once the animal is anesthetized, an area of skin around the incision site must be cleaned and disinfected to prevent postsurgical infection. An area must be shaved that is large enough to prevent contamination of the incision with the animals' hair. After removal of the hair, the skin should be thoroughly cleaned and disinfected with a surgical scrub solution containing such ingredients as chlorhexidine or povidone-iodine. The scrub solution may be rinsed off of the skin with sterile saline or alcohol. The area surrounding the incision should be draped adequately to prevent contamination of the surgical field.

Aseptic surgical technique must be used on rabbits and larger animals that undergo major survival surgery. Aseptic technique includes the use of sterile surgical gloves, gowns, caps, masks, and sterile instruments. Caution must be exercised to prevent any contamination from occurring during the surgery. Survival surgery on rodents requires the use of sterile surgical gloves and instruments and aseptic procedures.

Postsurgical care includes frequent monitoring of the animal to ensure an uncomplicated recovery. The animal should be observed until it is conscious and able to maintain a normal position. Supportive care may include fluids, analgesics, antibiotics, and supplemental heat and bedding to prevent hypothermia. Monitoring of the animal, generally twice daily until the skin sutures or wound clips are removed, is necessary to ensure complete recovery and healing of the incision. This usually requires 7 to 10 days.

ROUTINE RESEARCH PROCEDURES

In contrast to surgical procedures, routine research procedures are considerably easier to perform, although they are equally important to the outcome of the research. Procedures, such as animal identification, blood collection, and drug administration, may be performed several times daily and have the potential to ruin a study if incorrectly performed. The principal investigator must provide personnel with adequate training to ensure both scientific validity and humane care of the animals (67).

Animal Identification

Before animals are placed on a study, they should be individually identified. Most institutions provide cage identification cards. Information on the cards may include investigator's name, animal identification number, strain, stock, breed, or species, source of the animal, date of arrival, age or weight on arrival, and a protocol number. Because these cards may be easily lost or misplaced, individual animal identification is preferable.

Rodents usually are identified by ear punch, ear tags, dye, ear or tail tattoos, and electronic microchip implants. Tail tattoos generally are the most permanent method but require expertise and specialized equipment. The ear punch is permanent if the ear is not damaged, but interpretation of the code is not always consistent. Ear tags generally are easy to apply and to read but may become dislodged. Care should be taken not to place the ear tag too tightly because it will cause pressure necrosis of the skin. Dying the hair coat is effective for up to several months before the dye fades. Ear tags and hair coat dye are used also to identify rabbits.

For dogs, cats, and rabbits, an ear tattoo is the most common method of identification. It is permanent, easy to read, and does not harm the animal. Dogs and cats may be identified with tags on collars that may be useful when handling the animal, but care must be taken that nothing in the animal's pen can accidentally hook or catch the collar. Nonhuman primates are best identified with a tattoo on the chest or on the medial aspect of the forearm or thigh.

Blood Collection

A common technique in rodents is to collect a small amount of blood from the orbital sinus, which requires light anesthesia and does not affect the eye or the health of the animal. A glass capillary tube is used to gently penetrate the orbital conjunctiva at the medial canthus of the eye until the orbital sinus ruptures. Blood will fill the capillary tube, and the flow will cease when the tube is removed. Blood may be collected from the tail by amputation of the tip or laceration of the blood vessel. Placing the tail in a vacuum apparatus or slightly warming the tail to dilate blood vessels will increase the amount of blood collected before a clot forms. Samples may be collected by venipuncture of the tail vein using a 27-gauge needle and syringe. If xylene is used on the skin of the tail, it should be washed off immediately to prevent irritation and necrosis of the skin.

Cardiac puncture in rodents requires expertise to avoid accidentally lacerating the myocardium or large thoracic blood vessels. Cardiac puncture may be used only on anesthetized animals that preferably will not be allowed to recover. For mice, a 22-gauge or smaller needle is inserted just lateral and posterior to the xiphoid process and directed toward the heart. With the rat, a 20-gauge or smaller needle is inserted through the right thoracic wall at the point that the heart can be best palpated. Larger

serial samples of blood may be collected by surgically implanting a jugular catheter. Terminal blood samples may be collected by anesthetizing the animal and severing large vessels, such as the abdominal aorta, jugular vein, or brachial vessels. Another terminal blood collection method is to collect blood in a funnel after decapitation.

The most common site of collection in rabbits is the blood vessels of the ear. Volumes up to 50 ml can be collected from the central auricular artery or the marginal ear vein. The flow of blood may be increased by heating the ear slightly or by placing a small amount of xylene on the tip of the ear to increase vasodilation. Xylene must be quickly rinsed off the ear when finished to avoid skin irritation. Sedation and vasodilation of the ear blood vessels also can be produced by injecting a low intramuscular dose of droperidol/fentanyl. Blood may be collected from the auricular artery with the use of a miniperistaltic pump (68) or a vacuum apparatus (69). Large volumes may be collected by cardiac puncture in an anesthetized rabbit with an 18-gauge 1.5-inch needle and 50-ml syringe.

Blood can be collected from dogs and cats from the cephalic vein on the forelegs for small volumes and from the jugular vein for large volumes. Other less common sites include the metatarsal and femoral veins.

Nonhuman primates generally require sedation with drugs, such as ketamine or a tiletamine/zolazepan combination, for blood collection. The most common site for routine blood collection is the femoral vein within the femoral triangle. If the deeper femoral artery is punctured, pressure must be applied to prevent formation of a large hematoma. Small amounts of blood may be collected from the saphenous vein on the rear leg or larger volumes from the jugular vein.

Drug Administration

This section provides researchers with guidelines for the administration of maxi-

TABLE 5. *Dosage volume guidelines*

Species	Route (volume, ml/kg body weight)									
	Oral[a]		Intravenous[a]		Intraperitoneal[a]		Subcutaneous[b]		Intramuscular[b]	
	Ideal	Limit	Ideal	Limit	Ideal	Limit	Ideal	Limit	Ideal	Limit
Mouse	10.0	20.0	5.0	20.0	10.0	30.0	5.0	10.0	1.0	3.0
Rat	10.0	20.0[c]	5.0	20.0[d]	10.0	30.0[e]	2.0	10.0	0.2	2.0[f]
Hamster	10.0	20.0	5.0	20.0	10.0	30.0	2.0	10.0	0.2	2.0
Guinea pig	10.0	20.0[c]	5.0	20.0[d]	10.0	30.0[e]	2.0	10.0	0.1	2.0[f]
Rabbit	5.0	10.0	1.0	10.0	10.0	20.0	1.0	5.0	0.1	0.5
Dog	5.0	10.0	1.0	10.0	5.0	10.0	0.5	2.0	0.1	0.5[g]
Monkey	5.0	10.0	1.0	10.0	5.0	10.0	0.5	2.0	0.1	0.5[g]

The maximum intradermal dose for all species is 0.05–0.10 ml/site.

[a]Volumes listed are the maximum volume per administration or injection, assuming one administration per day. For two or three administrations per day, use a maximum of one half of the dose volume listed. For more than three administrations per day, consult a veterinarian.

[b]Volumes listed are the maximum volume per injection site. The maximum total daily s.c. volume is approximately 30 ml/kg.

The following limits supersede the maximum limits when dosing heavy animals.

[c]The maximum single oral dose for a rat or a guinea pig is 5.0 ml for animals greater than 0.25 kg.

[d]The maximum single i.v. dose for a rat or a guinea pig is 5.0 ml for animals greater than 0.25 kg.

[e]The maximum single i.p. dose for a rat or a guinea pig is 10.0 ml for animals greater than 0.35 kg.

[f]The maximum single i.m. dose for a rat or a guinea pig is 1.0 ml for animals greater than 0.50 kg.

[g]The maximum single i.m. dose for a dog or a monkey is 3.0 ml for animals greater than 6.0 kg.

mum dose volumes. Two volumes, an ideal and the limit, are provided in Table 5 for each species and route. The ideal volume should be considered the preferred maximum volume under normal circumstances. The limit is acceptable but should be used only when absolutely necessary. For large i.m. and s.c. injections, dividing the dose and injecting at two separate sites may be less irritating. For multidose studies, the same injection site should not be used for two consecutive administrations.

These guidelines apply generally for healthy, adult animals. If immature or debilitated animals are involved, consult a veterinarian. Administration of excessive dose volumes may produce pain, excitement, altered physiologic parameters (e.g., serum electrolyte imbalance or increased blood pressure or respiratory rate), and abnormal compound absorption. A large i.m. injection into a small muscle mass may force the dose into fascial planes and subcutaneous tissues and may accelerate lymphatic drainage.

It is equally important to ensure that the dose produces minimal irritancy and is concentrated, but not overly viscous, so that the minimum dose volume is administered. If a compound is a known irritant, volumes lower than those provided in Table 5 should be used.

If a constant i.v., i.m., or s.c. infusion is necessary, generally do not exceed 3% (30 ml/kg) of the animal's body weight in a 24-hour period. If the constant infusion is continued for more than 2 consecutive days, a lower rate should be used. Descriptions of dosing and cannulation techniques are available in references 67 and 70–72.

DRUG COMPLICATIONS

A commonly accepted tenet of drug testing involving animals is to avoid potential complications of study outcome by administering only the test compound without concurrent administration of other compounds. This section provides examples of complications that may occur with administration of drugs other than tranquilizers, anesthetics, and analgesics (36,65).

The drugs that are most likely to be used in case of illness are antibiotics. A few examples of direct pharmacologic interference with research are provided in addition to species-specific toxicities. Aminoglycoside antibiotics (e.g., neomycin, streptomycin, and gentamicin) affect the neuromuscular junction by inhibiting the release of acetylcholine. These agents may affect the development of muscle tension and enhance the effect of the anesthetics that act on the same junction (73,74). They also may exert a negative inotropic effect on the myocardium and alter the positive inotropic effects of norepinephrine (74). Dihydrostreptomycin has caused acute deaths within 2 hours of injection in Mongolian gerbils (75) and may produce neurotoxic effects on vestibular and auditory mechanisms of dogs (65). Nephrotoxicity is possible also with aminoglycoside antibiotic therapy.

Chloramphenicol may produce blood dyscrasia with prolonged use, but its primary effect on research is its interactions with other compounds. It should not be used with immunizing agents. It may lower prothrombin levels, inhibit biotransformation of drugs metabolized by hepatic microsomal enzymes (e.g., phenytoin, dicumarol, and pentobarbital), and prolong metabolism of local anesthetics (76–78).

Penicillin and other predominantly grampositive antibiotics have been associated with fatal *Clostridium difficile* enterocolitis in hamsters, guinea pigs, and rabbits (79,80). Gram-positive antibiotic therapy favors the overgrowth of *C. difficile* in the gastrointestinal tract, with subsequent toxin release. Several other examples of species-specific pharmacologic actions of agents have been reported that may affect certain studies. Hexachlorophene, a chlorinated phenol derivative, and disinfectants containing phenol are toxic to cats. Exposure may occur with dermal contact or by ingestion.

CONCLUSION

A complex array of factors exists that may affect the outcome of research involving animals. To assist investigators in improving the quality of their studies, examples of many of these factors are presented in this chapter. Simple changes, such as converting from the use of rodents infected with respiratory viruses to using pathogen-free rodents, typically have dramatic results. Investigators report improvements, such as greater reproducibility, decreased standard deviations of data, improved animal survival, decreased numbers of animals needed per study, and decreased time wasted repeating unsuccessful studies. It is unrealistic to assume that investigators have the time or energy to become knowledgeable in all the subjects covered in this chapter, but they can be aware of these issues. With the cooperation of laboratory animal veterinarians, animal care personnel, and trained technicians, the performance and outcome of research will be greatly enhanced.

ACKNOWLEDGMENTS

I gratefully acknowledge Julie Snider, Cindy Garland, and Patricia Fettgather for their assistance in the preparation of this chapter.

REFERENCES

1. Hottendorf G H. Species differences in toxic lesions. In: Roloff M V, Wilson A G E, Ribelin W E, Ridley W P, Ruecker F A, eds. *Human risk assessment—the role of animal selection and extrapolation*. London, Philadelphia: Taylor & Francis, 1987:87–93.
2. Cayen M N. Retrospective evaluation of appropriate animal models based on metabolism studies in man. In: Roloff M V, Wilson A G E, Ribelin W E, Ridley W P, Ruecker F A, eds. *Human risk assessment—the role of animal selection and extrapolation*. London, Philadelphia: Taylor & Francis, 1987:99–110.
3. Caldwell J. The current status of attempts to

predict species differences in drug metabolism. *Drug Metab Rev* 1981;12:221–237.

4. Walker C H. Species differences in microsomal monooxygenase activity and their relationships to biological half-lives. *Drug Metab Rev* 1978;7: 295–323.

5. Patterson R, Kelly J F. Animal models of the asthmatic state. *Annu Rev Med* 1974;25:53–68.

6. Haynes J D, Askenase P W. Cutaneous basophil responses in neonatal guinea pigs: active immunization, hapton-specific transfer with small amounts of serum, and preferential elicitation with phytohemagglutinin skin testing. *J Immunol* 1977;188:1063–1069.

7. *Animal models for biomedical research*, vols I–VI. Washington, DC: National Academy of Sciences, 1968–1971, 1973, 1976.

8. Andrews E J, Ward B C, Altman N H, eds. *Spontaneous animal models of human disease, vols I and II*. American College of Laboratory Animal Medicine Series. New York: Academic Press, 1979.

9. Baker H J, Lindsey J R, Weisbroth S H, eds. *The laboratory rat, vol IV, Research applications*. American College of Laboratory Animal Medicine Series. New York: Academic Press, 1980.

10. Cohen B J, ed. *Mammalian models for research on aging*. New York: Academic Press, 1981.

11. Desnick R J, Patterson D F, Scarpelli D G, eds. *Animal models of inherited metabolic diseases*. New York: Alan R. Liss, 1982.

12. Foster H L, Small J D, Fox J G, eds. *The mouse in biomedical research, vol IV, Experimental biology and oncology*. American College of Laboratory Animal Medicine Series. New York: Academic Press, 1982.

13. Jones T C, Copen C C, Hackel D B, Migaki G, eds. *A handbook: animal models of human disease*. Registry of Comparative Pathology. Washington, DC: Armed Forces Institute of Pathology, January 1972 to present.

14. Kawamata J, Melby E C, eds. *Animal models: assessing the scope of their use in biomedical research*. Progress in clinical and biological research, vol 229. New York: Alan R. Liss, 1987.

15. Makino S, Seko S, Nakao H, Mikazuki K. An epizootic of Sendai virus infection in a rat colony. *Exp Anim* 1972;22:275–280.

16. Coid C R, Wardman G. The effect of parainfluenza type 1 (Sendai) virus infection on early pregnancy in the rat. *J Reprod Fertil* 1971;24: 39–43.

17. Coid C R, Wardman G. The effect of maternal development and neonatal mortality in the rat. *Med Microbiol Immunol* 1972;157:181–185.

18. Parker J C, Whiteman M D, Richter C B. Susceptibility of inbred and outbred mouse strains to Sendai virus and prevalence of infection in laboratory rats. *Infect Immun* 1978;19:123–130.

19. Jakab G J. Interactions between Sendai virus and bacterial pathogens in the murine lung: a review. *Lab Anim Sci* 1981;31:170–177.

20. Jakab G J, Warr J A. Immune enhanced phago-

cytic dysfunction in pulmonary macrophages infected with parainfluenza 1 (Sendai) virus. *Am Rev Respir Dis* 1981;124:575–581.

21. Kay M M B. Long-term subclinical effects of parainfluenza (Sendai) infection on immune cells of aging mice. *Proc Soc Exp Biol Med* 1978; 158:326–331.

22. Kay M M B. Parainfluenza infection of aged mice results in autoimmune disease. *Clin Immunol Immunopathol* 1979;12:301–315.

23. Kay M M B, Mendoza J, Hausman S, Dorsey B. Age-related changes in the immune system of mice of eight medium and long-lived strains and hybrids. II. Short- and long-term effects of natural infection with parainfluenza type 1 virus (Sendai). *Mech Aging Dev* 1979;11:347–362.

24. Brownstein D G, Weir E C. Immunostimulation of mice infected with Sendai virus. *Am J Vet Res* 1987;12:1692–1696.

25. Wainberg M A, Israel E. Viral inhibition of lymphocyte mitogenesis. I. Evidence for the nonspecificity of the effect. *J Immunol* 1980;124: 64–70.

26. Roberts N J. Different effects of influenza virus, respiratory syncytial virus, and Sendai virus on human lymphocytes and macrophages. *Infect Immun* 1982;35:1142–1146.

27. Clark E A, Russell P H, Egghart M, Horton M A. Characteristics and genetic control of NK cell-mediated cytotoxicity activated by naturally acquired infection in the mouse. *Int J Cancer* 1979;24:688–699.

28. Streilein J, Stradduck J A, Pakes SP. Effects of splenectomy and Sendai virus infection on rejection of male skin isografts by pathogen-free C57BL/6 female mice. *Transplantation* 1981;32: 34–37.

29. Nettesheim P, Schreiber H, Cresia DH, Richter CB. Respiratory infections in the pathogenesis of lung cancer. *Recent Results Cancer Res* 1974;44:138–157.

30. Nettescheim P, Topping D C, Jambasi R. Host and environmental factors enhancing carcinogenesis in the respiratory tract. *Annu Rev Pharmacol Toxicol* 1981;21:133–163.

31. Parker J C. The possibilities and limitations of virus control in laboratory animals. In: Spiegel A, Erichsen S, Solleveld HA, eds. *Animal quality and models in research*. New York: Gustave Fischer Verlag, 1980:161–172.

32. Peck R M, Eaton G J, Peck E B, Litwin S. Influence of Sendai virus on carcinogenesis in strain A mice. *Lab Anim Sci* 1983;33:154–156.

33. Hall W C, Lubet R A, Henry C J, Collins Jr, M J. Sendai virus—disease processes and research complications. In: Hamm Jr, T E, ed. *Complications of viral and mycoplasmal infections in rodents to toxicology research and testing*. Washington, DC: Hemisphere Press, 1985:25–52.

34. Kenyon A J. Delayed wound healing in mice associated with viral alteration of macrophages. *Am J Vet Res* 1983;44:652–656.

35. Hsu C K. Genetic monitoring. In: Fox J G,

Cohen B J, Loew F M, eds. *Laboratory animal medicine.* New York: Academic Press, 1984:603–611.

36. Pakes, S P, Lu Y S, Meunier P C. Factors that complicate animal research. In: Fox J G, Cohen B J, Loew F M, eds. *Laboratory animal medicine.* New York: Academic Press, 1984:649–657.

37. Committee on Care and Use of Laboratory Animals of the Institute of Laboratory Animal Resources, Commission of Life Sciences, National Research Council. *Guide for the care and use of laboratory animals.* Bethesda, MD: National Institutes of Health, 1985.

38. Davis D E. Social behavior in a laboratory environment. In: *Symposium on laboratory animal housing.* Washington, DC: National Academy of Sciences, 1978:44–63.

39. Baker H J, Lindsey J R, Weisbroth S H. Housing to control research variables. In: Baker H J, Lindsey J R, Weisbroth S H, eds. *The laboratory rat.* New York: Academic Press, 1979:169–192.

40. Weihe W H. The effect of temperature on the action of drugs. *Annu Rev Pharmacol* 1973;13:409–425.

41. Weihe W H. Influence of light on animals. In: McSheehy I, ed. *Control of the animal house environment, lab animal handbook no. 7.* London: Laboratory Animals Ltd., 1976:63–76.

42. Scheving L E, Vedral D F, Pauly J E. A circadian susceptibility rhythm in rats to pentobarbital sodium. *Anat Rec* 1968;160:741–749.

43. Geber W F, Anderson T A, VanDyne B. Physiologic responses of the albino rat to chronic noise stress. *Arch Environ Health* 1966;12:751–754.

44. Nayfield K C, Besch E L. Comparative responses of rabbits and rats to elevated noise. *Lab Anim Sci* 1981;31:386–390.

45. Zondek B, Tamari I. Effect of audiogenic stimulation on genital function and reproduction. III. Infertility induced by auditory stimuli prior to mating. *Acta Endocrinol* 1964;45:227–234.

46. Peterson E A, Augenstein J S, Tanis D C, Augenstein D G. Noise raises blood pressure without impairing auditory sensitivity. *Science* 1981;211:1450–1452.

47. Iturian W B. Effect of noise in the animal house on experimental seizures and growth of weanling mice. In: *Defining the laboratory animal.* Washington, DC: National Academy of Sciences, 1971:332–352.

48. Vessel E S, Lang C M, White W J, et al. Environmental and genetic factors affecting the response of laboratory animals to drugs. *Fed Proc Fed Am Soc Exp Biol* 1976;35:1125–1132.

49. Conney A H, Burns J J. Metabolic interactions among environmental chemicals and drugs. *Science* 1972;178:576–586.

50. Broderson J R, Lindsey J R, Crawford J E. The role of environmental ammonia in respiratory mycoplasmosis in rats. *Am J Pathol* 1976;85:115–130.

51. Owen P R. Turbulent flow and particle deposition in the trachea. In: Wolstenholme G E W,

Knight J, eds. *Circulation and respiratory mass transport.* Ciba Foundation Symposium 1969:236–255.

52. Shapiro R. Chemical contamination of drinking water: what it is and where it comes from. *Lab Anim* 1980;9:45–51.

53. Newberne P M, McConnell R G. Dietary nutrients and contaminants in laboratory animal experimentation. *J Environ Pathol Toxicol* 1980;4:105–122.

54. Edwards G S, Fox J G, Policastro P, Goff U, Wolf M H, Fine D H. Volatile nitrosamine contamination of laboratory animal diets [Letter]. *Cancer Res* 1979;39:1857–1858.

55. Kopp S J, Glanek T, Erlanger M, Perry E F, Barany M, Perry H M. Altered metabolism and function of rat heart following chronic low level cadmium/lead feeding. *J Mol Cell Cardiol* 1980;12:1407–1425.

56. Perry H M, Erlanger M W. Metal-induced hypertension following chronic feeding of low levels of cadmium and mercury. *J Lab Clin Med* 1974;83:541–547.

57. Cook J A, Hoffman E O, DiLuzio N R. Influence of lead and cadmium on the susceptibility of rats to bacterial challenge. *Proc Soc Exp Biol Med* 1975;150:741–747.

58. Koller L D. Effects of environmental contaminants on the immune system. *Adv Vet Sci Comp Med* 1979;23:267–295.

59. Gerber S B, Leonard A, Jacquet P. Toxicity, mutagenicity, and teratogenicity of lead. *Mutat Res* 1980;76:115–141.

60. Degraeve N. Carcinogenic, teratogenic, and mutagenic effects of cadmium. *Mutat Res* 1981;86:115–135.

61. Cunliffe-Beamer T L, Freeman L C, Myers D D. Barbiturate sleeptime in mice exposed to autoclaved or unautoclaved wood beddings. *Lab Anim Sci* 1981;31:672–675.

62. Andrews E J, Bennett B J, Clark J D, et al. 1993 Report of the AVMA panel on euthanasia. *J Am Vet Med Assoc* 1993;202:229–249.

63. Clifford D H. Preanesthesia, anesthesia, analgesia, and euthanasia. In: Fox J G, Cohen B J, Lowe F M, eds. *Laboratory animal medicine.* New York: Academic Press, 1984:528–561.

64. Flecknell P A. *Laboratory animal anesthesia.* New York: Academic Press, 1987.

65. Booth N H, McDonald L E, eds. *Veterinary pharmacology and therapeutics, 5th ed.* Ames, Iowa: Iowa State University Press, 1982.

66. Papaioannou V E, Fox J G. Efficacy of tribromoethanol anesthesia in mice. *Lab Anim Sci* 1993;43:189–192.

67. Bivin W S, Smith G D. Techniques of experimentation. In: Fox J G, Cohen B J, Loew F M, eds. *Laboratory animal medicine.* New York: Academic Press, 1984:564–588.

68. Stickrod G, Ebaugh T, Garnett C. Use of a mini-peristaltic pump for collection of blood from rabbits. *Lab Anim Sci* 1981;31:87–88.

69. Hoppe P C, Laird C W, Fox R R. A simple technique for bleeding the rabbit ear vein. *Lab Anim Care* 1969;19:524–525.

70. Flecknell P A. *Laboratory animal anesthesia, an introduction for research workers and technicians.* Orlando, FL: Academic Press, 1987.

71. Lang C M, ed. *Animal physiologic surgery,* 2nd ed. New York: Springer-Verlag, 1982.

72. Waynforth H. *Experimental and surgical technique in the rat.* Orlando, FL: Academic Press, 1980.

73. Wright J M, Collier B. Inhibition by neomycin of acetylcholine release and ^{45}Ca accumulation in the superior cervical ganglion. *Pharmacologist* 1974;16:285.

74. Adams H R. Antibiotic-induced alterations of cardiovascular reactivity. *Fed Proc Fed Am Soc Exp Biol* 1976;35:1148–1150.

75. Wightman S R, Mann P C, Wagner J E. Dihydrostreptomycin toxicity in the mongolian gerbil *Meriones unguiculatus. Lab Anim Sci* 1980;30:71–75.

76. Adams H R. Prolongation of barbiturate anesthesia by chloramphenicol in laboratory animals. *J Am Vet Med Assoc* 1972;157:1908–1913.

77. Adams H R, Dixit B N. Prolongation of pentobarbital anesthesia by chloramphenicol in dogs and cats. *J Am Vet Med Assoc* 1970;156:902.

78. Teske R H, Carter G G. Effect of chloramphenicol on pentobarbital-induced anesthesia in dogs. *J Am Vet Med Assoc* 1971;159:777.

79. Lowe B R, Fox J G, Bartelett J G. *Clostridium difficule*-associated cecitis in guinea pigs exposed to penicillin. *Am J Vet Res* 1980;41:1277–1279.

80. LaMont J T, Sonnenblink E B, Rothman S. Role of clostridial toxin in the pathogenesis of clindamycin colitis in rabbits. *Gastroenterology* 1979;76:356–361.

Anesthetic Toxicity, edited by
Susan A. Rice and Kevin J. Fish.
Raven Press, Ltd., New York © 1994.

3

Principles of Epidemiology for Evaluation of Anesthetic Toxicity

Kristie L. Ebi

*EMF Health Studies Program, Environment Division, Electric Power Research Institute,
Palo Alto, California 94304*

Epidemiology is the study of the distributions and determinants of health effects and injuries in human populations. This chapter discusses the epidemiologist's approach and tools used in studying suspected beneficial and adverse health effects. The areas discussed include measurement of event rates, measurement of the association between an exposure and an event, sources of error, study design, assessment of exposure and other factors, interpretation of results, and screening for disease. The terminology used is defined. The discussions assume that the time periods are defined over which an exposure and an event occur.

Epidemiologists studying the toxicity of anesthetic agents concern themselves with the frequency of beneficial and adverse health effects and with the factors that influence the distribution of these effects in populations. The study of anesthetic toxicity can be approached from two different perspectives. Epidemiologists can begin by identifying individuals with an adverse health effect or with an anesthetic exposure.

When working from the perspective of an adverse effect, the frequency of occurrence for that effect is compared among population subgroups to determine whether the frequency is higher in some subgroups. These subgroups are then studied to determine the factors associated with the adverse effect. In the case of anesthetics, the factors could include the agents used, the exposure concentration, or the circumstances of exposure. Identification of the most closely associated factors ultimately may be used to prevent or to control the adverse health effects.

When working from the perspective of the exposure, epidemiologists study exposed populations to determine what adverse health effects are evident following short-term or long-term exposure. Both perspectives have been used in studying the toxicity of anesthetics.

DEFINITIONS

Most epidemiologic research focuses on the factors associated with adverse health effects. Adverse health effects encompass a broad range of biologic responses from decreased fertility to increased mortality. For the purposes of this discussion, adverse health effects are called "events." The number of discrete events counted in a study is not necessarily the same as the number of individuals studied. For example, several studies counted the number of spontaneous abortions as a measure of adverse reproductive and developmental outcomes following occupational exposure to anesthetics. Obviously, over a multiyear study period, one woman may have more than one spontaneous abortion. This example raises an important issue in counting events vs counting individuals. Some individuals may have characteristics that predispose them to repeated events. These characteristics will be overrepresented if the study focuses on events. This can lead to the study results not accurately reflecting the true association between the exposure and the event.

Generally, epidemiologic studies collect information on individuals with an event (cases) and on individuals without the event (controls or the comparison group). The epidemiologic definition of a case is "a person in the population or study group identified as having the particular disease, health disorder, or condition under investigation" (1). For example, Hemminki et al. (2) defined cases in their 1985 study of spontaneous abortion as nurses with pregnancies that ended in a spontaneous abortion during 1973–1979 and who were employed during the first trimester in an anesthesia, surgery, intensive care, operating room, or internal medicine department of a general hospital. The controls were nurses employed in the same general hospital who were within 1.5 years of age of the cases, gave birth to a healthy infant during 1973–1979, never had a malformed child, and did not have a spontaneous abortion during the study period (that is, cases were excluded from controls).

A population is the total number of individuals from which a study sample may be chosen; the sample should be representative of the total population of interest. For example, the population could be all anesthetic nurses. Within a study sample may be various subgroups with defined characteristics in common. For example, one subgroup could be all married anesthetic nurses employed in a particular hospital who work 20 or more hours per week.

A Dictionary of Epidemiology, 2nd edition, edited by John M. Last (1), is a good source of definitions used in epidemiology.

MEASUREMENT OF EVENT RATES

Fundamental to the evaluation of an association between an exposure and an event is the comparison of the frequency of the event among groups. Rates measure the frequency at which events occur in the study population. Rates relate the number of cases or events to the total number of people in the population, to an exposure period, or to some other denominator. A rate is a fraction whose numerator equals the number of events and whose denominator equals the number of people in the population at risk of such events during a specified time period.

Mathematically all rates are ratios (that is, are calculated by dividing a numerator by a denominator). Epidemiology defines rates as proportions when individuals counted for the numerator come from the population counted for the denominator. Everyone in the denominator is at risk of experiencing the event and, thus, of entering the numerator. Only those at risk of entering the numerator are in the denominator. Incidence and prevalence rates (discussed later) are proportions. For example, when calculating the rate of spontaneous abortion (sa), the denominator should include only fertile women at risk of pregnancy during the specified time period.

$$Rate_{sa} = \frac{\text{Number of women experiencing a spontaneous abortion}}{\text{Number of women capable of bearing children}}$$

In practice, it is generally not possible to identify only women who can actually conceive. When the numerator and denominator come from different populations, the number calculated is called a ratio and not a rate. If the denominator in the example given includes all women of childbearing age, the number calculated is the spontaneous abortion ratio.

Incidence rates estimate the probability that a healthy person will suffer the event;

they are defined per unit population over specified time periods. The numerator of an incidence rate includes only new cases or events, and the denominator includes only the population at risk of the event during a defined time period. Mortality rates are examples of incidence rates.

Prevalence rates estimate the number of existing cases or events per unit population for a defined time period. The numerator of a prevalence rate includes all current cases or events, and the denominator includes the total population at risk at the specified time. In practice, some prevalence rates include the total population in the denominator, not just the population at risk. Prevalence rates calculated this way will be smaller than the true rates because the denominator includes individuals who cannot enter the numerator. For example, prevalence rates could be calculated from a survey of the number of cases of heart disease in the study population.

The prevalence rate of a disease is related both to the incidence and to the duration of the disease; that is, the number of existing cases depends on how frequently new cases develop and on how long the disease lasts. For example, the incidence rate of pancreatic cancer is close to the prevalence rate because the duration of the disease tends to be short, but the incidence of type II diabetes is smaller than the prevalence rate because the duration of the disease is long.

Incidence and prevalence rates usually are calculated for the entire study population and for specific subgroups. Rates calculated from the raw data are called "crude rates" and are useful to summarize the experience of the population. However, these rates may be misleading if some subgroups experience substantially higher or lower rates of events than the total study population. For example, although the crude birth rate in the United States in 1989 was 69.2 per 1000 women, it was 116.6 for women aged 25 to 29 years and 5.2 for women aged 40 to 44 years (3).

Central to evaluating an association between an exposure and an event is the comparison of rates of events among populations exposed and not exposed to the factor of interest. Ideally, the only difference between the exposed and unexposed populations is the exposure, and the populations are similar in all other factors that could influence the rate of the exposure or the event. This rarely occurs in practice. Generally, populations differ in a number of ways other than the presence of exposure, and these differences can skew the comparisons of rates. In order to minimize the effect of these differences, the rates need to be adjusted using statistical techniques. For example, the crude birth rate in many developing countries is substantially higher than the rate in the United States. This is at least partly due to differences in the age distributions. If an investigator wanted to examine crude birth rates among several nations and wanted to eliminate the effect of age on the rates, the data would need to be age-adjusted before comparing the rates. Because age is an important factor in many events, rates often are adjusted for differing age distributions. Rates also can be adjusted for other factors.

Two commonly used adjustment techniques are direct and indirect standardization. Age is used as an example of the factor to be adjusted. Both methods calculate summary rates that minimize the differences in age distributions between the study populations. To calculate a directly standardized age-adjusted rate, the age distribution of a standard population is determined. The age-specific event rates observed in the study populations are applied to this standard population. To calculate an indirectly standardized rate, the age distributions of the study populations are determined. The age-specific event rates in a standard population are applied to the study populations to calculate expected event rates for the study populations that are compared with the observed rates. Both directly and indirectly standardized rates are summary measures that can be compared among the study subgroups. The disadvantages of standardized rates include that the rates no longer directly express the experience of the study subgroups, the values of the calculated rates depend on the standard population chosen, and the statistical methods summarize over other factors that may influence the rates of the event.

TABLE 1. *Association between an exposure and an event*

| Exposure | Event | | Total |
	Yes	No	
Yes	a	b	a + b
No	c	d	c + d
Total	a + c	b + d	a + b + c + d

MEASUREMENT OF THE ASSOCIATION BETWEEN AN EXPOSURE AND AN EVENT

Generally, epidemiologic studies are designed to determine whether there is an association between an exposure and an event. If there is an association, it is important to determine the strength of that association. Underlying this determination is one of two assumptions about how the exposure influences the rate of the event: either the exposure multiplies the risk of the event (multiplicative model), or the exposure adds to the risk of the event (additive model). Statistically, there are a variety of methods for calculating the strength of an association between an exposure and an event. The basic measures of association are calculated from data collected for Table 1.

If a is the number of new cases of the event from the exposed population a + b, then a/(a + b) is the rate of the event in the exposed population (Re). If c is the number of new cases of the event from the unexposed population c + d, then c/(c + d) is the rate of the event in the unexposed population (Ru). The rate ratio (also called the risk ratio or the relative risk, RR) compares the rate of the event in the exposed to the rate of the event in the unexposed.

$$RR = Re/Ru$$

Rate ratios can be thought of as the ratio of two incidence rates. Rate ratios can be calculated from data collected in prospective and cross-sectional studies.

For example, the rate of congenital abnormalities in one group is 5.0%. To evaluate whether that rate is approximately what would be expected, more than expected, or less than expected, the rate of congenital abnormalities in the comparison group must be determined and the RR calculated. The RR is based on a multiplicative model of the effect of the exposure on the rate of the event. An RR of 10.0 means that the exposed population had 10 times the rate of disease as the unexposed population. The RR is the measure of association used most frequently and is one of the measures used when evaluating whether an association is likely or not to be causal. An RR of 2.0 or less generally is considered evidence of a weak association between an exposure and an event.

In case-control studies, the total population at risk for the event may not be known. Although it may not be possible to determine accurately both Re and Ru, the ratio of these rates usually can be estimated. In case-control studies, the number of individuals with and without the event is usually determined by the investigator. For example, a case-control study of factors associated with congenital abnormalities identified 50 infants with and 50 infants without congenital abnormalities; that is, the addition of the sums (a + c) and (b + d) equals 50. Re and Ru are fixed for the study and may be different from the population Re and Ru. Thus, an RR cannot be calculated. The measure of association calculated for case-control studies is the odds ratio (OR). An OR is the ratio of two ratios whose exact probabilities are defined according to the specifics of the study design. In the example of congenital abnormalities, the OR is the ratio of the odds that the infants with congenital abnormalities had the exposure under investigation to the odds that the infants without congenital abnormalities had the exposure. Mathematically, the OR = $(a * d)/(b * c)$.

The OR is a good approximation of the RR if the event is rare (often considered as an incidence of less than about 2%) in a stable population, if cases are representative of all individuals with the event, and if controls are representative of all individuals without the event. If these conditions are not met, the OR tends to be larger than the RR that would be calculated if the appropriate data were available. For example, the OR may not be a good approximation of the RR for spontaneous abortions because spontaneous abortions are not rare.

The rate difference (sometimes called the attributable risk) is based on an additive model of the affect of the exposure on the rate of the event; exposure adds to the risk of the event. It is a measure of the excess rate of the event in the exposed population. Using the incidence rates calculated for the RR, the rate difference is defined as Re − Ru. It is assumed that except for the factor of interest, all other causes of the event act equally in the exposed and unexposed populations. The rate difference is useful for determining the impact of an event on a population. The RR indicates the magnitude of the risk for the exposed, and the rate difference indicates the number of exposed who will suffer the event due to the exposure (and not due to other factors). Other additive measures of association can be calculated (for further discussion, see ref. 4).

SOURCES OF ERROR

In an ideal study, data are collected on every member of the population, and the calculated measure of association between an exposure and an event is the true value for the population. In the real world, epidemiologists must take samples from the total population and calculate estimates from these samples of the true measure of association between an exposure and an event. Epidemiologists strive to obtain measures of association that are as close to the true values as possible; that is, they try to obtain accurate measures of association.

The accuracy of a measure of association depends on its precision and validity. The analogy of shooting darts or arrows often is used to explain precision and validity. Each dart or arrow represents one measure of association calculated for a sample drawn from the population to evaluate the effect of an exposure on the rate of an event. A precise measure of association means that all the darts or arrows are grouped tightly together. However, although the measures of association are close in absolute value, they may or may not be close to the true measure of association for the population. For example, all the darts might be together but still far from the bull's-eye.

A valid measure of association means that all the darts are centered around the bull's-eye. The darts may or may not be scattered all over the target. Although the measures of association are, on average, close to the true measure of association for the population, any one measure of association may be far from the bull's-eye. A measure of association may be precise but not valid, valid but not precise, both, or neither.

The measures of association calculated from an epidemiologic study can be no more accurate than the data collected. Inaccurate results can be caused by systematic or random errors that cause the measure of association calculated from the study data to deviate from the true value for the population. Precision (or reproducibility) is the absence of random errors. Validity is the absence of systematic errors. In designing a study to describe the relationship between an exposure and an event (one that is unlikely to be explained by differences between the study groups other than the exposure of interest), the investigator needs to consider sources of variation in the characteristics of the study groups that relate either to the risk of the exposure or the risk of the event.

Random errors occur in all studies and are generally due to chance. These errors do not result from the measurements taken or the variables studied. Random errors arise because studies are based on a limited number of observations. Increasing the number of study subjects decreases random error.

Systematic errors arise either because of deficiencies in study design or in data quality, or because of factors that are related to both the exposure and the event. Systematic errors may result in overestimation or underestimation of the measure of association. There are a variety of ways of categorizing systematic errors. Selection bias, observer bias, recall bias, misclassification, and confounding are discussed later. Additional biases may be present in epidemiologic studies (for definitions, see ref. 1, and for a more thorough discussion, see ref. 4).

Selection bias arises from systematic differences in the characteristics of those studied from those not studied. Selection bias may result from flaws in the study design, from nonresponse of study subjects during data collection, from loss of respondents to follow-up, or from selective survival. Of particular concern is differential nonresponse or loss to follow-up among study groups. Selection bias will cause an overestimation of the measure of association if the exposed cases and unexposed controls are overrepresented in comparison with the unexposed cases and exposed controls. Selection bias is of particular concern in case-control studies because the selection of cases and controls may be influenced by their exposure status. For example, selection bias is of particular concern in studies of hospital patients because there

may be different probabilities of hospital admission for individuals with and without the exposure of interest. Current users of intrauterine devices may be more likely than nonusers to be admitted to the hospital following the diagnosis of pelvic inflammatory disease.

Selection bias is of concern in many studies of reproductive and developmental outcomes following occupational exposure to anesthetics because of the generally low response rates to postal questionnaires. Nonrespondents may differ from respondents in a number of ways that can bias the results. Investigators rarely achieve a response rate of 100%. The higher the response rate, the greater the assurance that any systematic differences between the study populations are minimized. For example, Axelsson and Rylander (5) found that the spontaneous abortion rates for the gestational period up to 16 weeks were 15.8% among women working in areas with high exposure to anesthetics and 8.0% among women not exposed ($p < 0.05$). An important part of the study was the collection of information on pregnancy outcomes among nonrespondents. A detailed follow-up of nonrespondents had not been done in earlier studies of the reproductive effects of anesthetics. A bias was found among the nonrespondents with respect to place of employment during pregnancy and pregnancy outcome. All women experiencing a spontaneous abortion at the same time as exposure to anesthetics at their worksite reported both their exposure and the spontaneous abortion. Among nonrespondents, only two thirds of all spontaneous abortions were reported by women not exposed to anesthetics during pregnancy. When the 113 spontaneously aborted pregnancies among the nonrespondents were added to the data collected from the original questionnaire, the spontaneous abortion rate for the period up to 16 weeks of gestation became 15.1% among women employed in high exposure areas and 9.9% among women not exposed to anesthetics.

The difference was not statistically significant.

A bias closely related to selection bias is ascertainment bias, which is a systematic failure to represent all subgroups equally. The measure of association may be spuriously elevated if, for example, exposed cases have a greater likelihood than unexposed cases of being diagnosed and selected for the study because they receive more thorough medical follow-ups than individuals not exposed.

Observer bias arises from systematic differences between the true value of a datum point and the value actually reported by the observers. Observer bias may result from consistent differences among observers (interobserver variation) or from differences in readings by the same observer on different occasions (intraobserver variation). For example, observers may ask questions in slightly different manners, resulting in different responses, or one observer may not consistently ask questions in the same manner. This is the reason why it is so important to train staff to collect data properly.

Recall bias arises from systematic differences in accuracy or completeness of recalling and reporting prior events or experiences. Recall bias is particularly important for studies of reproductive and developmental outcomes because mothers of infants with adverse outcomes are more likely than mothers of healthy infants to recall details of possible exposures during gestation. In addition, mothers of infants with adverse outcomes may recall events inaccurately and report them as occurring following exposures when they actually occurred at other times. To reduce recall bias, data on exposures should be collected as close in time as possible to the event. Some of the studies of reproductive and developmental outcomes following occupational exposure to anesthetics asked respondents about exposures and outcomes for as many as 20 years before the questionnaire date. It is

likely that recall bias would affect the data collected for the earlier time periods.

Misclassification bias is the erroneous classification of an individual to an exposure or an event category. It arises because of flaws in measuring the presence of either an exposure or an event. The probability of misclassification may be the same in all groups (nondifferential misclassification) or may be different for different groups (differential misclassification). Misclassification of the presence of an exposure can result in either an underestimation or overestimation of the association between an exposure and an event. Misclassification of the presence of an event can cause cases to be classified as controls or controls to be classified as cases. For example, individuals with preclinical disease may be erroneously categorized as controls. This misclassification generally results in an underestimate of the association between an exposure and an event.

Confounding arises when both the event and the exposure of interest are associated with another factor. The presence of confounding generally results in a stronger measure of association between an exposure and an event than actually exists. The presence of confounding is determined by comparing the crude measure of association with a measure adjusted for the confounding factors. Confounding is present when the crude measure differs substantially from the adjusted measure. For example, the crude RR is 4.0, but the RR adjusted for confounding is 1.5. Risk factors in the study population and factors unique to the particular study can result in confounding. For example, assume that cigarette smoking is associated with certain adverse pregnancy outcomes and with alcohol consumption. If a study reports an association between alcohol consumption and adverse pregnancy outcomes but does not ascertain smoking habits, the reported association between adverse pregnancy outcome and alcohol consumption could come from the confounding influence of smoking habits.

STUDY DESIGN

There are two basic study designs in epidemiology: observational and experimental. The main difference between them is that the investigator can specify the study conditions in an experimental study but cannot specify the study conditions in observational studies. Most animal studies and clinical trials are experimental studies. In these studies, the objective is to determine the effect of exposure alone while keeping other conditions and characteristics constant. In clinical trials, this is accomplished by the random assignment of individuals with similar characteristics to the exposed or the nonexposed study groups. When an experimental design is not feasible, an observational study is designed to approximate an experimental study. Observational studies take advantage of natural conditions and situations that simulate the conditions of an experiment. Observational studies include cross-sectional, cohort, and case-control study designs. Studies can be categorized in a variety of ways from the way data are collected to how the data are analyzed. Nearly all epidemiologic studies of anesthetic toxicity are categorized as retrospective studies because data were collected for previous time periods.

Cross-sectional studies examine the prevalence of an event in relation to an exposure of interest in a defined population at a particular moment in time. Such studies are similar to taking a snapshot because they provide a picture of conditions at one moment. A cross-sectional study examines either an entire population or a representative sample. Data are collected on the presence or absence of both the exposure and the event. History of exposure can be determined by questionnaire, but not necessarily accurately. Comparisons can be made of the prevalence of an event among exposed groups or the prevalence of an exposure among groups with the event. The temporal relationship between an exposure and an event cannot necessarily be determined. Serial cross-sectional studies, for example the Census, are useful for evaluating whether the prevalence rate of an event is changing over time.

Cohort studies are the best design for establishing the temporality of an association between an exposure and an effect. An exposed cohort is a subgroup of a defined population that has been exposed, is currently being exposed, or is likely to be exposed to the factor of interest in the future. An unexposed cohort is comparable except for exposure. All cohort studies determine the presence of the exposure before recording of the event. The cohort is followed over time to determine the incidence of the event within each exposure category. Because of this, cohort studies are less liable than other observational study designs to a variety of systematic errors.

Cohort studies may be conducted prospectively or retrospectively; that is, data on events may be collected from a certain time forward, or data may be collected from records or questionnaires or events that occurred in the past. For prospective cohort studies, exposure may be in the past, concurrent with the study, on in the future. Studies on acute exposures are designed so that members of the cohort enter the study after an appropriate period following exposure. It is more difficult to define the entry point for cohort members when exposures are chronic.

Most studies of adverse health effects following exposure to anesthetics are retrospective cohort studies. Both the exposure to anesthetics and the adverse health effect occurred in the past. Many of the studies had relatively low response rates to the postal questionnaires used to collect data on the exposure and the events. This raises the potential problem of selection bias because respondents may have differed from nonrespondents in ways that influenced the event rates. Most studies collected data by self-administered questionnaire. This raises the potential problem of recall bias. Respondents who experienced an adverse health effect may be more likely to report both the exposure and the event. The design and execution of prospective cohort studies are particularly appropriate for the study of reproductive and developmental outcomes following occupational exposure to anesthetics. Large groups can be identified readily for study, and environmental monitoring can be instituted before recording the events. This could eliminate many of the problems with selection and recall bias.

Case-control studies often are used when the event is relatively rare because it would be very time consuming and expensive to follow a cohort large enough to identify a sufficient number of cases. Case-control studies start with the identification of individuals with (cases) and without (controls) the event of interest. The frequency of exposure to the studied risk factors is compared between the case and control groups. Such studies usually are retrospective because they start after exposure and the onset of the event, but cases and their controls can be accumulated prospectively. One of the main considerations in case-control studies is the selection of an appropriate control group. Ideally, a control group is similar to the case group in all characteristics except the exposure or risk factor of interest. In practice, cases and controls may differ in a number of ways that can influence the study results. Cases may differ from controls in age, socioeconomic characteristics, and smoking habits. For example, Hemminki et al. (2) studied spontaneous abortions and congenital abnormalities in infants of Finnish nurses who worked in selected departments of general hospitals. Cases were selected from registry data. This method reduces the possibility of selection and recall bias, although cases not registered obviously would be missed. To make the control group similar to the cases, controls were chosen from normal births to hospital nurses. To control for the effects of age and hospital of employment, controls were matched to cases on age and hospital. Exposure information was obtained from head nurses. This method reduces the possibility of recall bias.

ASSESSMENT OF EXPOSURE AND OTHER FACTORS

Once an epidemiologic study design is selected, the type of data required to answer the study hypothesis and the best way to collect that data accurately must be considered. Data are collected on the occurrence of the event, the exposure of interest, and related factors. Data collection instruments may be designed from scratch or may use portions of published instruments, taking into account characteristics of the study population. Questionnaires are commonly used instruments to collect data on exposure and on a large number of other factors. An epidemiologist specializing in questionnaire design should be consulted on the design, execution, and analysis of questionnaires. Certain data also may be collected from registry and other publicly available data files. A register is a data file that includes all cases of an event in a defined population, such as a cancer register.

Epidemiologic studies of occupational exposure to anesthetics frequently collected data by postal questionnaires. Postal questionnaires have the advantage of being a relatively cost-effective method of contacting large numbers of individuals. The disadvantage is that the response rates tend to be low, even when nonrespondents are contacted repeatedly, which can result in selection bias.

Interviewing is another commonly used method of data collection. Interviews and self-administered questionnaires are necessary to collect certain data, such as early spontaneous abortions and smoking habits. A potential bias in collecting data by interview is the interviewers themselves. Interviewers need to be unaware of the event status of the study subjects. Otherwise, the interviewers may pursue exposure information more vigorously for known cases than for controls. Information gathered by trained interviewers may be more reliable than information collected by self-administered questionnaire because interviewers try to assure accurate interpretation of the question asked. Accurate assessment of both the exposure and the event is very important.

In toxicology, the term "dose" is used to refer to the amount of a substance administered. In epidemiology, the actual dose of a substance that an individual received is generally unknown. The term "exposure" is used in epidemiology to represent an estimate of the dose. Exposure may be substantially different from the amount of the substance absorbed into the body or by the target organ. Epidemiologic studies should aim to assess exposure in quantitative terms to allow the derivation of exposure–effect relationships. Specific study designs are associated with particular problems related to the accurate assessment of exposure. Prospective studies are designed to collect accurate data on exposure before the occurrence of the event, whereas that may not be possible for a retrospective study.

Many epidemiologic studies are initiated because there is a perception that one group has a higher rate of an event than another group. Initial studies explore whether the rate is elevated and if there are exposures or other risk factors that might explain the increase. Generally, the measurement of exposure in these studies is fairly crude, for example, whether employment in a certain department or group is associated with the event. In this case, employment is a surrogate measure for the exposure of interest. The actual risk factor associated with the event may be environmental (for example, one of a number of chemicals used in the department), related to the work situation (for example, stress or rotating shifts), characteristics of the individuals in the department (for example, smoking habits), or some other factor. Even in early studies, it is important that the intensity, duration, and frequency of the suspected exposure be defined as specifically as possible. For example, the number of hours worked per day in the department, the number of days worked per week, the number of days worked per year, and the total number of years worked.

The accuracy of measurement of the exposure should increase with increasing information about the exposure and the population groups at risk. If earlier studies suggest that a risk factor for an event may be exposure to a particular chemical, follow-up studies should be designed to measure that exposure as accurately as possible. In the case of anesthetics, air concentrations in the working environment need to be measured to assess reported associations between exposure and various adverse health effects. In some cases, it may be possible to measure concentrations of the chemical of interest in the ambient air or in biologic fluids. In other cases, the exposure or absorbed dose may be quantitatively assessed via biomarkers. Unfortunately, many epidemiologic studies of anesthetic toxicity have poor measurements of exposure (see chapter by Ardies).

When designing the measurement of exposure for a particular chemical, it is necessary to take into consideration information about the population being studied, the natural history of the event, and the chemical under investigation. If the event being studied is an adverse health effect with a short latency period, it would be appropriate to measure exposure at approximately the same time as recording the occurrences of the event. For example, a study of the relationship between exposure to nitrous oxide and the rate of spontaneous abortion should measure air concentrations of nitrous oxide concurrent with collecting information on the occurrences of spontaneous abortions. Concentrations should be measured frequently during the study period. However, if the adverse health effect has a long latency period, current concentrations of the chemical of interest may not reflect the concentrations that existed during the critical time period of exposure. Any decreases over time in the air concentrations of the chemical of interest must be taken into account in the study design or in the analysis to the degree possible. Similarly, other considerations are work practices, environmental controls, and other factors that may have changed over time and could have changed the extent or duration of exposure.

The most commonly used method of quantitatively assessing exposure is environmental monitoring, the systematic collection of environmental samples for the analysis of pollutant concentrations. In the case of anesthetics, environmental monitoring consists of taking air samples in which the concentration of each anesthetic in the work environment is measured. When designing a monitoring program, the following points need to be considered: what chemicals need to be sampled, how long and how often should the samples be taken, where should the samples be taken, and what analytic techniques should be used.

INTERPRETATION OF RESULTS

Most epidemiologic studies are designed to investigate the causes of events. Epidemiologic evidence alone is not sufficient to establish that an exposure causes an event. The following formal criteria are widely accepted to evaluate the likelihood that an association is causal: strength of the association, dose–response relationship, specificity of the association, appropriate temporal association, consistency of the association across multiple studies, biologic plausibility, and coherence of the evidence. Ideally, all criteria are fulfilled to determine that an association is causal. Practically, most of the criteria have to be fulfilled. None of these criteria are sufficient in and of themselves to conclude that an association is causal.

The strength of the association refers to the size of the RR or OR. The larger the ratio, the more likely that the association is causal. Related to the strength of the association is an evaluation of whether there is a dose–response relationship between the extent of the exposure and the development of the event. The specificity of the association refers to whether there is a one-to-one correspondence between the exposure and the event; this applies more often in evaluating causality for infectious diseases. To be causal, the exposure must occur before the event and before any induction or latency periods. In addition, the reported strength and direction of the association should be relatively consistent across studies. The likelihood of a causal relationship between the exposure and the adverse health outcome is increased if the relationship is biologically plausible. However, this depends on the state of scientific knowledge at the time. In addition, the associations reported from epidemiologic studies should be coherent with the known facts of the natural history and biology of the event. Very few events have one and only one cause; each event usually is associated with multiple etiologies. A given cause may be necessary (must always be present before the adverse health effect), sufficient (always initiates or produces an effect), both, or neither (for further discussion, see ref. 4).

The conclusion that a relationship is causal is reached more easily when a majority of the criteria are met. The decision on causality is more difficult when the measures of association are weak and where information is lacking for many of the criteria. For example, the chapter by Ebi and Rice summarizes the epidemiologic evidence of an association between occupational exposure to anesthetics and adverse reproductive and developmental outcomes. Approximately one half of the studies reported an association between occupational exposure to anesthetics and congenital abnormalities. However, most of the studies used a retrospective cohort study design that is subject to both selection and recall bias. Generally, data were collected by self-administered questionnaire without verification of either the exposure or the outcome, so the temporality of the reported association in relation to gestational age was not assured. None of the studies reported measurements of air anesthetic concentrations. Exposure was generally measured by employment status. It could not be determined whether the association was specific to an individual anesthetic or to some other factor related to the work environment (e.g., other exposures) or to the study respondents (e.g., experience of degree of stress). The presence of a dose–response relationship could not be evaluated. The associations were not strong and were not consistent among studies, and there was no pattern to the specific abnormalities reported. Thus, the human data are too weak to conclude that there is a causal association between occupational exposure to anesthetics and congenital abnormalities.

SCREENING FOR DISEASE

Screening tests generally are aimed at detecting chronic diseases in apparently healthy individuals not currently under treatment for those diseases or at detecting individuals at high risk for development of disease. Screening was defined in 1951 by the U.S. Commission on Chronic Illness (cited in ref. 1) as

> The presumptive identification of unrecognized disease or defect by the application of tests, examinations or other procedures which can be applied rapidly. Screening tests sort out apparently well persons who probably have a disease from those who probably do not. A screening test is not intended to be diagnostic. Persons with positive or suspicious findings must be referred to their physicians for diagnosis and necessary treatment.

The following characteristics of screening tests are described: sensitivity, specific-ity, and predictive values of positive and negative tests.

The validity of a screening test is measured by its sensitivity and specificity. The sensitivity of a screening test is defined as the ability of the test to correctly identify those individuals with the disease; that is, sensitivity is the probability that a diseased individual will be correctly identified. Specificity is defined as the ability of a test to correctly identify those individuals without the disease; that is, specificity is the probability that a nondiseased individual will be correctly identified. Sensitivity and specificity are determined by comparing the results of the screening test with a definitive diagnostic procedure, or gold standard. True positives are those individuals whom the screening test correctly identifies as having the disease. False positives are those individuals whom the screening test incorrectly identifies as having the disease. Similarly, true negatives are those individuals whom the screening test correctly identifies as not having the disease, and false negatives are those individuals whom the screening test incorrectly identifies as not having the disease. Sensitivity equals the number of true positives divided by the number of true positives plus false negatives (i.e., the true number of individuals with the disease).

$$\text{Sensitivity} = \frac{\text{True positives}}{\substack{\text{Number of individuals} \\ \text{with disease}}} \times 100$$

Specificity equals the number of true negatives divided by the number of true negatives plus false positives (i.e., the true number of individuals without the disease).

$$\text{Sensitivity} = \frac{\text{True negatives}}{\substack{\text{Number of individuals} \\ \text{without disease}}} \times 100$$

The ability to predict that a given individual is a true positive or a true negative depends on the prevalence of the disease as well as the sensitivity and the specificity of the screening test. The predictive value of a positive test equals the number of true positives divided by the number of true positives plus the number of false positives (or the total number tested positive). The higher the prevalence, the more likely that a positive test is predictive of the disease.

$$\text{Predictive value} \atop \text{(positive test)} = \frac{\text{True positives}}{\text{Number of individuals} \atop \text{tested positive}} \times 100$$

The predictive value of a negative test equals the number of true negatives divided by the number of true negatives plus the number of false negatives (or the total number tested negative).

$$\text{Predictive value} \atop \text{(negative test)} = \frac{\text{True negatives}}{\text{Number of individuals} \atop \text{tested negative}} \times 100$$

SUMMARY

Epidemiologic studies are initiated because there is a perception that the rate of an event is higher in one group than in another. The first step in investigating this perception is formulation of a study hypothesis. Next, the most appropriate study design is chosen to address the hypothesis. The study designs that have been used most commonly in studying the toxicity of the anesthetics in humans are cohort and case-control studies. Cohort studies have the advantage of usually establishing that exposure occurred before the event, and case-control studies have the advantage of requiring fewer study subjects when the event is rare. The choice of study design is often based on these and other considerations. As discussed, prospective cohort studies are particularly appropriate for the study of reproductive and developmental outcomes following occupational exposure to anesthetics because large groups can be identified readily for study, and environmental monitoring can be instituted before recording the events. This study design could

eliminate many of the problems with selection bias and recall bias.

Once the study design is chosen, the investigator determines the type of data on the occurrence of the event and on the exposure necessary to answer the study hypothesis and the best way to collect that data. The study population is chosen and the data collection instrument is designed, taking into account characteristics of the study population. The exposure is measured, and data are collected on the occurrence of the event. The data are analyzed in reference to the study hypothesis. The analyses used depend on the study design. Various measures of association are calculated, taking into account confounding influences. The measures of association are evaluated and put in context with other published results to determine whether the association between the exposure and the event is likely to be causal.

Epidemiology provides powerful tools for the identification and evaluation of factors associated with beneficial and adverse health events. The results of epidemiologic studies complement both clinical and laboratory animal studies. The combined and often iterative use of these study approaches ultimately can answer questions of whether a particular factor causes an event.

REFERENCES

1. Last J M, ed. *A dictionary of epidemiology,* 2nd ed. New York: Oxford University Press, 1988.
2. Hemminki K, Kyyronen P, Lindbohm M L. Spontaneous abortions and malformation in the offspring of nurses exposed to anaesthetic gases, cytostatic drugs, and other potential hazards in hospitals, based on registered information of outcome. *J Epidemiol Community Health* 1985;39: 141–147.
3. U.S. Bureau of the Census. *Statistical abstract of the United States: 1992,* 112th ed. Washington, DC, 1992.
4. Rothman K J. *Modern epidemiology.* Boston: Little, Brown and Company, 1986.
5. Axelsson G, Rylander R. Exposure to anaesthetic gases and spontaneous abortion: response bias in a postal questionnaire study. *Int J Epidemiol* 1982;11:250–256.

Anesthetic Toxicity, edited by
Susan A. Rice and Kevin J. Fish.
Raven Press, Ltd., New York © 1994.

4

Metabolism of the Volatile Anesthetics

Lucy Waskell

*Department of Anesthesia, University of California,
San Francisco, California 94143 and Anesthesiology Service,
Veterans Affairs Medical Center, San Francisco, California 94121*

This chapter presents a broad overview of the pathways and enzymology of anesthetic metabolism, with emphasis on the currently used volatile anesthetics. The focus is a basic understanding of modern drug metabolism research so that the metabolism and toxicity of drugs in clinical use today can be readily understood and those introduced in the future can be predicted by anesthesiologists. In addition, the material discussed provides a basis for understanding (a) the 40-fold variation in the ability of normal human subjects to metabolize a given drug and (b) why one drug will have an impact on the metabolism, clinical effect, and toxicity of another.

The armamentarium of drugs available to physicians is dwarfed by the number of known chemical compounds. The Chemical Abstracts Service lists 8 million unique structures, and the number is growing at a rate of 7000/week. More than 63,000 chemical compounds are in common use, and about 11,500 of them are ingested as additives to food or pharmaceutical preparations (1). There are thousands of potentially toxic compounds produced naturally by plants that are consumed in the daily diet. It is widely believed that the enzymes thought of today as drug-metabolizing enzymes evolved millions of years ago to detoxify and metabolize chemical compounds in the diet to assure that such compounds did not accumulate. Thus, it is no coincidence that human drug-metabolizing enzymes can metabolize a large number of structurally diverse compounds (2). The drug-metabolizing enzymes may protect us against foreign chemicals in the same way the immune system protects us against foreign pathogens.

Drug metabolism is primarily a hepatic event, although it also occurs to some extent in the blood, intestine, kidney, lung, skin, and all other organs in the body. The major function of the drug-metabolizing enzymes is to convert fat-soluble compounds to water-soluble compounds that can be excreted by the kidney in the urine. The numerous enzymes that catalyze the metabolism of lipophilic xenobiotics are most abundant in the endoplasmic reticulum of the liver. Perhaps another reason for the predominant role of the liver in the metabolism of xenobiotics, most of which typically would be taken orally, is its immediate access to compounds absorbed via the intestine. In the course of converting fat-soluble compounds to water-soluble excretable compounds, the drug-metabolizing enzymes may detoxify drugs, but they may also convert a pro-drug to a drug (i.e., codeine is converted to morphine; enalapril is deacetylated to the active drug) or may activate a nontoxic compound to a toxic (halothane is converted to trifluoroacetyl chloride) or carcinogenic one.

BIOTRANSFORMATION REACTIONS

The major enzymatic reactions of drug metabolism are oxidation, reduction, hydrolysis, and conjugation. A complete review of these reactions has been published (1). Synthetic (i.e., conjugation) reactions involve the enzymatic addition of an activated endogenous compound, such as glucuronic acid or sulfate, to a drug. Frequently, a drug will undergo oxidation, reduction, or hydrolysis, and a reactive group, such as an acid, amine, or hydroxyl group, will be generated. The product of this reaction can then be conjugated with, for example, glucuronic acid. The conjugated compound will generally, but not always, be water-soluble and inactive.

Oxidation

The superfamily of mixed function oxidases known as cytochrome P450 catalyze at least one step in the metabolism of the majority of drugs used by anesthesiologists. Humans are estimated to have 50 to 200 different cytochromes P450. To date, 30 different human cytochromes P450 have been characterized, and collectively they are probably the most significant enzymes involved in the metabolism of drugs, carcinogens, and steroids (3). These enzymes are found in highest concentration in the endoplasmic reticulum of the liver, where they may account for up to 10% of the protein in this organelle. They also occur in all other organs of the body, typically at lower concentrations than that found in the liver. However, depending on the particular form of cytochrome P450, the aggregate amount of extrahepatic cytochrome P450 may be greater than that found in the liver (4).

A number of apparently different reactions are catalyzed by cytochrome P450. The less common reactions catalyzed by cytochrome P450, such as oxidation of ethylenes and aromatic ring systems, have been reviewed (5–7). By far, the single most commonly catalyzed reaction of the approximately 200 cytochromes P450 known at this time (8,9) is the monooxidation of substrates (i.e., the insertion of an atom of oxygen into the carbon hydrogen bond of the substrate). The overall reaction catalyzed by a cytochrome P450 requires oxygen and NADPH and can be represented as follows.

$$SH + NADPH + O_2 + H^+ \rightarrow$$
$$SOH + NADP^+ + H_2O$$

where SH is the substrate and SOH is the oxidized product. As can be seen from the equation, a diatomic molecule of oxygen is activated and subsequently split, with one atom of oxygen being incorporated into the substrate and the second atom of oxygen being incorporated into a water molecule. The flow of electrons proceeds from NADPH to the flavoprotein NADPH-cytochrome P450 reductase, which then transfers the electrons to the heme group of cytochrome P450 one at a time (Fig. 1). The cytochromes P450 do not catalyze the insertion of oxygen into carbon–halogen bonds.

In vivo cytochrome P450 exists in the ferric (Fe^{3+}) state in the hepatic endoplasmic reticulum. The first step in the cytochrome P450 reaction cycle is the binding of substrate. This promotes rapid transfer of the first electron from cytochrome P450 reductase, resulting in the reduction of the heme iron to the ferrous (Fe^{2+}) form. In the absence of oxygen, it is the reduced ferrous (Fe^{2+}) form of cytochrome P450 that can react with alkyl halide substrates, such as halothane, to generate a free radical (Fig. 2). The reduced form (i.e., Fe^{2+}) of cytochrome P450 binds oxygen, giving rise to oxycytochrome P450. It should be noted that as with myoglobin, hemoglobin, and cytochrome oxidase, only the ferrous form of the heme protein binds oxygen. The reduced form of cytochrome P450 binds very tightly to carbon monoxide (CO). The stable ferrous cytochrome P450 CO complex gives rise to the characteristic 450 nm ab-

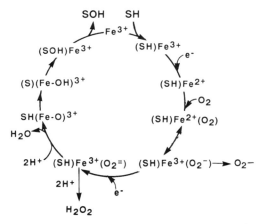

FIG. 1. Reaction cycle of cytochrome P450. SH represents the substrate, and SOH is the oxidized product.

sorption peak. When CO is bound to ferrous cytochrome P450, it prevents oxygen from binding and thereby inhibits the activity of cytochrome P450.

The oxycytochrome P450 can break down to regenerate the ferric form of cytochrome P450 with the formation of a superoxide anion free radical (O_2^-). This side reaction can be observed during the *in vitro* metabolism of the volatile anesthetics and many other substrates by cytochrome P450 (10). Its significance *in vivo* remains to be elucidated. The oxyferrous substrate-bound form of cytochrome P450 next accepts a second electron, usually from cytochrome P450 reductase. However, there are a number of drugs, such as lidocaine, nifedipine, enflurane, halothane, methoxyflurane, and sevoflurane, and endogenous compounds, such as prostaglandins, whose metabolism proceeds much more rapidly when the second electron comes from cytochrome b_5 (4,11,12). Oxygen may dissociate from cytochrome P450 at this stage to regenerate the ferric (Fe^{3+}) cytochrome P450 and the two electron reduced-oxygen species, hydrogen peroxide.

The next step in the reaction cycle is cleavage of the oxygen–oxygen bond with concurrent incorporation of an oxygen atom

into a molecule of water. The remaining activated oxygen atom is bound to the heme iron as a formal $(FeO)^{3+}$ complex. This is the form of cytochrome P450 that has been hypothesized to be the active oxidizing species that functions in catalysis to abstract a hydrogen atom from the substrate. The resulting hydroxyl radical collapses with the substrate carbon radical to generate the product alcohol. The final step is dissociation of the oxidized substrate and regeneration of the oxidized ferric (Fe^{3+}) form of the enzyme (6,13). The details of the cytochrome P450 reaction cycle have been discussed to enable the reader to follow the subsequent discussion of the biodegradation of the individual anesthetics by cytochrome P450 and to predict the metabolism of newer anesthetics as they are introduced into clinical practice. For further information on this subject and its relevance to anesthesiology, the reader is referred to a review about the prediction of rates of drug clearance and drug interactions (14).

ISOZYMES OF CYTOCHROME P450 THAT METABOLIZE ANESTHETICS

Cytochrome P450-2E1

In the cytochrome P450 nomenclature, the first Arabic numeral following P450 denotes the cytochrome P450 family. This is followed by a letter designating the subfamily, which in turn is followed by an Arabic numeral representing the gene within the subfamily. Cytochrome P450-2E1 is a member of the cytochrome P450-2 family, a very diverse, large family that metabolizes a vast number of drugs and endogenous compounds. There is greater than 67% amino acid sequence homology among the subfamilies within the family. An important characteristic of the cytochromes P450-2E is that they metabolize small, rather polar molecules, including the anesthetics (halothane, enflurane, sevoflurane, and methoxyflurane) and halogenated hydrocarbons (chloroform, vinyl chloride, ethylene dibromide, trichloroethylene, and 1,1,1,2-tetrafluoroethane) to a greater extent than do other cytochromes P450 (10,15). Cytochrome P450-2E1 is among the best-conserved forms of cytochrome P450 in different animal species. Hence, experimental results in animals are more likely to be extrapolatable to humans. A complete list of the known substrates for cytochrome P450-2E1 is provided by Koop (15). Other frequently encountered compounds oxidized by this cytochrome P450 are aniline, ethanol, acetaminophen, acetone, benzene, diethyl ether, and a number of carcinogenic nitrosamines. The ability of cytochrome P450-2E1 to be induced by and to metabolize acetone suggests that ketone disposition and gluconeogenesis, particularly during starvation and in untreated diabetes, may represent the physiologic functions of the enzyme (16). Pantuck et al. (17) demonstrated the physiologic relevance of this reaction with the metabolism of enflurane, which was stimulated in the presence of untreated diabetes in rats. Insulin treatment promptly abolished the enhanced enflurane metabolism.

Because cytochrome P450-2E1 plays an important role in anesthetic metabolism, the mechanisms involved in its regulation are of interest to anesthesiologists. Indeed, the enhanced bioactivation of anesthetics noted after exposure to drugs, such as isoniazid and ethanol, stems from elevation of hepatic levels of this enzyme. The intracellular cytochrome P450-2E1 concentration, in contrast to some of the other cytochromes P450, is subject to tight control at the level of transcription, translation, and degradation. There is still disagreement among researchers in the field as to the role of each factor in a specific set of circumstances.

The proposed regulatory mechanisms include (a) increases in cytochrome P450-2E1 mRNA resulting from transcriptional activation or mRNA stabilization, (b) enhanced protein synthesis, and (c) diminished enzyme degradation. The three mechanisms may act individually or in concert to increase the cytochrome P450-2E1 content in the liver (10). Which of the mechanisms predominates depends on a number of factors, including the animal species, the particular inducing agent, the duration of exposure (acute or chronic) to the inducer, and the concentration of the inducer (10,18). For example, ethanol increases cytochrome P450-2E1 concentration by elevating mRNA concentration when blood ethanol levels are high (300 mg/dl) and by stabilizing the protein against proteolytic degradation at low ethanol concentrations (18–20). On withdrawal of ethanol, the activity of the protein declines more rapidly than the immunodetectable cytochrome P450-2E1, suggesting that this cytochrome is inactivated before degradation (21). On the other hand, acetone and starvation increase cytochrome P450-2E1 concentration by markedly inhibiting its degradation. Compared to most other cytochromes P450, cytochrome P450-2E1 has a short half-life, 7 to 8 hours, versus 24 hours for most other cytochromes P450 (22). The numerous, complex, and rapidly acting mechanisms that regulate the cellular levels of cytochrome P450-2E1 are consistent with its purported role in the metabolism of endogenous ligands, such as acetone and acetol (15).

The highest concentrations of cytochrome P450-2E1 are found in the liver. Both before and after induction, cytochrome P450-2E1 expression is maximal in perivenular hepatocytes in humans and animals (18,23). The preferential expression of cytochrome P450-2E1 in the perivenular area of the liver may explain the enhanced susceptibility of these cells to damage from hepatotoxins, including halogenated hydrocarbons (10). Immunochemical procedures also have shown cytochrome P450-2E1 to be present and inducible in extrahepatic tissues, such as rat kidney, lung, nasal epithelia, duodenal and jejunal villous cells, and epithelial cells derived from the cheek mucosa, tongue, esophagus, forestomach, and colon (24). In rabbits, ethanol-inducible cytochrome P450 is found in kidney, nasal mucosa, and, interestingly, bone marrow. The extrahepatic distribution of cytochrome P450-2E1 has not been studied in humans, although most investigators would be surprised if there were not great similarities in the tissue distribution between animals and humans. In mice, in contrast to rats and rabbits, cytochrome P450-2E1 is regulated in a sex-dependent manner. Male mice but not female or immature animals exhibit significant levels of cytochrome P450-2E1 in their kidneys. This most likely explains the kidney damage observed in male but not female mice after exposure to chloroform (10,25). Available evidence suggests that cytochrome P450 concentrations in humans are for the most part not sex dependent.

Two allelic polymorphisms are associated with the cytochrome P450-2E1 gene with a frequency of 10 percent and 24 percent. The ramifications of these polymorphisms for protein expression and function are not known, although it has been reported that susceptibility to lung cancer is associated with the polymorphism that has an incidence of 24% (10,26). Conceivably, these polymorphisms or other yet to be identified polymorphisms in the cytochrome P450-2E1 gene may explain some of the great variability found in the metabolism of the volatile anesthetics by humans. Polymorphisms also have been found in the promoter region of the gene. The promoter region of a gene is a regulatory DNA sequence upstream (at the 5' end) of the actual gene that influences the rate at which the gene is expressed. Two polymorphisms in the promoter region of the cytochrome P450-2E1 gene have been described that increase the expression of a reporter gene by 10-fold (27). If the polymorphisms are found actually to influence in vivo expression of the cytochrome P450-2E1 structural gene itself, individuals possessing such a polymorphism will express more hepatic protein and be capable of enhanced anesthetic metabolism (10).

The activity of cytochrome P450-2E1 or any cytochrome P450 can be decreased in the presence of inhibitors. Such compounds if present in the appropriate concentration in vivo could result in decreased anesthetic metabolism. The two major types of inhibitors are (a) competitive inhibitors that act by preventing the anesthetic from occupying the substrate-binding site of the cytochrome P450 and (b) suicide inhibitors that mediate inhibition by first undergoing activation by cytochrome P450 to a reactive compound that then combines with the cytochrome P450 and destroys the enzyme. A competitive inhibitor may or may not be a substrate for the cytochrome P450 isozyme. It is, therefore, not surprising that the anesthetics and ethanol would mutually inhibit one another's metabolism. A number of suicide inhibitors of cytochrome P450-2E1 are known. Dihydrocapasaicin, a natural product from red peppers used in the treatment of neuralgias, is a suicide inhibitor of cytochrome P450-2E1 and irreversibly inactivates cytochrome P450-2E1 by an incompletely understood mechanism. Diethyldithiocarbamate, the reductive metabolite of disulfiram, and phenethylisothiocyanate, a constituent of cabbage and brussels sprouts, illustrate the diverse sources of inhibitors in our environment and remind us that diet can influence the activity of drug-metabolizing enzymes (15).

Cytochrome P450-2E1, as well as most other cytochromes P450, catalyzes reductive reactions at the ferrous iron of the heme before oxygen binding (Fig. 1). Reductive substrates for cytochrome P450-2E1 include carbon tetrachloride, lipid hydroperoxides, and probably halothane (15). This reaction is discussed in the section, Halothane Metabolism. In conclusion, the regulation of the activity of the enzymes that catalyze anesthetic metabolism and determine anesthetic toxicity is influenced by a myriad of factors that are incompletely understood and warrant further investigation.

Cytochromes P450-2B and P450-3A

The cytochrome P450-2B subfamily prefers globular molecules (i.e., phenobarbital, benzphetamine, and DDT). It also will oxidize methoxyflurane and halothane, but P450-2B does not really specialize in the metabolism of these molecules as does cytochrome P450-2E1 (28). Phenobarbital induces many members of the 2B subfamily of cytochromes P450 in animals. These enzymes have been characterized and studied extensively. This information is currently guiding us in our study of the human enzymes (29). In humans, the 2B subfamily is poorly understood due to its low concentration in human liver and lack of known inducers (14,30). A moderately specific inhibitor of rabbit cytochrome P450-2B4 is phencyclidine, which is better known as a drug of abuse.

The cytochrome P450-3A family in human liver accounts for 60% of the total P450 in some individuals. It has an affinity for large nonplanar substrates (e.g., erythromycin, cyclosporine, ergotamine derivatives, some steroids, alfentanil, nifedipine, midazolam, lidocaine, and aflatoxin) (14,28, 31). At least four very closely related genes are found in humans in the cytochrome P450-3A family. Although the rat cytochrome P450-3A isozyme metabolizes isoflurane (32), it is not known whether this occurs also in humans. The cytochromes P450-3A are inducible by rifampicin, glucocorticoids, such as pregnenolone-16α-carbonitrile, antibiotics, such as erythromycin, and antiseizure medications, such as phenytoin, phenobarbital, and carbamazepine (2). In addition to being an inducer of cytochrome P450-3A, erythromycin is a suicide substrate for this protein. Its net effect is to inhibit the metabolism of the normal substrates of the cytochrome, such as alfentanil, theophylline, carbamazepine, cyclosporine, and midazolam (33–35). At present, no polymorphism has been demonstrated in the cytochrome P450-3A family. Therefore, the interindividual variabil-

ity in the metabolism of substrates of this enzyme is most likely due to variations in the hepatic concentration of cytochrome P450-3A.

Effect of Obesity on Anesthetic Metabolism

One fourth of the adult population of the United States is reported to be more than 20% above the normal weight, and 3% to 5% of the population is morbidly obese, i.e., twice the ideal body weight (36,37). The large number of patients with obesity suggests it is important to know whether these patients metabolize anesthetics in the same manner as nonobese patients. Obese patients produce higher serum concentrations of metabolites, especially inorganic fluoride ion, after administration of halothane (38,39), methoxyflurane (39), or enflurane (40). In contrast, fluoride concentrations are not significantly elevated in obese individuals who have received sevoflurane or isoflurane (41,42). What accounts for the increased metabolism of some of the volatile anesthetics in obese individuals? An early study with halothane and methoxyflurane in obese patients suggested that metabolism of these rather lipid-soluble drugs may have been enhanced because of their extensive absorption into adipose tissue and the subsequent release of this reservoir of drug on discontinuation of the anesthetic. This mechanism provides a greater amount of anesthetic to be metabolized. Another possible mechanism for increased fluoride concentration in obese patients is an increased rate of hepatic biotransformation by cytochrome P450. Salazar et al. demonstrated an increase in hepatic microsomal cytochrome P450-2E1 in obese overfed rats (43), and it is possible that obese humans also have elevated levels of the homologous cytochrome P450. Steroid-metabolizing enzymes, which are known to be increased in obesity, also may metabolize the anesthetics. The small volatile anesthetics may be able to gain entrance to the active site of the steroid-metabolizing enzymes and undergo oxidation. Cytochrome P450 aromatase, which converts androgens to estrogens, is found in low concentrations in adipose tissue (44,45). If adipose tissue were increased by 100 kg as it often is in morbid obesity, the total body content of cytochrome P450 aromatase would be substantially increased and potentially could augment hepatic anesthetic metabolism significantly.

If anesthetic metabolism is increased in human obesity because cytochrome P450-2E1 is increased, the metabolism of sevoflurane also should be increased because human cytochrome P450-2E1 metabolizes sevoflurane (46). The lack of enhanced sevoflurane metabolism in obese patients suggests that cytochrome P450-2E1 may not be increased in obese humans in contrast to the obese overfed rat. It also demonstrates that cytochrome P450 aromatase and the cortisol-metabolizing cytochrome P450 do not metabolize sevoflurane. Thus, the most likely explanation for the enhanced metabolism of the lipid-soluble anesthetics, halothane, methoxyflurane, and enflurane but not the relatively insoluble sevoflurane in obese patients is that the lipid-soluble drugs dissolve in the adipose tissue and release anesthetic for continued metabolism long after the drug has been discontinued.

With the preceding information as a background, the metabolism of the individual anesthetics can be discussed. An excellent review of the metabolism of all the volatile anesthetics has been written by Baden and Rice (47). It should be consulted, particularly for information regarding the nonclinically used anesthetics. The following discussion deals primarily with understanding the metabolism of the volatile anesthetics as it relates to the recent research on the molecular biology, structure, and function of the cytochromes P450. Except for the conjugation of the sevoflurane metabolite, hexafluoroisopropranol, these oxidases catalyze virtually all volatile anesthetic metabolism.

Halothane

Oxidative Metabolism

The oxidative and reductive pathways of halothane metabolism are illustrated in Figure 2A,B. Halothane has a carbon–hydrogen bond that is susceptible to oxidation by cytochrome P450. When this carbon–hydrogen bond is replaced by a deuterium–carbon bond, the deuterated halothane is more slowly metabolized, indicating that cleavage of the carbon–hydrogen bond is a determinant of the rate-limiting step in halothane metabolism (48). The product of halothane oxidation by cytochrome P450 is 1,1,1-trifluoro-2-chloro-2-bromoethanol, which is unstable and rapidly decomposes *in vivo* to produce hydrogen bromide and trifluoroacetyl chloride, which is also a chemically reactive compound that spontaneously breaks down in the presence of water to produce trifluoroacetic acid. Trifluoroacetic acid is readily quantitated in the blood and urine (49–51). Bromide ion is easily measured. However, it is an inaccurate index of the amount of halothane metabolized because bromide excretion is markedly dependent on hydration and anion balance (50,51). Because approximately 25% to 46% of the halothane absorbed by the body in the course of an anesthetic is metabolized to trifluoroacetyl chloride, several grams of it are expected to be generated during the course of a halothane anesthetic (52,53). It is thus a metabolite whose chemical reactivity and abundance suggest it may be toxic *in vivo*. In fact, the trifluoroacetyl moiety does covalently react with the microsomal membrane lipid, phosphatidyl ethanolamine, which is degraded to the urinary metabolite, N-trifluoroacetyl-2-aminoethanol (54,55). Although the immunogenicity of trifluoroacetyl phosphatidylethanolamine has never been demonstrated, some N-substituted derivatives of phosphatidylethanolamine are immunogenic (56). These two incidental observations are quite intriguing and lead one to

OXIDATIVE METABOLISM OF HALOTHANE

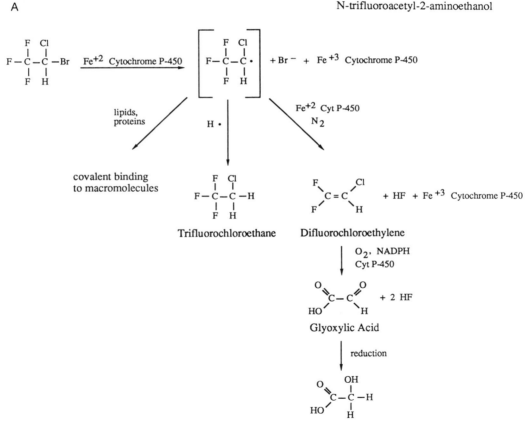

FIG. 2. A. Oxidative metabolism of halothane. B. Reductive metabolism of halothane. Fe^{2+} cytochrome P450, and Fe^{3+} cytochrome P450 refer to ferrous (Fe^{2+}) cytochrome P450 and ferric (Fe^{3+}) cytochrome P450, respectively.

wonder whether trifluoroacetyl phosphatidylethanolamine might play a role in halothane hepatitis.

Trifluoroacetyl chloride also reacts with the amino group of lysines on intracellular proteins but does not significantly bind to cellular RNA or DNA (57–60). It has been demonstrated that humans with halothane hepatitis produce antibodies to trifluoroacetylated rabbit serum albumin and have trifluoroacetylated protein adducts in their liver. The presumed antigens for these antibodies are the hepatic trifluoroacetylated-protein adducts (59,61–63). Patients who recently have received halothane harbor trifluoroacetylated protein adducts in their liver, regardless of whether or not halothane hepatitis eventually develops. These trifluoroacetylated proteins from humans and animals crossreact with antibodies in the sera from patients with halothane hepatitis (59,61,62,64). Despite this circumstantial evidence, a direct role for such antibodies in mediating hepatic injury has not been demonstrated and is clearly the missing link in proving an immunologic etiology for halothane hepatitis. One study by Callis et al. (65) appears to suggest that antibodies may not have a role in halothane hepatitis. Rabbits were immunized with trifluoroacetylated rabbit serum albumin and developed high antibody titers. The antibodies to trifluoroacetylated rabbit serum albumin are known to crossreact with liver antigens of rats and rabbits exposed to halothane and, surprisingly, with antigens in animals that have never been exposed to halothane (63). However, rabbits with high antibody titers were not more prone to halothane-induced hepatotoxicity. The protein that molecularly mimics the trifluoroacetylated protein adducts recently has been identified as the dihydrolipoamide acetyltransferase subunit of the pyruvate dehydrogenase enzyme, which is localized to the cytosol. Free lipoic acid, the prosthetic group of the pyruvate dehydrogenase complex, can competitively inhibit the interaction of the pyruvate dehydrogenase complex and trifluoroacetylated-protein adducts with the antitrifluoroacetylated rabbit serum albumin antibody. These data suggest that lipoic acid, whose structural similarity to trifluoroacetylated lysine was unappreciated until this study, molecularly mimics trifluoroacetylated protein adducts (63).

At present, the direct toxicologic consequences of trifluoroacetylated protein adduct formation within the liver are unclear. However, these data suggest alternative mechanisms for halothane hepatitis. For instance, it might be possible for a standard amount of trifluoroacetylation to inactivate a critical mutant cellular protein, rendering it inactive and ultimately culminating in the appearance of hepatic necrosis. Another possibility is that a rare individual may have an extraordinary capacity for halothane oxidation and, therefore, generate a toxic amount of trifluoroacetylated protein adducts. For example, a mutation in the promoter region of the cytochrome P450 gene could lead to overproduction of the protein that catalyzes halothane oxidation. For additional details and discussion about halothane hepatitis, see the chapter by Baker and Van Dyke.

Reductive Metabolism

Of the halothane absorbed during the course of an anesthetic, it has been estimated both in children and adults that 0.1% to 0.64% is metabolized via a reductive pathway to fluoride ion (Fig. 2b) (51,66–68). Because of the numerous inherent inaccuracies in measuring low levels of fluoride ion excretion (e.g., urine volume, bone absorption) and the fact that fluoride is the end product of only one of the reactions of the trifluoro-chloroethane radical, this value is probably low. Nonetheless, it is clearly the minor pathway of halothane metabolism under normal clinical conditions. The 1,1,1-trifluoro-2-chloroethane free radical is the primary product of the reductive metabolism of halothane. This reaction was first described about 20 years ago and is simply the reduction of an alkyl halide by a reduced heme protein. The caveat is that the alkyl halide must be able to gain access to the iron of the heme protein and must possess a good leaving group (i.e., bromide) (69–74). These early studies have been confirmed using halothane and hemin, hemoglobin, and cytochrome P450 (75). Typically, the products resulting from the reaction of a reduced (Fe^{2+}) heme protein and alkyl halide are the ferric (Fe^{3+}) heme protein, an alkyl free radical, and a halide ion. In the reaction cycle of cytochrome P450 depicted in Figure 1, this reaction occurs after introduction of the first electron but before oxygen binds. Once oxygen binds, the reaction cycle will proceed to undergo oxidation and to forgo reduction. Thus, it is easy to understand why this reaction is favored in the absence of oxygen (76–78). If this free radical diffuses out of the active site of the cytochrome P450 where it was generated, it can abstract a hydrogen free radical from a cellular molecule, possibly an unsaturated lipid, to yield the volatile compound 1,1,1-trifluoro-2-chloroethane, which is excreted into the breath of both animals and humans (79,80). The free 1,1,1-trifluoro-2-chloroethane radical also has been shown to covalently react with unsaturated lipids (81). The third reaction the 1,1,1-trifluoro-2-chloroethane free radical may undergo is further reduction by either the same or another molecule of cytochrome P450 to yield the CF_3CClH^- carbanion, which then decomposes to 1,1-difluoro-2-chloroethylene by beta elimination of fluoride (82–84). Glyoxylic acid, glycolic acid, and fluoride are products of the *in vitro* metabolism of 1,1-difluoro-2-chloroethylene by rat cytochrome P450 (85). During the reductive metabolism of halothane, cytochrome P450 may undergo irreversible inactivation and destruction of its heme prosthetic group. This process is known as suicide inactivation and presumably is due to the activated halothane molecule react-

ing with the heme group of cytochrome P450 (86).

Although it is not known which isozymes of human cytochrome P450 metabolize halothane, it has been demonstrated that the purified phenobarbital- and ethanol-induced forms of cytochrome P450 from the rabbit readily metabolize halothane to trifluoroacetic acid (12). In the current nomenclature, cytochrome P450-2B4 and P450-2E1 are the phenobarbital- and ethanol-inducible forms of rabbit cytochrome P450, respectively. They were known formerly as cytochromes P450-LM2 and P450-3a (9,87). The purified cytochrome P450-2E1 is 2.5-fold more active in metabolizing halothane than is cytochrome P450-2B4, the phenobarbital-inducible form of cytochrome P450. In humans, there is a cytochrome P450 that is homologous to the animal ethanol-inducible cytochromes P450. The human ethanol-inducible cytochrome P450 has 88% of its amino acids identical to the rabbit protein and 78% identical to the rat protein (88,89). It is, therefore, likely that human cytochrome P450-2E1 will also metabolize halothane (10). The clinical implications of the metabolism of halothane by the ethanol-inducible form of cytochrome P450 are unknown at this time. In humans, this form of cytochrome P450 is induced by isoniazid and ethanol (90). However, it should be remembered that the intracellular level of this cytochrome P450 is very highly regulated (91). High levels of this protein exist in the presence of ethanol. Under these conditions, halothane metabolism would be expected to be competitively inhibited by the ethanol. As the ethanol concentrations fell, there would be a window of time, approximately 8 to 12 hours, during which the cytochrome P450 level still would be high and the ethanol concentration would be low if not absent, and, thus, halothane metabolism would occur very rapidly and perhaps have toxicologic consequences (92). Additional research into the relationship between halothane metabolism and the cellular concentrations of the ethanol-inducible cytochrome P450 would be most interesting and might provide insights into the mechanism of halothane hepatitis.

Enflurane

Enflurane is much less readily metabolized than halothane. The consensus is that 2% to 8% of the enflurane taken up during the course of an anesthetic is metabolized (52,93). Knowing that cytochrome P450 metabolizes enflurane and, further, that cytochrome P450 oxidizes carbon–hydrogen bonds, not carbon–halogen bonds, one can predict both of the pathways of enflurane metabolism shown in Figure 3. Cytochrome P450 attacks both of the hydrogen bonds of enflurane, giving rise to reactive intermediates that spontaneously break down. The quantum chemical calculations performed by Loew et al. (94) correctly predict the relative susceptibility of the three ether anesthetics—enflurane, methoxyflurane, and isoflurane—to biodegradation. At present, it is not possible to predict with any accuracy which carbon–hydrogen bond on a molecule will be preferentially oxidized. This is because one of the major determinants of which carbon–hydrogen bond will be oxidized is the proximity of a given bond to the active oxygen species in the ac-

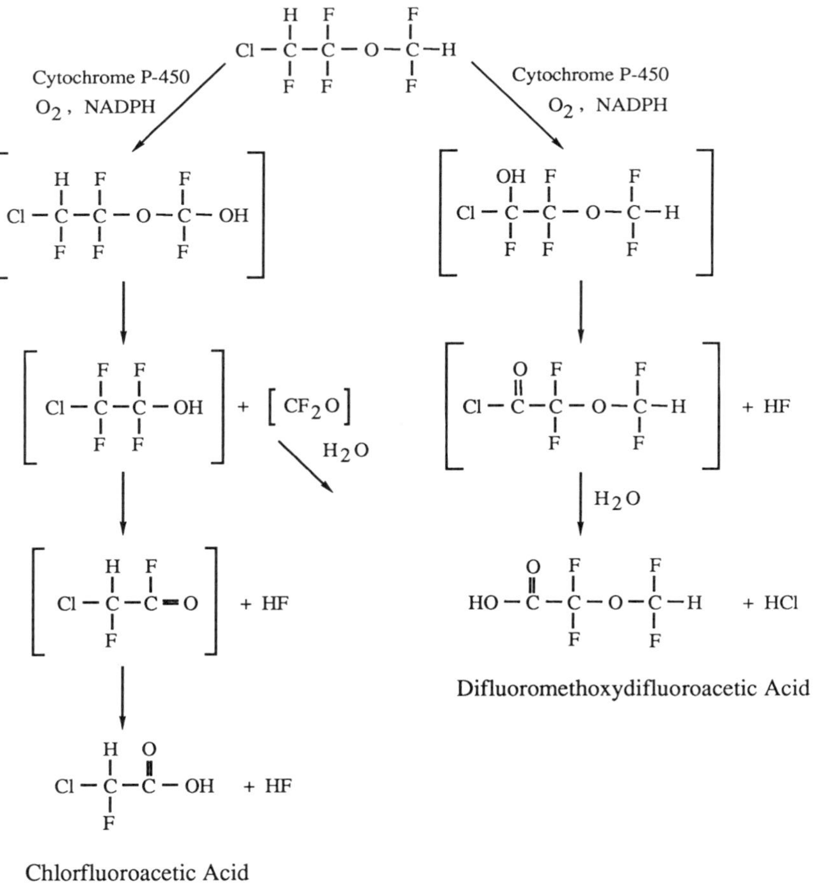

FIG. 3. Metabolism of enflurane.

tive site of cytochrome P450 (7). All other things being equal, the carbon–hydrogen bond closest to the active oxygen will be preferentially attacked. Until the high-resolution structure of the active sites of the different cytochromes P450 can be determined either by x-ray crystallography or model building, it will not be possible to know in advance with any accuracy which part of the molecule will be most susceptible to oxidation. The x-ray crystal structures of two different cytochromes P450 have been determined (95–102), and they have been used as a template to build models of additional mammalian microsomal cytochromes P450 (103–107). A remarkable discovery is that although the amino acid sequences of the cytochromes P450 can have less than 10% homology, their overall three-dimensional structure is well conserved (108). This has enabled researchers to construct a model of some cytochromes P450 and predict which amino acids near the substrate binding site of a particular cytochrome P450 might regulate the regioselectivity of a given substrate (109,110).

Replacement of the hydrogens in enflurane with deuterium decreases the metabolism of enflurane as expected (111). The experiments of Burke et al. have revealed that the majority of enflurane metabolism occurs via oxidation of the CHClF group to form CHF_2OCF_2COOH and chloride and fluoride ions (112). In contrast, the CHF_2 group does not appear to be appreciably susceptible to metabolic oxidative dehalogenation. Insufficient amounts of fluoride are generated during the course of long enflurane anesthetics or in patients taking the cytochrome P450-2E1 inducer isoniazid to lead to clinical evidence of significant renal toxicity secondary to fluoride (113–118), (see chapter by Fish).

Is enflurane hepatotoxic? The consensus is that there is no compelling evidence to seriously incriminate enflurane or to formulate firm clinical guidelines (see chapter by Baker and Van Dyke) (119). In spite of the lack of clinical evidence for enflurane hepatitis, Christ et al. proposed a plausible molecular mechanism for such hepatotoxicity (120,121). These investigators demonstrated that enflurane metabolism produces covalently bound liver adducts that are recognized by antibodies from patients with halothane hepatitis. The proposed enflurane protein adduct is CF_2HOCF_2CONH-protein. Because the antibodies to halothane-protein adducts in halothane hepatitis patients have not been shown to play a role in halothane hepatitis in humans, the clinical significance of this finding in patients receiving enflurane is unknown at present. Along this same line is the fact that hydrochlorofluorocarbons, in particular 2,2-dichloro-1,1,1-trifluoroethane (CF_3CCl_2H), which are being developed as substitutes for the ozone-depleting chlorofluorocarbons, also generate trifluoroacetylated lysine adducts in the liver, kidney, and heart of exposed rats. Such adducts crossreact with a polyclonal antibody to trifluoroacetylated rabbit serum albumin (122,123). The authors of these articles suggest that humans exposed to hydrochlorofluorocarbons may be at risk of developing an immunologically mediated hepatitis.

Phenobarbital pretreatment of rats has been observed by some but not all investigators to at most double the rate of enflurane metabolism by rat liver microsomes (124–126). Liver microsomes from rabbits pretreated with phenobarbital did not metabolize enflurane any faster than microsomes from untreated animals (Waskell, unpublished data). Humans chronically taking barbiturates also did not have higher serum fluoride levels following administration of enflurane (113,127). Thus, the bulk of the evidence suggests that enflurane metabolism is not induced by the barbiturates.

A case report of an isoniazid-treated patient who developed a high serum fluoride ion level and a transient urinary concentrating defect following enflurane anesthesia provided the first clue that isoniazid might be a cytochrome P450 inducer in humans (115). Subsequent studies in rats (126), rabbits (11), and humans (90,114) have supported these preliminary findings. Isoniazid induces the same cytochrome P450-2E1 that is induced by ethanol. This protein is capable of metabolizing the four ether anesthetics (11,126) and halothane (12) and, hence, is of particular interest to anesthesiologists. One curious observation was made by Mazze et al. (114) in their study of enflurane metabolism in patients taking isoniazid. Only one half of the patients who were allegedly taking isoniazid experienced elevated levels of serum fluoride ion following enflurane administration. The authors speculated that this somehow might be related to the acetylator phenotype of the individual (114). Ethanol also induces cytochrome P450-2E1 and enhances enflurane metabolism (92,128,129). Experiments using purified cytochrome P450-2E1 from rabbits and humans have confirmed the results of studies that used microsomes (11,130) and have demonstrated that cytochrome P450-2E1 is the predominant, if not the exclusive, enzyme catalyzing enflurane defluorination in human liver.

Isoflurane

In early clinical trials, isoflurane, an isomer of enflurane, was shown to be physically stable and minimally susceptible to biodegradation. It, therefore, was a great surprise when Corbett reported that it was carcinogenic in mice (131). Isoflurane was withdrawn until a further extensive study indicated that isoflurane was not carcinogenic (132). The explanation for Corbett's original findings of the carcinogenicity of isoflurane is that the animal feed was inadvertently contaminated with mutagenic polybrominated biphenyls during an episode of foodstuff contamination in Michigan in 1975. Resolution of the carcinogenic potential of isoflurane permitted its reintroduction into clinical practice where, until the recent introduction of desflurane, it was the

most slowly metabolized of the fluorinated volatile anesthetics. A mere 0.2% of the isoflurane absorbed during the course of an anesthetic is metabolized to trifluoroacetic acid and fluoride ion (Fig. 4). The rest is exhaled unchanged. In humans, peak serum fluoride concentrations average 4.4 μM following 1.2 to 5.3 MAC-hours of isoflurane. This value is twice the preanesthetic value and well below the nephrotoxic threshold (133). Recent studies by Murray and Trinick with 19.2 MAC-hours of isoflurane found peak serum fluoride ion concentrations of 50 μM, far higher than previously realized (134). Although no clinical or biochemical evidence was found to suggest postoperative renal dysfunction, caution was advised when using isoflurane for such prolonged periods.

As with its isomer enflurane, the difluoromethyl group of isoflurane is relatively resistant to attack by cytochrome P450. Note that trifluoroacetic acid is a metabolite of both halothane and isoflurane metabolism (133,135,136). The initial attack on the isoflurane molecule occurs at the hydrogen-bearing carbon on the ethyl group and results in the formation of the reactive intermediate, trifluoroacetyl chloride. It is the identical reactive intermediate generated during the course of halothane metabolism. This intermediate will also trifluoroacetylate amino groups on proteins, but because of the 100-fold lesser amount of metabolism of isoflurane, the reaction is believed to be quantitatively inconsequential. Nonetheless, Christ et al. were able to detect low levels of trifluoroacetylated liver microsomal protein adducts that were recognized by antibodies to trifluoroacetylated rabbit serum albumin, when rats were given isoflurane (121). These data suggest there may be some crossreaction between isoflurane and halothane. The labeling produced by isoflurane was much lower than that produced by halothane, and, hence, the immunogenic potential is considered to be lower. Christ et al. (121) have stated that the risk cannot be considered trivial because

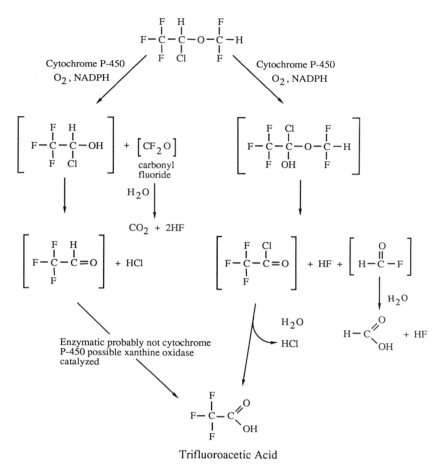

FIG. 4. Metabolism of isoflurane.

the degree of haptenic alteration necessary to provoke an immune response in a sensitized individual is unknown. In 1987, the Anesthetic and Life Support Advisory Committee concluded that "current evidence does not indicate a reasonable likelihood of an association between the use of isoflurane and the occurrence of postoperative hepatic dysfunction" (137).

As previously stated, both isoniazid and ethanol induced the metabolism of isoflurane (126,128,138), suggesting that isoflurane is also metabolized by the ethanol-inducible cytochrome P450-2E1. Isoflurane metabolism is stimulated by pretreating rats

with phenobarbital and pregnenolone-16α-carbonitrile (PCN) but not by pretreating animals with β-napthoflavone (32). The major forms of rat cytochrome P450 induced by phenobarbital are cytochrome P450-2B1 and P450-2B2, whereas PCN induces two proteins from another gene family, cytochrome P450-3A. Cytochrome P450-3A appears to be more active in metabolizing isoflurane than cytochromes P450-2B1 and P450-2B2 (32). The cytochrome P450-3A family also plays an important role in humans in metabolizing a number of other drugs, for example, midazolam, alfentanil, erythromycin, testosterone, nifedipine, and cyclosporine (9). Isoflurane can be expected to inhibit the metabolism of these drugs.

Methoxyflurane

Prior to the studies by Van Dyke et al. in 1964, the volatile anesthetics were considered to be biochemically inert (139). These investigators demonstrated the existence of radioactive metabolites of methoxyflurane in the exhaled breath and urine of animals receiving the radioactively labeled anesthetic. The following year, it was shown that anesthetic biodegradation was carried out primarily by hepatic microsomes (140). Fluoride ion was first documented as a metabolite of methoxyflurane metabolism by Taves et al. (141) using the recently developed fluoride ion electrode. In patients who had received methoxyflurane, fluoride ion was shown to be markedly elevated in serum. The elevated levels were associated with a polyuric, vasopressin-resistant, renal failure that was first reported by Goldemburg in patients receiving i.v. injections of sodium fluoride for treatment of thyrotoxicosis (142). A dose–response study of methoxyflurane published in 1973 lead Cousins and Mazze to recommend that the use of methoxyflurane in clinical anesthesia should be restricted to situations where it offers specific advantages and where dosages less than 2.5 MAC-hours can be attained (143) (see chapter by Fish).

The molecular mechanism by which fluoride ion causes nephrotoxicity is unknown. (Oxalic acid has been shown not to be the etiologic agent of methoxyflurane renal failure [144]). Fluoride ion may cause renal damage simply because of the higher concentration achieved in the renal tubule than in other organs of the body. Concentrations of 1000 μM, which are readily achieved *in vivo* in the renal tubule, are toxic to cells *in vitro* (141). Studies by Edwards et al. (145) have shown that fluoride ion can bind to arginine-48 at the active site of cytochrome c

peroxidase and markedly alter the structure and function of this protein. This example raises the possibility that fluoride ion may be binding to an arginine on a critical molecule in the renal tubules, perhaps the antidiuretic hormone receptor. A second possibility is that fluoride ion may disrupt the activity of a critical intracellular nucleotide-binding protein. It is known, for example, that millimolar concentrations of fluoride in conjunction with aluminum and beryllium alter the activity of a number of important nucleotide-binding proteins, such as transducin, mitochondrial ATPase, tubulin, muscle adenylate kinase, actin, and myosin (146).

The two predicted pathways of methoxyflurane biodegradation are shown in Figure 5. Replacement of the hydrogen atoms of methoxyflurane with deuterium decreases metabolism at the predicted carbon–deuterium bond. Deuteration of the ethyl portion of methoxyflurane enhances oxidation at the unsubstituted methyl group (111,147). These data indicate that the active oxygen species of cytochrome P450 is irreversibly committed to catalysis, and when one bond is difficult to oxidize, it will simply attack an adjacent bond. Because of its extensive metabolism, readily quantifiable metabolites, and requirement for cytochrome b_5 in addition to cytochrome P450, methoxyflurane is an excellent model of drug metabolism and has been studied extensively both *in vivo* and *in vitro*. It has been estimated that 70% to 75% of the methoxyflurane taken up by humans is metabolized (52,135,148). Methoxydifluoroacetic acid is the major metabolite both *in vivo* in humans and *in vitro* (135; Gruenke and Waskell, unpublished data). It is nontoxic and soluble in water. The purified phenobarbital-inducible rabbit cytochrome P450-2B4 attacks the carbon–hydrogen bond on the ethyl group of methoxyflurane approximately seven times faster than it attacks the methyl group. The reaction stoichiometry depicted in Figure 5 has in fact been observed (149; Gruenke and Waskell, unpublished data). In both re-

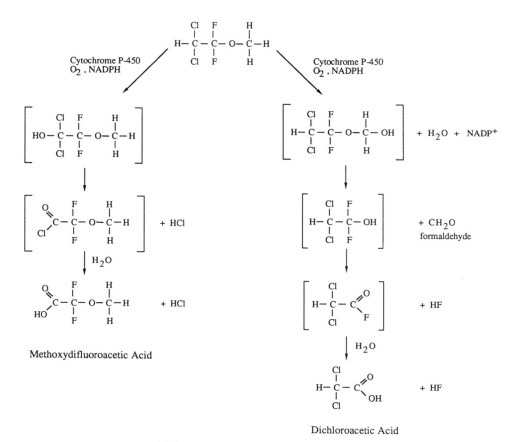

FIG. 5. Metabolism of methoxyflurane.

actions, only cytochrome b_5 can provide the second electron (Fig. 1). Thus, in the absence of functional cytochrome b_5, methoxyflurane metabolism is minimal both in hepatic microsomes and with purified cytochrome P450 (150–152). Why cytochrome P450 reductase is unable to provide the second electron to cytochrome P450-2B4 during methoxyflurane metabolism is a mystery with unknown but potentially interesting physiologic consequences. It should be noted that this phenomenon is not restricted to the metabolism of methoxyflurane by cytochrome P450-2B4 but also can be observed with methoxyflurane metabolism by cytochrome P450-4B1 (LM5) and

the cytochrome P450-2E1-catalyzed oxidations of halothane and enflurane (11,12,152).

Cytochrome b_5 normally functions to provide electrons for fatty acid desaturation and cholesterol biosynthesis and is required for the metabolism of some prostaglandins by cytochrome P450 (150). *In vivo* cytochrome b_5 receives its electrons from NADH, in contrast to cytochrome P450, which receives its reducing equivalents from NADPH. This suggests that the relative intracellular levels of NADH and NADPH may regulate critical cellular homeostatic processes that might be disrupted when an anesthetic requiring cytochrome b_5 for metabolism is administered. In rare instances, perhaps in someone with a genetic defect in lipid biosynthesis, such an interaction might serve as a mechanism by which halothane metabolism, for example, diverts electrons away from critical biochemical reactions, thereby augmenting hepatotoxicity.

Methoxyflurane administration is not associated with hepatotoxicity. Methoxyflurane is metabolized by the two purified phenobarbital-inducible cytochromes P450-2B4 and P450-4B from rabbit liver (152) and the ethanol-inducible cytochrome P450-2E1 (11). Methoxyflurane metabolism also is enhanced by pretreatment of rats and rabbits with phenobarbital, phenytoin, ethanol, diazepam, and isoniazid (153–156).

Desflurane

Desflurane, which differs from isoflurane by having a fluorine instead of a chlorine atom on the ethyl group, was introduced into clinical practice in the United States in 1993. It is a very stable molecule and undergoes significantly less metabolism than isoflurane. It presumably is oxidized in a manner analogous to isoflurane to trifluoroacetic acid and fluoride ion (157). When administered to patients (3.1 MAC-hours) and volunteers (7.35 MAC-hours), postanesthesia serum fluoride ion concentrations did not differ from background fluoride ion concentrations. Trifluoroacetic acid levels in the serum and urine are elevated over control values, but they are approximately 10-fold less than levels seen after exposure to isoflurane.

Sevoflurane

Sevoflurane is a fluorinated inhaled anesthetic currently undergoing clinical trials in the United States, whereas it is already in clinical use in Japan. It is a moderately chemically unstable molecule both *in vivo* and in the presence of soda lime and bara-

lyme. In addition to methanol, five compounds are formed as degradation products of the reaction between sevoflurane and soda lime in a glass flask (158). However, during circulation of sevoflurane in a closed anesthesia circuit for 8 hours, one major and one minor degradation product were detected. The major product is called compound A ($CF_2 = C(CF_3)OCH_2F$), and the minor product is known as compound B ($CH_3OCF_2CH(CF_3)OCH_2F$). Compound A presumably arises by abstraction of a proton from the hydrogen on the isopropyl groups of sevoflurane by the base, soda lime. The negatively charged product then eliminates a fluoride ion to yield compound A, which is toxic at levels twice those found in the anesthesia circuit of patients receiving sevoflurane (133,159). Recall that halothane also is deprotonated in soda lime and yields difluorobromochloroethylene ($CF_2 = CClBr$), which is then conjugated with cysteine (54, 80). Compound B presumably results from addition of the methoxide anion (CH_3O^-) to the CF_2 group of compound A. The methoxide is formed by abstraction of a proton from methanol by the base, soda lime. Interestingly, this addition of an alcohol to a haloethylene is similar to the reaction used to synthesize the ethyl methyl ether anesthetic, methoxyflurane (160). Compound B, which is saturated, is not toxic. In light of the toxicity of compound A and the fact that the nontoxic volatile anesthetics desflurane and isoflurane are clinically available, Mazze has recommended that more research be done on the toxicity of sevoflurane before it is released for clinical practice in the United States (161).

In humans, sevoflurane, which possesses a low blood-gas partition coefficient (0.6), undergoes limited biotransformation, 1% to 4% of the absorbed dose (162) (Fig. 6). Accordingly, sevoflurane is similar to enflurane with respect to biotransformation in humans. In rats and in humans, the products of sevoflurane metabolism are fluoride ion, formic acid, and hexafluoroisopro-

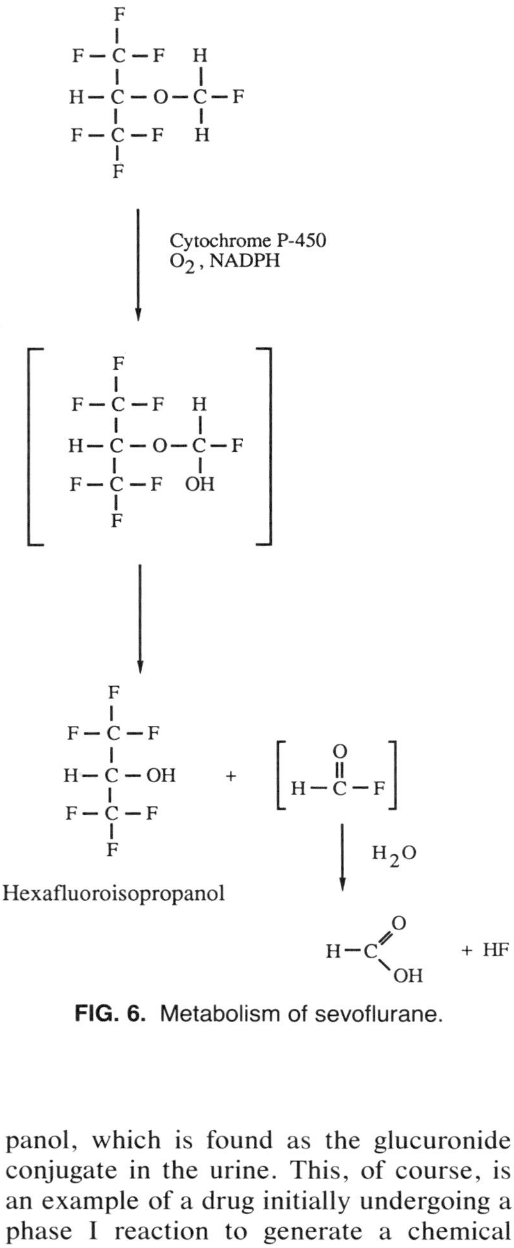

FIG. 6. Metabolism of sevoflurane.

bonds in sevoflurane can be oxidized by cytochrome P450. Because attacks at both the methyl and dichloroethyl positions would result in the same final product, only the oxidation considered most likely is illustrated (Fig. 6). After 1 MAC-hour exposure to sevoflurane, the serum fluoride concentration is 22.1 μM. Longer periods of administration have resulted in peak concentrations of approximately 50 μM, which have not been associated with clinical evidence of renal toxicity (166,167). Fluoride concentrations fall rapidly on discontinuation of sevoflurane due to the low tissue solubility. Consequently, most biotransformation occurs during exposure, in contrast to the very lipid-soluble anesthetic methoxyflurane, where most of the metabolism occurs postexposure as fat depots release the stored anesthetic. It thus appears that both the peak concentration of fluoride and the length of time it is sustained are determinants of renal toxicity.

Sevoflurane metabolism is increased in hepatic liver microsomes from rats pretreated with phenobarbital and dilantin (155) but not in hepatic microsomes from rabbits pretreated with phenobarbital (11). It is unknown if this is also true in humans. Isoniazid, ethanol, and imidazole pretreatment of rats and rabbits results in enhanced metabolism of sevoflurane due to induction of cytochrome P450-2E1 (11,126,129,138). Purified rabbit cytochrome P450-2E1 metabolized sevoflurane. Addition of cytochrome b_5 to the reaction mixture enhances sevoflurane defluorination 6-fold. As discussed in the methoxyflurane section, the physiologic significance of the role of cytochrome b_5 in *in vivo* anesthetic metabolism is unknown and poses a very interesting clinical question (11).

SUMMARY

The recent introduction of desflurane into the clinical practice of anesthesiology is the culmination of a three decades long

panol, which is found as the glucuronide conjugate in the urine. This, of course, is an example of a drug initially undergoing a phase I reaction to generate a chemical group that subsequently can be conjugated and converted to a water-soluble compound (162–164). The median lethal dose of hexafluoroisopropanol in mice is 300 to 600 mg/kg, far greater than amounts expected from sevoflurane biotransformation in humans, even during long anesthetics (165). Theoretically, both of the carbon–hydrogen search for an anesthetic that is clinically stable and nontoxic. The need for such a compound arose out of research demonstrating that the toxicity of the volatile anesthetics could be attributed to their metabolism to chemically reactive metabolites.

REFERENCES

1. Vessey D. Metabolism of drugs and toxins by human liver. In: Zakim D, Boyer T, eds. *Hepatology: A textbook of liver disease.* Philadelphia: WB Saunders, 1990:196–234.
2. Watkins P. Role of cytochromes P450 in drug metabolism and hepatotoxicity. *Semin Liver Dis* 1990;10:235–250.
3. Guengerich F. Human cytochrome P450 enzymes. *Life Sci* 1992;50:1471–1478.
4. Peyronneau M-A, Renaud J, Truan G, Urban P, Pompon D, Mansuy D. Optimization of yeast-expressed human liver cytochrome P450-3A4 catalytic substrates by coexpressing NADPH cytochrome P450 reductase and cytochrome b₅. *Eur J Biochem* 1992;207:109–116.
5. Guengerich P. Bioactivation and detoxification of toxic and carcinogenic chemicals. *Drug Metab Disp* 1993;21:1–6.
6. Ortiz de Montellano P, Reich N. Inhibition of cytochrome P450 enzymes. In: Ortiz de Montellano P, ed. *Cytochrome P450 structure, mechanism and biochemistry.* New York, London: Plenum Press, 1986:273.
7. Ortiz de Montellano P. Cytochrome P450 catalysis: radical intermediates and dehydrogenation reactions. *Trends Pharmacol Sci* 1989;10:354–359.
8. Nebert D. Proposed role of drug-metabolizing enzymes: regulation of steady-state levels of the ligands that affect growth, homeostasis, differentiation and neuro-endocrine functions. *Mol Endocrinol* 1991;5:1203–1214.
9. Gonzalez F. The molecular biology of cytochrome P450s. *Pharmacol Rev* 1989;40:243–288.
10. Raucy J, Kraner J, Lasker M. Bioactivation of halogenated hydrocarbons by cytochrome P450-2E1. *Crit Rev Toxicol* 1993;23:1–20.
11. Hoffman J, Konopka K, Buckhorn C, Koop D, Waskell L. Ethanol-inducible cytochrome P450 in rabbits metabolizes enflurane. *Br J Anaesth* 1989;63:103–108.
12. Gruenke L, Konopka K, Koop D, Waskell L. Characterization of halothane oxidation by hepatic microsomes and purified cytochrome P450 using a gas chromatographic mass spectrometric assay. *J Pharm Exp Ther* 1988;246:454–459.
13. White R, Coon M. Oxygen activation by cytochrome P450. *Annu Rev Biochem* 1980;49:315–356.
14. Gonzalez F. Human cytochromes P450: prob-

lems and prospects. *Trends Pharmacol Sci* 1992;13:346–352.
15. Koop D. Oxidative and reductive metabolism by cytochrome P450-2E1. *FASEB J* 1992;6:724–730.
16. Koop D, Casazza J. Identification of the ethanol-inducible P450 isozyme 3a as the acetone and acetol monooxygenase of rabbit microsomes. *J Biol Chem* 1985;260:13607–13612.
17. Pantuck E, Pantuck C, Conney A. Affect of streptozotocin-induced diabetes in the rat on the metabolism of fluorinated volatile anesthetics. *Anesthesiology* 1987;66:24–28.
18. Takahashi T, Lasker J, Rosman A, Lieber C. Induction of cytochrome P450-2E1 in the human liver by ethanol is caused by a corresponding increase in encoding messenger RNA. *Hepatology* 1993;17:236–245.
19. Eliasson E, Johansson I, Ingelman-Sundberg M. Substrate-, hormone-, and cAMP-regulated cytochrome P450 degradation [published erratum appears in *Proc Natl Acad Sci USA* 1990;87:5232]. *Proc Natl Acad Sci USA* 1990;87:3225–3229.
20. Badger T, Huang J, Ronis M, Lumpkin C. Induction of cytochrome P450-2E1 during chronic ethanol exposure occurs via transcription of the CYP 2E1 gene when blood alcohol concentrations are high. *Biochem Biophys Res Commun* 1993;190:780–785.
21. Johansson I, Ekstrom G, Scholte B, Puzycki D, Jornvall H, Ingelman-Sundberg M. Ethanol-, fasting-, and acetone-inducible cytochromes P450 in rat liver: regulation and characteristics of enzymes belonging to the IIB and IIE gene subfamilies. *Biochemistry* 1988;27:1925–1934.
22. Tierney D, Haas A, Koop D. Degradation of cytochrome P450-2E1: selective loss after labilization of the enzyme. *Arch Biochem Biophys* 1992;293:9–16.
23. Johansson I, Lindros K, Eriksson H, Ingelman-Sundberg M. Transcriptional control of CYP-2E1 in the perivenous liver region and during starvation. *Biochem Biophys Res Commun* 1990;173:331–338.
24. Shimizu M, Lasker J, Tsutsumi M, Lieber C. Immunohistochemical localization of ethanol-inducible P450-IIE1 in the rat alimentary tract. *Gastroenterology* 1990;99:1044–1053.
25. Pohl L, George J, Satoh H. Strain and sex differences in chloroform-induced nephrotoxocity. Different rates of metabolism of chloroform to phosgene by the mouse kidney. *Drug Metab Disp* 1984;12:304–308.
26. Uematsu F, Kikuchi H, Motomiya M, et al. Association between restriction fragment length polymorphism of the human cytochrome P450-IIE1 gene and susceptibility to lung cancer. *Jpn J Cancer Res* 1991;82:254–256.
27. Hayashi S, Watanabe J, Kawajiri K. Genetic polymorphisms in the 5'-flanking region change transcriptional regulation of the human cytochrome P450-IIE1 gene. *J Biochem* 1991;110:559–565.
28. Parke D, Ioannides C, Lewis D. The 1990

Pharmaceutical Manufacturers Association of Canada keynote lecture. The role of the cytochromes P450 in the detoxication and activation of drugs and other chemicals. *Can J Physiol Pharmacol* 1991;69:537–549.

29. Porter T, Coon M. Cytochrome P450. Multiplicity of isoforms, substrates, and catalytic and regulatory mechanisms. *J Biol Chem* 1991; 266:13469–13472.

30. Guengerich F. Characterization of human cytochrome P450 enzymes. *FASEB J* 1992;6:745–748.

31. Yun C, Wood M, Wood A, Guengerich F. Identification of the pharmacogenetic determinants of alfentanil metabolism: cytochrome P450-3A4. *Anesthesiology* 1992;77:467–474.

32. Bradshaw J, Ivanetich K. Isoflurane: a comparison of its metabolism by human and rat hepatic cytochrome P450. *Anesth Analg* 1984;63: 805–813.

33. Bartkowski R, Goldberg M, Larijani G, Boerner T. Inhibition of alfentanil metabolism by erythromycin. *Clin Pharmacol Ther* 1989;46: 99–102.

34. Echizen H, Kawasaki H, Chiba K, Tani M, Ishizaki T. A potent inhibitory effect of erythromycin and other macrolide antibiotics on the mono-N-dealkylation metabolism of disopyramide with human liver microsomes. *J Pharm Exp Ther* 1993;264:1425–1431.

35. Hiller A, Olkkola K, Isohanni P, Saarnivaara L. Unconsciousness associated with midazolam and erythromycin. *Br J Anaesth* 1990;65: 826–828.

36. Abraham S, Johnson C. Prevalence of severe obesity in adults in the United States. *Am J Clin Nutr* 1980;33:364–369.

37. Lardy H, Shrago E. Biochemical aspects of obesity. *Annu Rev Biochem* 1990;59:689–710.

38. Bentley J, Vaughan R, Gandolfi A, Cork R. Halothane biotransformation in obese and nonobese patients. *Anesthesiology* 1982;57:94–97.

39. Young S, Stoelting R, Peterson C, Madura J. Anesthetic biotransformation and renal function in obese patients during and after methoxyflurane or halothane anesthesia. *Anesthesiology* 1975;42:451–457.

40. Bentley J, Vaughan R, Miller M, Calkins J, Gandolfi A. Serum inorganic fluoride levels in obese patients during and after enflurane anesthesia. *Anesth Analg* 1979;58:409–412.

41. Strube P, Hulands G, Halsey M. Serum fluoride levels in morbidly obese patients: enflurane compared with isoflurane anaesthesia. *Anaesthesia* 1987;42:685–689.

42. Frink E Jr, Malan T Jr, Brown E, Morgan S, Brown B Jr. Plasma inorganic fluoride levels with sevoflurane anesthesia in morbidly obese and nonobese patients. *Anesth Analg* 1993;76: 1337–1337.

43. Salazar D, Sorge C, Corcoran G. Obesity as a risk factor for drug-induced organ injury. VI. Increased hepatic P450 concentration and microsomal ethanol oxidizing activity in the obese overfed rat. *Biochem Biophys Res Commun* 1988;157:315–320.

44. Mahendroo M, Means G, Mendelson C, Simpson E. Tissue-specific expression of human P450AROM. The promoter responsible for expression in adipose tissue is different from that utilized in placenta. *J Biol Chem* 1991;266: 11276–11281.

45. Garces L, Kenny F, Drash A, Taylor F. Cortisol secretion rate during fasting of obese adolescent subjects. *J Clin Endocrinol Metab* 1968; 28:1843–1847.

46. Kharasch E, Thummel K. Human liver volatile anesthetic defluorination: role of cytochrome P450-IIE1. *Anesthesiology* 1991;75:A350.

47. Baden J, Rice S. Metabolism and toxicity. In: Miller R, ed. *Anesthesia*. New York: Churchill-Livingstone, 1990:135–170.

48. Lind R, Gandolfi A, Hall P. The role of oxidative biotransformation of halothane in the guinea pig model of halothane-associated hepatotoxicity. *Anesthesiology* 1989;70:649–653.

49. Gruenke L, Waskell L. A gas chromatographic mass spectrometric method for the analysis of trifluoroacetic acid: application to the metabolism of halothane by in vitro preparations. *Biomed Environ Mass Spec* 1988;17:471–475.

50. Maiorino R, Gandolfi A, Spies I. Gas-chromatographic method for the halothane metabolites, trifluoroacetic acid and bromide in biological fluids. *J Anal Toxicol* 1980;4:250–254.

51. Wark H, Earl J, Chau D, Overton J. Halothane metabolism in children. *Br J Anaesth* 1990;64: 474–481.

52. Carpenter R, Eger E 2d, Johnson B, Unadkat J, Sheiner L. The extent of metabolism of inhaled anesthetics in humans. *Anesthesiology* 1986;65:201–205.

53. Cohen E. Metabolism of the volatile anesthetics. *Anesthesiology* 1971;35:193–202.

54. Cohen E, Trudell J, Edmunds H, Watson E. Urinary metabolites of halothane in man. *Anesthesiology* 1975;43:392–401.

55. Müller R, Stier A. Modification of liver microsomal lipids by halothane metabolites: a multinuclear NMR spectroscopic study. *Arch Pharmacol* 1982;321:234–237.

56. Uemura K-I, Nicolotti R, Six H, Kinsky S. Antibody formation in response to liposomal model membranes sensitized with N-substituted phosphatidylethanolamine derivatives. *Biochemistry* 1974;13:1572–1578.

57. Edmunds H, Trudell J, Cohen E. Low-level binding of halothane metabolites to rat liver histones *in vivo*. *Anesthesiology* 1981;54:298–304.

58. Gandolfi A, White R, Spies I, Pohl L. Bioactivation and covalent binding of halothane in vitro: studies with [^{3}H]- and [^{14}C] halothane. *J Pharmacol Exp Ther* 1980;214:721–725.

59. Kenna J, Neuberger J, Williams R. Identification by immunoblotting of three halothane-induced liver microsomal polypeptide antigens recognized by antibodies in sera from patients

with halothane-associated hepatitis. *J Pharm Exp Ther* 1987;242:733–740.

60. Kenna J, Satoh H, Christ D, Pohl L. Metabolic basis for a drug hypersensitivity: antibodies in sera from patients with halothane hepatitis recognize liver neoantigens that contain the trifluoroacetyl group derived from halothane. *J Pharm Exp Ther* 1988;245:1103–1169.

61. Satoh H, Gillette J, Davies H, Schulick R, Pohl L. Immunochemical evidence of trifluoroacetylated cytochrome P450 in the liver of halothane-treated rats. *Mol Pharmacol* 1985; 28:468–474.

62. Kenna J. The molecular basis of halothane-induced hepatitis. *Biochem Soc Trans* 1991;19: 191–195.

63. Christen U, Jenö P, Gut J. Halothane metabolism: the dihydrolipoamide acetyltransferase subunit of the pyruvate dehydrogenase complex moleculary mimics trifluroacetyl-protein adducts. *Biochemistry* 1993;32:1492–1499.

64. Kenna J, Neuberger J, Williams R. Evidence for expression in human liver of halothane-induced neoantigens recognized by antibodies in sera from patients with halothane hepatitis. *Hepatology* 1988;8:1635–1641.

65. Callis A, Brooks S, Waters S, et al. Evidence for a role of the immune system in the pathogenesis of halothane hepatitis. In: Roth S, Miller K, eds. *Molecular and cellular mechanisms of anesthetics.* New York: Plenum, 1986; 443–453.

66. Widger L, Gandolfi A, Van Dyke R. Hypoxia and halothane metabolism *in vivo:* release of inorganic fluoride and halothane metabolite binding to cellular constituents. *Anesthesiology* 1976;44:197–201.

67. Gallagher T, Black G. Uptake of volatile anaesthetics in children. *Anaesthesia* 1985;40: 1073–1077.

68. Sakai T, Takaori M. Biodegradation of halothane, enflurane and methoxyflurane. *Br J Anaesth* 1978;50:785–791.

69. Wade R, Castro C. Oxidation of heme proteins by alkyl halides. *J Am Chem Soc* 1973;95:231–234.

70. Wade R, Castro C. Oxidation of iron (II) porphyrins by alkyl halides. *J Am Chem Soc* 1973;95:226–230.

71. Bartnicki E, Belser N, Castro C. Oxidation of heme proteins by alkyl halides: a probe for axial inner sphere redox capacity in solution and in whole cells. *Biochemistry* 1978;17:5582–5586.

72. Castro C. Biodehalogenation. *Environ Health Perspect* 1977;21:279–283.

73. Castro C. The rapid oxidation of iron (II) porphyrins by alkyl halides. A possible mode of intoxication of organisms by alkyl halides. *J Am Chem Soc* 1964;86:2310–2314.

74. Castro C, Wade R, Belser N. Biodehalogenation: reactions of cytochrome P450 with polyhalomethanes. *Biochemistry* 1985;24:204–210.

75. Baker M, Nelson R, Van Dyke R. The release of inorganic fluoride from halothane and halo-

thane metabolites by cytochrome P450, hemin, and hemoglobin. *Drug Metab Dispos Biol Fate Chem* 1983;11:308–311.

76. Nastainczyk W, Ullrich V. Effect of oxygen concentration on the reaction of halothane with cytochrome P450 in liver microsomes and isolated perfused rat liver. *Biochem Pharmacol* 1978;27:387–392.

77. Lind R, Gandolfi A, Sipes I, Brown B Jr, Waters S. Oxygen concentrations required for reductive defluorination of halothane by rat hepatic microsomes. *Anesth Analg* 1986;65:835–839.

78. Knights K, Gourlay G, Cousins M. Changes in rat hepatic microsomal mixed function oxidase activity following exposure to halothane under various oxygen concentrations. *Biochem Pharmacol* 1987;36:897–906.

79. Mukai S, Morior M, Fujii K, Hanaki C. Volatile metabolites of halothane in the rabbit. *Anesthesiology* 1977;47:248–251.

80. Sharp J, Trudell J, Cohen E. Volatile metabolites and decomposition products of halothane in man. *Anesthesiology* 1979;50:2–8.

81. Trudell J, Bösterling B, Trevor A. 1-Chloro-2,2,2-trifluoroethyl radical: formation from halothane by human cytochrome P450 in reconstituted vesicles and binding to phospholipids. *Biochem Biophys Res Commun* 1981;102:372–377.

82. Ahr H, King L, Nastaincyzk W, Ullrich V. The mechanism of reductive dehalogenation of halothane by liver cytochrome P450. *Biochem Pharm* 1982;31:383–390.

83. Baker M, Bates J, Van Dyke R. Stabilization of the reduced halocarbon-cytochrome P450 complex of halothane by N-alkanes. *Biochem Pharmacol* 1987;36:1029–1034.

84. Ruf H, Ahr H, Nastainczyk W, et al. Formation of a ferric carbanion complex from halothane and cytochrome P450: electron spin resonance, electronic spectra and model complexes. *Biochemistry* 1984;23:5300–5306.

85. Baker M, Vasquez M, Bates J, Chiang C. Metabolism of 2-chloro-1,1-difluoroethene to glyoxylic and glycolic acid in rat hepatic microsomes. *Drug Metab Disp: Biol Fate Chem* 1990;18:753–758.

86. Manno M, Ferrara R, Cazzaro S, Rigotti P, Ancona E. Suicidal inactivation of human cytochrome P450 by carbon tetrachloride and halothane *in vitro*. *Pharmacol Toxicol* 1992;70:13–18.

87. Nebert D, Nelson D, Coon M, et al. The P450 superfamily: update on new sequences, gene mapping, and recommended nomenclature. *DNA Cell Biol* 1991;10:397–398.

88. Khani S, Zaphiropoulos P, Fujita V, Porter T, Koop D, Coon M. cDNA and derived amino acid sequence of ethanol-inducible rabbit liver cytochrome P450 isozyme 3a (P450-ALC). *Proc Natl Acad Sci USA* 1987;84:638–642.

89. Song B, Gelboin H, Park S, Yang C, Gonzalez F. Complementary DNA and protein sequences

of ethanol-inducible rat and human cytochrome P450s. Transcriptional and posttranscriptional regulation of the rat enzyme. *J Biol Chem* 1987;261:16689–16697.

90. Wrighton S, Thomas P, Molowa D, et al. Characterization of ethanol-inducible human liver N-nitrosodimethylamine demethylase. *Biochemistry* 1986;25:6731–6735.

91. Ronis M, Johansson I, Hultenby K, Lagercrantz J, Glaumann H, Ingelman-Sundberg M. Acetone-regulated synthesis and degradation of cytochrome P450-2E1 and cytochrome P450-2B1 in rat liver. *Eur J Biochem* 1991;198:383–389.

92. Pantuck E, Pantuck C, Ryan D, Conney A. Inhibition and stimulation of enflurane metabolism in the rat following a single dose or chronic administration of ethanol. *Anesthesiology* 1985;62:255–262.

93. Chase R, Holaday D, Fiserova-Bergerova V, Saidman L, Mack F. The biotransformation of ethrane in man. *Anesthesiology* 1971;35:262–267.

94. Loew G, Motulsky H, Trudell J, Cohen E, Hjelmeland L. Quantum chemical studies of the metabolism of the inhalation anesthetics methoxyflurane, enflurane, and isoflurane. *Mol Pharmacol* 1974;10:406–418.

95. Ravichandran K, Boddupalli S, Hasermann C, Peterson J, Deisenhofer J. Crystal structure of the hemoprotein domain of P450BM3, a prototype for microsomal P450's. *Science* 1993;261:731–736.

96. Poulos T. Modeling of mammalian P450 on the basis of P450 camphor x-ray structure methods. *Methods Enzymol* 1991;206:11–30.

97. Poulos T, Howard A. Crystal structure of metyrapone- and phenylimidazole-inhibited complexes of cytochrome P450cam. *Biochemistry* 1987;26:8165–8174.

98. Poulos T, Raag R. Cytochrome P450cam crystallography, oxygen activation, and electron transfer. *FASEB J* 1992;6:674–679.

99. Poulos T, Finzel B, Howard A. Crystal structure of substrate-free *Pseudomonas putida* cytochrome P450. *Biochemistry* 1986;25:5314–5322.

100. Poulos TL, Finzel BC, Howard AJ. High-resolution crystal structure of cytochrome P450cam. *J Mol Biol* 1987;195:687–700.

101. Poulos T, Finzel I, Gunsalus I, Wagner G, Kraut J. The 2.6-Å crystal structure of *Pseudomonas putida* cytochrome P450. *J Biol Chem* 1985;260:16122–16130.

102. Raag R, Poulos T. Crystal structure of the carbon monoxide–substrate–cytochrome P450cam ternary complex. *Biochemistry* 1989;28:7586–7592.

103. Laughton C, Neidle S. A molecular model for the enzyme cytochrome P450 17α, a major target for the chemotherapy of prostate cancer. *Biochem Biophys Res Commun* 1990;171:1160–1167.

104. Laughton C, Zvelebil M, Neidle S. A detailed molecular model for human aromatase. *J Steroid Biochem Molec Biol* 1993;44:399–407.

105. Zvelebil M, Wolf C, Sternberg M. A predicted three-dimensional structure of human cytochrome P450: implications for substrate specificity. *Protein Eng* 1991;4:271–282.

106. Chen S, Zhou D. Functional domains of aromatase cytochrome P450 inferred from comparative analyses of amino acid sequences and substantiated by site-directed mutagenesis experiments. *J Biol Chem* 1992;267:22587–22594.

107. Koymans L, Vermeulen N, van Acker S, et al. A predictive model for substrates of cytochrome P450-debrisoquine (2D6). *Chem Res Toxicol* 1992;5:211–219.

108. Lewis D, Moereels H. The sequence homologies of cytochrome P450 and active-site geometries. *J Comp Aided Mol Design* 1992;6:235–252.

109. Johnson E. Mapping determinants of the substrate selectivities of P450 enzymes by site-directed mutagenesis. *Trends Pharmacol Sci* 1992;13:122–126.

110. Iwasaki M, Darden T, Pedersen L, et al. Engineering mouse P450coh to a novel corticosterone 15-alpha-hydroxylase and modeling steroid-binding orientation in the substrate pocket. *J Biol Chem* 1993;268:759–762.

111. McCarty L, Malek R, Larsen E. The effects of deuteration on the metabolism of halogenated anesthetics in the rat. *Anesthesiology* 1979;51:106–110.

112. Burke T Jr, Branchflower R, Lees D, Pohl L. Mechanism of defluorination of enflurane. Identification of an organic metabolite in rat and man. *Drug Metab Disp: Biol Fate Chem* 1981;9:19–24.

113. Dooley J, Mazze R, Rice S, Borel J. Is enflurane defluorination inducible in man? *Anesthesiology* 1979;50:213–217.

114. Mazze R, Woodruff R, Heerdt M. Isoniazid-induced enflurane defluorination in humans. *Anesthesiology* 1982;57:5–8.

115. Cousins M, Greenstein L, Hitt B, Mazze R. Metabolism and renal effects of enflurane in man. *Anesthesiology* 1976;44:44–53.

116. Mazze R, Calverley R, Smith N. Inorganic fluoride nephrotoxicity: prolonged enflurane and halothane anesthesia in volunteers. *Anesthesiology* 1977;46:265–271.

117. Mazze R, Sievenpiper T, Stevenson J. Renal effects of enflurane and halothane in patients with abnormal renal function. *Anesthesiology* 1984;60:161–163.

118. Fish K, Sievenpiper T, Rice S, Wharton R, Mazze R. Renal function in Fischer 344 rats with chronic renal impairment after administration of enflurane and gentamicin. *Anesthesiology* 1980;53:481–488.

119. Kline M. Enflurane-associated hepatitis. *Gastroenterology* 1980;79:126–127.

120. Christ D, Satoh H, Kenna J, Pohl L. Potential metabolic basis for enflurane hepatitis and the

apparent cross-sensitization between enflurane and halothane. *Drug Metab Disp* 1988;16:135–140.

121. Christ D, Kenna J, Kammerer W, Satoh H, Pohl L. Enflurane metabolism produces covalently bound liver adducts recognized by antibodies from patients with halothane hepatitis. *Anesthesiology* 1988;69:833–838.

122. Harris J, Pohl L, Martin J, Anders M. Tissue acylation by the chlorofluorocarbon substitute 2,2-dichloro-1,1,1-trifluoroethane. *Proc Natl Acad Sci USA* 1991;88:1407–1410.

123. Huwyler J, Gut J. Exposure to the chlorofluorocarbon substitute 2,2-dichloro-1,1,1-trifluoroethane and the anesthetic agent halothane is associated with transient protein adduct formation in the heart. *Biochem Biophys Res Commun* 1992;184:1344–1349.

124. Greenstein L, Hitt B, Mazze R. Metabolism in vitro of enflurane, isoflurane, and methoxyflurane. *Anesthesiology* 1975;42:420–424.

125. Mazze R, Hitt B. Effects of phenobarbital and 3-methylcholanthrene on anesthetic defluorination in Fischer 344 rats. *Drug Metab Disp* 1978;6:680–681.

126. Rice S, Talcott R. Effects of isoniazid treatment on selected hepatic mixed-function oxidases. *Drug Metab Disp* 1979;7:260–262.

127. Maduska A. Serum inorganic fluoride levels in patients receiving enflurane anesthesia. *Anesth Analg* 1974;53:351–353.

128. Van Dyke R. Enflurane, isoflurane, and methoxyflurane metabolism in rat hepatic microsomes from ethanol-treated animals. *Anesthesiology* 1983;58:221–224.

129. Rice S, Dooley J, Mazze R. Metabolism by rat hepatic microsomes of fluorinated ether anesthetics following ethanol consumption. *Anesthesiology* 1983;58:237–241.

130. Thummel K, Kharasch E, Podoll T, Kunze K. Human liver microsomal enflurane defluorination catalyzed by cytochrome P450-2E1. *Drug Metab Disp* 1993;21:350–357.

131. Corbett T. Cancer and congenital anomalies associated with anesthetics. *Ann NY Acad Sci* 1976;271:58–66.

132. Eger E 2d, White A, Brown C, Biava C, Corbett T, Stevens W. A test of the carcinogenicity of enflurane, isoflurane, halothane, methoxyflurane, and nitrous oxide in mice. *Anesth Analg* 1978;57:678–694.

133. Mazze R, Cousins M, Barr G. Renal effects and metabolism of isoflurane in man. *Anesthesiology* 1974;40:536–542.

134. Murray J, Trinick T. Plasma fluoride concentrations during and after prolonged anesthesia: a comparison of halothane and isoflurane. *Anesth Analg* 1992;74:236–240.

135. Holaday D, Fiserova-Bergerova V, Latto I, Zumbiel M. Resistance of isoflurane to biotransformation in man. *Anesthesiology* 1975;43:325–332.

136. Hitt B, Mazze R, Cousins M, Edmunds H, Barr G, Trudell J. Metabolism of isoflurane in Fischer 344 rats and man. *Anesthesiology* 1974;40:62–67.

137. Stoelting R, Blitt C, Cohen P, Merin R. Hepatic dysfunction after isoflurane anesthesia. *Anesth Analg* 1987;66:147–153.

138. Rice S, Sbordone L, Mazze R. Metabolism by rat hepatic microsomes of fluorinated ether anesthetics following isoniazid administration. *Anesthesiology* 1980;53:489–493.

139. Van Dyke R, Chenoweth M, Van Poznik A. Metabolism of volatile anesthetics—I. Conversion *in vivo* of several anesthetics to $^{14}CO_2$ and chloride. *Biochem Pharm* 1964;13:1239–1247.

140. Van Dyke R, Chenoweth M. The metabolism of volatile anesthetics—II. *In vivo* metabolism of methoxyflurane and halothane in rat liver slices and cell fractions. *Biochem Pharm* 1965;14:603–609.

141. Taves D, Fry B, Freeman R, Gillies A. Toxicity following methoxyflurane anesthesia. II. Fluoride concentrations in nephrotoxocity. *JAMA* 1970;214:91–95.

142. Goldemberg L. Tratamiento de la enfermedad de Basedow del hipertiroidismo por fluor. *Rev Soc Med Int Soc Tisiol* 1931;6:217–242.

143. Cousins M, Mazze R. Methoxyflurane nephrotoxicity: a study of dose–response in man. *JAMA* 1973;225:1611–1616.

144. Cousins M, Mazze R, Kosek J, Hitt B, Love F. The etiology of methoxyflurane nephrotoxicity. *J Pharmacol Exp Ther* 1974;190:530–541.

145. Edwards S, Poulos T, Kraut J. The crystal structure of fluoride-inhibited cytochrome c peroxidase. *J Biol Chem* 1984;259:12984–12988.

146. Garin J, Vignais P. Characterization of the inhibition of rabbit muscle adenylate kinase by fluoride and berylium ions. *Biochemistry* 1993;32:6821–6827.

147. Hitt B, Mazze R, Denson D. Isotopic probe of the mechanism of methoxyflurane defluorination. *Drug Metab Disp* 1979;7:446–447.

148. Yoshimura N, Holaday D, Fiserova-Bergerova V. Metabolism of methoxyflurane in man. *Anesthesiology* 1976;44:372–379.

149. Waskell L, Gonzales J. Dependence of microsomal methoxyflurane O-demethylation on cytochrome P450 reductase and the stoichiometry of fluoride ion and formaldehyde release. *Anesth Analg* 1982;61:609–613.

150. Canova-Davis E, Waskell L. The identification of the heat-stable microsomal protein required for methoxyflurane metabolism as cytochrome b_5. *J Biol Chem* 1984;259:2541–2546.

151. Canova-Davis E, Chiang JYL, Waskell L. Obligatory role of cytochrome b5 in the microsomal metabolism of methoxyflurane. *Biochem Pharm* 1985;34:1907–1912.

152. Waskell L, Canova-Davis E, Philpot R, Parandoush Z, Chiang J. Identification of the enzymes catalyzing metabolism of methoxyflurane. *Drug Metab Disp* 1986;14:643–648.

153. Son S, Colella J Jr, Brown B Jr. The effect of phenobarbitone on the metabolism of methoxy-

flurane to oxalic acid in the rat. *Br J Anaesth* 1972;44:1224–1228.

154. Biermann J, Rice S, Gallagher E, West J. Effect of diazepam treatment on hepatic microsomal anesthetic defluorinase activity. *Arch Int Pharm Ther* 1986;283:181–192.

155. Caughey G, Rice S, Kosek J, Mazze R. Effect of phenytoin (DPH) treatment on methoxyflurane metabolism in rats. *J Pharmacol Exp Ther* 1979;210:180–185.

156. Berman M, Lowe H, Bochantin J, Hagler K. Uptake and elimination of methoxyflurane as influenced by enzyme induction in the rat. *Anesthesiology* 1973;38:352–357.

157. Koblin D. Characteristics and implications of desflurane metabolism and toxicity. *Anesth Analg* 1992;75:S10–S16.

158. Hanaki C, Fujii K, Morio M, Tashima T. Decomposition of sevoflurane by soda lime. *Hiroshima J Med Sci* 1987;36:61–67.

159. Morio M, Fujii K, Satoh N, et al. Reaction of sevoflurane and its degradation products with soda lime. *Anesthesiology* 1992;77:1155–1164.

160. Tarrant P, Brown H. The addition of alcohols to some 1,1-difluoroethylenes. *J Am Chem Soc* 1951;73:1781.

161. Mazze R. The safety of sevoflurane in humans [Editorial; Comment]. *Anesthesiology* 1992;77:1062–1063.

162. Holaday D, Smith F. Clinical characteristics and biotransformation of sevoflurane in healthy human volunteers. *Anesthesiology* 1981;54:100–106.

163. Kikuchi H, Morio M, Fujii K, et al. Clinical evaluation and metabolism of sevoflurane in patients. *Hiroshima J Med Sci* 1987;36:93–97.

164. Martis L, Lynch S, Napoli M, Woods E. Biotransformation of sevoflurane in dogs and rats. *Anesth Analg* 1981;60:186–191.

165. Crank G, Harding D, Szinai S. Perfluoroalkyl carbonyl compounds. 2. Derivatives of hexafluoroacetone. *J Med Chem* 1970;13:1215–1217.

166. Frink E Jr, Ghantous H, Malan T, et al. Plasma inorganic fluoride with sevoflurane anesthesia: correlation with indices of hepatic and renal function. *Anesth Analg* 1992;74:231–235.

167. Kobayashi Y, Ochiai R, Takeda J, Sekiguchi H, Fukushima K. Serum and urinary inorganic fluoride concentrations after prolonged inhalation of sevoflurane in humans. *Anesth Analg* 1992;74:753–757.

Anesthetic Toxicity, edited by
Susan A. Rice and Kevin J. Fish.
Raven Press, Ltd., New York © 1994.

5

Hepatotoxicity of Halogenated Anesthetics

Max T. Baker and *Russell A. Van Dyke

Department of Anesthesia, University of Iowa, Iowa City, Iowa 52242
*Department of Anesthesiology, Henry Ford Hospital, Detroit, Michigan 48202

Toxicity to the liver resulting from the exposure of individuals to the halogenated anesthetics is a side effect that was linked to halogenated anesthetic exposure almost since their use as anesthetics began. Cases of jaundice and death following chloroform administration were reported as early as 1848 (1), and in 1850 it was determined experimentally that chloroform could cause biochemical changes in the livers of rats (2). Not until the turn of the century was the seriousness of this side effect fully appreciated when it was confirmed that chloroform (2,3) and carbon tetrachloride (4), the latter of which was used as an anesthetic for a short period, caused massive liver necrosis and delayed death in a large number of patients administered these compounds.

During the early use of the chlorocarbon anesthetics, it was believed, and for the most part correctly, that breakdown or metabolism of these compounds to other substances in the body played a role in their liver toxicity. The carbon–fluorine bond was known to be stronger than the carbon–chlorine bond (5). Therefore, in the search for better and safer anesthetics, compounds with fluorine substituents subsequently were synthesized, tested, and developed. Those that came into commercial use, including methoxyflurane, halothane, fluroxene, enflurane, isoflurane, desflurane, and sevoflurane, are chemically more stable and metabolize at rates much lower than the chlorocarbon an-

esthetics, chloroform, carbon tetrachloride, and trichloroethylene.

Liver toxicity initially appeared to be non-existent with the fluorinated anesthetics, but as their use increased, nearly all the fluorinated anesthetics have become associated with liver toxicity to various degrees. For some, such as fluroxene, hepatotoxicity has been firmly demonstrated in experimental animals (6), and its use as an anesthetic has been discontinued. Even though halothane is a very poor liver toxin, enough evidence has accumulated to clearly associate a low incidence of jaundice (7) and rare cases of fulminant liver failure to anesthesia with this agent (8). For others, such as isoflurane and enflurane, relationships are very tenuous. In fact, in many clinical cases, it has been debated whether the hepatotoxic effects attributed to these anesthetics were due to the anesthetic *per se* or to organ manipulation or liver hypoxia or both occurring during surgical procedures (4,9).

Because severe illness and death are a final outcome of liver failure and fluorinated anesthetics are administered to a large number of people, many studies have been undertaken to elucidate the course of events leading to anesthetic-associated liver damage. Complicating such studies, however, is the very low incidence of human hepatotoxicity and the difficulty in establishing an animal model that appropriately mimics human toxicity. With a focus on halothane, the following discussion summarizes the evidence for anesthetic interactions with the hepatocyte and highlights the latest theories by which the fluorinated anesthetics are thought to cause damage to the liver.

HALOTHANE HEPATITIS

Without a doubt, the anesthetic that has received the greatest attention in regard to anesthetic-associated hepatotoxicity is halothane. Halothane was introduced in 1956 (10) and gained widespread popularity because of its nonflammability (a major advance at the time) and desirable anesthetic properties. When halothane was introduced, it was believed to be resistant to metabolism and, therefore, nontoxic to the liver. Over the years, however, clinical cases of halothane-associated hepatic necrosis (or halothane hepatitis) began to surface (11–14), and controversy ensued as to whether the anesthetic was truly hepatotoxic or if liver toxicity was coincident to surgical procedures. Reasons for the debate were that the incidence of toxicity was low, changes in liver function are not uncommon following surgical procedures, and many other concomitantly administered drugs were known to produce liver damage. The diagnosis of halothane hepatitis is by necessity based on the exclusion of other causes of hepatitis because no positive diagnostic tests have been developed that conclusively identify the syndrome.

Clinical symptoms observed in halothane-associated liver toxicity are the same as those that result from hepatitis caused by other processes. These include fever, jaundice (increase in blood and tissue bilirubin concentration), and, in some cases, rash and eosinophilia. More specific indicators of liver injury include elevated concentrations of serum enzymes, such as serum aspartate aminotransferase (AST) and serum alanine aminotransferase (ALT), which are released from the damaged hepatocyte (7).

Measurement of serum glutathione-S-transferase (GST) (15,16) has been used in recent years in humans and is thought to be a more sensitive indicator in evaluating mild liver damage. Because liver disease can be caused by other factors, such as viral infection (halothane hepatitis is morphologically similar to the necrosis caused by infection with the hepatitis B virus), diagnosis of halothane hepatitis includes rigorous exclusion of viral infection. Histologic study of livers from patients with fatal halothane hepatitis shows a pathologic status much like that seen with ethanol or hypoxic centrilobular necrosis, so that histologic diagnosis is not conclusive.

The National Halothane Study (8), which was undertaken to retrospectively examine liver toxicity in patients exposed to halothane from 1959 to 1962, estimated that the incidence of unexplained massive liver necrosis following halothane anesthesia was 1 in 35,000. Other reports of liver toxicity following halothane use revealed a mild type of liver damage with no clinical symptoms and only evidenced by increases in serum aminotransferases (17). When the more sensitive GST assay was used, it was found that 50% of patients had increased GST after halothane, 20% following enflurane, and 11% following isoflurane (16). The milder halothane toxicity thought to occur in 20% of those patients exposed to halothane is reversible (7). On the other hand, in the small group in which fulminant hepatic necrosis develops, mortality is high.

Apparent risk factors for halothane hepatitis were addressed previously and are briefly discussed here. The ratio of female to male patients with fulminant hepatitis attributed to halothane anesthesia was reported to be 1.6 : 1 in one study, indicating that females are more susceptible (18). Other studies put the ratio at 2 : 1 (19). Observations also revealed that obesity is a contributing factor, since more individuals diagnosed were overweight (20,21). Although adults are susceptible to halothane hepatitis, it is very rare in children (22), so

oxygen use. A particular problem in differentiating the effects of hypoxia from halothane reductive metabolism in the pathogenesis of halothane-induced hepatotoxicity in whole animals is that lowering liver oxygen always causes the rates of halothane reduction to increase (30).

Whether or not liver hypoxia is the primary cause of hepatotoxicity in the rat, specific mechanisms by which halothane produces vasoconstriction are of interest. Two possible mechanisms are (a) halothane enhances catecholamine release, and (b) halothane may decrease release of the endogenous vasodilator, nitric oxide (NO), or interfere with its vasodilating effect. If it is assumed that vasomotor tone is controlled by the opposing actions of catecholamines as vasoconstrictors and nitric oxide as a vasodilator, a change in either would produce a corresponding change in vasomotor tone. Halothane has been reported to increase circulating plasma catecholamines (68), and although attempts to purposely raise or lower catecholamines have received only minimal study, preliminary studies suggested that raising catecholamines increases halothane toxicity in the rat. Decreasing circulating catecholamines abolishes the hepatotoxicity. Not surprisingly, animals stressed before or during anesthetic exposure may be more susceptible to hepatotoxic injury, with the presumption being that this is the consequence of higher circulating catecholamine levels.

The role of NO in modulating liver vasomotor tone during halothane exposure raises the possibility of several mechanisms for interaction. Nitric oxide synthetase, a cytochrome P450-like enzyme that forms NO from arginine (69), and guanylate cyclase, which is activated by NO, both contain a heme moiety that functions in the reduced state (70). It is well known that halothane directly interacts with and is reduced by ferrous heme (71). The possibility exists that halothane can inhibit NO formation or block its effect on guanylate cyclase by interacting with the heme component of these enzymes. The action of halothane as well as other halocarbons on the effects of NO requires further study.

Possible Role of Calcium

Calcium undoubtedly plays a vital role in the regulation of biochemical processes in the cell. Ca^{2+} is a second messenger capable of activating many other enzymes, such as kinases and phosphorylases (72). Homeostasis requires calcium concentrations to be held extracellularly at about 10^{-3} M and intracellularly at 10^{-7} M. These gradients are maintained by regulatory sites located primarily on the membranes. Calcium enters the cell by voltage-sensitive channels and receptor-activated channels and by permeation through the plasma membrane (73). Calcium is removed from the cell by an ATP-dependent calcium pump and an Na^+-Ca^{2+} exchange mechanism (74). Intracellularly, calcium is pumped into the mitochondria and sequestered in the endoplasmic reticulum and proteins on the plasma membrane. When calcium homeostasis is sufficiently disrupted, cell death occurs (72).

There has been interest in the hypothesis that altered calcium homeostasis could be involved in hepatocyte injury by halogenated hydrocarbons (75,76). Hepatocyte exposure to halocarbons related to the anesthetics, including carbon tetrachloride, chloroform, and 1,1-dichloroethylene, has been linked to increases in cytoplasmic calcium by impairment of intracellular calcium sequestration (77–79). Studies of the volatile anesthetics, isoflurane, enflurane, halothane, and sevoflurane, at anesthetic concentrations have shown that each will cause a release of stored calcium into the intracellular fluid in isolated hepatocytes within seconds of their administration (80,81). The initial response may be followed by a greater, more sustained calcium release into the intracellular fluid that is more likely to cause cell death than rapid fluxes. Farrell et al. (82) found increases in ionized intra-cellular calcium in the livers of guinea pigs 24 hours after halothane exposure. The increase in release of calcium was proportional to the severity of the liver necrosis, and it was suggested that halothane-altered calcium homeostasis was due to impaired microsomal calcium uptake.

Altered calcium flux may be operative in the interaction of hypoxia and anesthetics in regard to hepatocyte toxicity. Hypoxia itself will cause the cell to release intra-cellular calcium into the cytoplasm (83). Therefore, hypoxia in combination with halothane exposure may produce an intra-cellular calcium concentration great enough that the hepatocyte is not able to survive. Because enflurane and isoflurane cause a much smaller release of calcium (80), this interactive mechanism is in keeping with the fact that halothane is more hepatotoxic than enflurane or isoflurane.

Role of the Immune System

Although a strong case can be made for a mechanism of hepatotoxicity that relies on deficiencies of cellular energy supplies and a relatively weak case for direct toxicity of its metabolites, another mechanism has been gaining support. Concurrent with the development of the hypoxic rat model, data were being gathered that supported a role of the immune system in halothane liver toxicity in humans. The evidence that the incidence of severe halothane hepatitis is greater in patients who receive more than one exposure to halothane (19) suggested to some that halothane liver injury was the result of sensitization or an immune response mechanism.

Vergani et al. (84) found antibodies in the serum of patients with severe halothane-associated hepatitis that reacted with hepatocytes from halothane-treated rabbits (84,85). Serum from patients who did not have halothane hepatitis or those who had acetaminophen-induced hepatocellular ne-

crosis did not show reactivity. Likewise, there was no reactivity between antibodies in serum from patients with halothane hepatitis and hepatocytes from diethyl ether-treated rabbits. Such data were highly suggestive that specific antibodies were formed as a result of halothane exposure in humans. Although it was considered that halothane, without undergoing metabolism, might disrupt the hepatocyte membrane to expose specific antigenic determinants, it was more correctly postulated that halothane was metabolized to products that bind to membrane components that were responsible for antigen formation (84). Formation of antibodies against halothane itself was not likely because of the small size of the molecule.

In related studies, Neuberger et al. (86) attempted to answer the question whether the oxidative or reductive pathway of halothane metabolism was responsible for expression of the hepatocyte antigen recognized by human antisera. Hepatocytes from rabbits exposed to halothane under various oxygen tensions were incubated with sera from patients with halothane hepatitis and with normal lymphocytes from healthy patients. Cytotoxicity occurred in hepatocytes from rabbits treated with the cytochrome P450 inducer, β-napthoflavone, and exposed to halothane in 99% oxygen. Hepatotocytes from rabbits exposed to halothane under low oxygen tensions, conditions where halothane oxidation is reduced and reduction is increased, were much less susceptible to cytotoxicity. Therefore, oxidative metabolism of halothane to macromolecular adducts expressed on the cellular membrane appeared to be the mechanism for this cellular-mediated toxic immune response.

The discovery of the specific antibodies in a high percentage (67%) of patients with halothane hepatitis (87) and the evidence in animals that it was a TFA adducted protein appeared to open important avenues in halothane hepatitis research. These included the use of antibody screens as diagnostic tools for halothane hepatitis in humans (88) and investigation of events that might lead to cell death by the proposed immune response mechanism. The latter area of investigation has involved primarily identification of specific halothane antigen or antigens formed in rat liver and factors that modulate their formation.

Because halothane is oxidized by cytochrome P450 to the reactive intermediate, trifluoroacetyl chloride, which binds to protein (89), Satoh et al. (90) synthesized and immunized rabbits with a trifluoroacetyl-adducted rabbit serum albumin (TFA-RSA). (Trifluoroacetyl chloride reacts with the amino residue of lysine to form TFA-L-lysine.) These investigators, using immunofluorescence techniques, found circulating IgG antibodies in rabbits that reacted with rat hepatocytes from phenobarbital-treated rats exposed to halothane. Deuteration inhibits the oxidation of halothane but has no effect on its reductive metabolism (89). Exposure of rats to deuterated halothane resulted in less antibody reactivity with the rat hepatocytes. This confirmed the importance of the oxidative pathway for halothane-mediated antigen formation.

Initially, there was evidence that human anti-TFA antibodies reacted to a microsomal 54 kDa protein from rat liver thought to be a form of cytochrome P450 (90). Subsequent studies with immunoblotting techniques showed that anti-TFA antibodies from patients with halothane hepatitis could recognize other rat liver hepatocyte proteins as well. These halothane-labeled antigens ranged in molecular weight from 54 to 100 kDa (91,92) and had in common that they were trifluoroacetylated as a result of halothane oxidation. Treatment of rat liver microsomes with piperidine, which cleaves the trifluoroacetyl group from the adducted proteins, significantly decreased binding. Antigenic proteins identified include a 59 kDa antigen from rat liver microsomes, shown to be a microsomal carboxylesterase (93), a phosphatidylinositol-specific phospholipase C-alpha (58 kDa)

(94), calreticulin (63 kDa) (95), and possibly disulfide isomerase (57 kDa) (96). Interestingly, a 100 kDa labeled protein was identified as a stress-inducible protein (97).

Such findings raised intriguing questions. Is there a particular antigen among those identified that is ultimately responsible for an immune toxic response, and how were proteins labeled intracellularly with the TFA moiety expressed on the surface of the hepatocyte? The process of expression of antigens on the cell surface is not a trivial issue because halothane is primarily metabolized to reactive intermediates on the outer lumen of the smooth endoplasmic reticulum by cytochrome P450, and antigens must be present on the cellular surface to be recognized by the immune system.

Kenna et al. (98) investigated the topography of the antigenic proteins in the rat liver and provided evidence that most (57 kDa, 59 kDa, 76 kDa, and 100 kDa) were resident in the lumen of the endoplasmic reticulum, whereas the 54 kDa antigen, which is likely a cytochrome P450 form, was integrated into the membrane of the endoplasmic reticulum. It has been proposed that the process of labeling proteins in the lumen of the endoplasmic reticulum involves partitioning of trifluoroacetyl chloride into the lumen rather than into the cytoplasm due to the lipophilicity of trifluoroacetyl chloride (98). Once labeled, the TFA proteins may translocate to the hepatocellular membrane by migration along intracellular membranes to the plasma membrane. They may possibly become incorporated into the major histocompatibility complex. Many questions about this process remain to be answered.

It has been suggested that the epitope recognized by the anti-TFA antibodies includes the TFA moiety plus specific structural features of the TFA-bound proteins (98). This may explain why no antigens have been found that result from halothane–protein binding via reductive halothane metabolism (44). Binding of both the trifluorochloroethyl radical resulting from halothane reduction and binding of the tri-fluoroacetyl chloride intermediate resulting from halothane oxidation produce a protein-bound 2,2,2-trifluoroethyl moiety. The reductive radical intermediate would likely react with different amino acid residues at different portions of the protein molecule that may not be recognized readily by the immune system. Recently, however, serum antibody(s) from one patient with halothane hepatitis was found to recognize a protein from rat liver that was altered by halothane exposure but was not trifluoroacetylated. It was postulated that the protein was modified by a reductive metabolite of halothane (99).

Because adducts occur through a reaction of the trifluoroacetyl chloride with the amide group of the amino acid lysine, it is expected that TFA adduct formation should be proportional to the number of lysine residues. Although this may be the case, it has been reported that the antigenicity of proteins labeled with TFA is not necessarily related to the number of adducts per molecule. For example, a 59 kDa protein that has been isolated and purified with TFA adducted to it is known to contain a relatively large quantity of TFA-bound moiety, but of the TFA adducted proteins isolated, it is not as antigenic as others with lesser bound TFA. This can be interpreted to mean that the specific protein portion of the antigen is of equal or greater importance as an epitope than the TFA adduct, or antibody formation is not directly related to the development of the toxicity.

The guinea pig model might be expected to exhibit dissimilarities to the rat model. Halothane induces hepatotoxicity in each species, yet the fact that the guinea pig does not require phenobarbital treatment or exposure to halothane and low inspired oxygen tensions to develop halothane-induced liver damage suggests that mechanisms may differ. There is evidence, however, that guinea pigs, like rats, produce antibodies that recognize TFA-bound protein. Siadat-Pajouh et al. (100) demonstrated that anti-TFA antibodies occurred in three strains of guinea pigs following multiple exposures to halothane. The Hartley strain had considerably higher levels than strain 2 or the Amana strain. Correlations between antigen formation and increases in the serum alanine aminotransferase, however, were not clearly evident. Hubbard et al. (101) localized antigens with anti-TFA antibodies and found that halothane-exposed guinea pigs expressed antigen in the centrilobular area (around the central vein). Two or three exposures caused the greatest antigen formation. Consistent with the theory that oxidative halothane metabolism is involved, exposure to deuterated halothane resulted in production of less antigenic determinants in the guinea pig liver.

TFA antigens in the livers of guinea pigs exposed to halothane were identified as having molecular weights ranging from 51 kDa to 97 kDa (102), which are similar in size to the TFA antigens in the rat liver. Use of guinea pig liver slices incubated with ^{14}C-halothane to assay for the formation of halothane protein adducts showed that halothane bound to cytosolic proteins of 26 and 27 kDa that were glutathione-S-transferases (103). Antigens from microsomal proteins of higher molecular weights that appear to be important in rats were not preferentially labeled with ^{14}C-halothane in guinea pig liver slices. This suggests, as discussed previously, that there is a lack of direct correlation between the degree of protein labeling and antigenicity.

There is no doubt that a hypersensitivity reaction does occur involving halothane exposure in animals and humans. However, the involvement of antigen-antibody reactions in cell death is not clear. Immunotoxic reactions can be of the cellular-mediated type (sensitized T lymphocytes vs target cells) or of the humoral type involving circulating antibodies. Both types of reactions may cause cell death, but antibody-antigen reactions on the cellular membrane *per se* do not necessarily cause cell toxicity.

There are a number of complicating factors in studies of the immunopathology of halothane hepatitis. Antigenic determinants can arise as a consequence of cell death and may not be involved in the initial toxic process. Further, although anti-TFA antibodies usually recognize TFA-adducted proteins, there have been cases where anti-TFA antibodies react with certain proteins in liver tissue from animals and humans not exposed to halothane (104). This suggests that one or more of the proteins that react with anti-TFA antibodies may be unlabeled constitutive proteins in nonexposed animals. Other evidence of nonspecificity of antibody reactivity toward antigens is shown by the fact that exposure of rats to enflurane and isoflurane produces proteins that crossreact with anti-TFA antibodies. Lastly, as noted, not all patients with halothane hepatitis have circulating antibodies that recognize TFA antigens. For these reasons and others, precise immunopathologic mechanisms in halothane hepatitis have yet to be confirmed.

The role of stress proteins in adduct formation and toxicity is of particular interest because of the apparent role of stress proteins in cellular function and the relationship of their presence to the damaged hepatocyte. These proteins are largely inducible, although some are constitutive. The molecular masses very closely mimic some of those found as TFA adducts (70 to 100 kDa). The stress proteins have functions associated with defense or repair processes, as their name implies (105). For example, the origin of the name, heat-shock protein, was applied to these proteins because in various cells, including hepatocytes, they were induced following exposure to nonfatal elevated temperatures (40°C). On subsequent exposures of these cells to even higher temperatures that are normally fatal, the cells were able to survive. Studies on the intracellular function of these proteins have indicated that they act as chaperones to assist in proper protein folding and most recently have been found to function in the immune response. They actually may be responsible for certain of the autoimmune reactions. In addition to these functions, all of the heat-shock pro-

teins identified have been found to be ATPases and require ATP for normal functions (105).

Studies have shown that the specific treatment of rats required to produce halothane hepatitis (i.e., phenobarbital pretreatment, hypoxia, and halothane exposure) will result in the induction of a series of the stress proteins. Further, the distribution of these stress proteins in the rat liver, as determined by antistress protein antibody reactions, is exactly superimposable on the halothane-induced lesion that develops around the central vein (106). The relationship between the TFA-labeled proteins and the stress proteins has not been identified at the molecular level, yet there appears to be a relationship of these proteins and anesthetic-induced hepatocyte damage.

HEPATOTOXICITY OF OTHER ANESTHETIC AGENTS

Methoxyflurane

Methoxyflurane was introduced 3 years after halothane, yet the concern over fluoride-induced renal toxicity by methoxyflurane metabolism tended to overshadow investigations of its potential hepatotoxic properties. However, Joshi and Conn (107) reviewed 24 cases of hepatitis in patients previously anesthetized with methoxyflurane for which no other causes could be found. They concluded that a methoxyflurane hepatitis-related syndrome was evident. Similar to the halothane hepatitis syndrome, postoperative fever as well as jaundice occurred in a high number of patients. Two thirds were women, many of whom were obese. As with halothane, a sensitization process was suggested because the onset of hepatitis occurred more rapidly in patients who had been exposed previously to methoxyflurane or halothane. Methoxyflurane metabolism to toxic intermediates as a causative event cannot be ruled out. Although methoxyflurane has not been investigated in regard to reactive metabolite formation, it is metabolized more extensively than other anesthetics, such as halothane and enflurane (108). It is likely that on oxidation of the dichloro-β-carbon of methoxyflurane, a reactive acyl chloride is formed analogous to that formed from halothane that may adduct with protein.

Enflurane

Enflurane also has been investigated for liver toxic effects. Although it is considered less toxic than halothane, there is evidence that in humans the features of this injury are similar to those of halothane. After excluding other potential causes, Lewis et al. (109) analyzed 24 cases of enflurane-associated liver injury. The presenting features were postoperative fever and jaundice. A prospective study by Fee et al. (17) indicated that repeat exposures to enflurane or halothane increased the incidence of the liver toxic effects, and the incidence of liver injury was greater after halothane exposure compared to enflurane exposure. The consensus is that enflurane has less hepatotoxic potential than either halothane or methoxyflurane but nevertheless possesses hepatotoxic properties.

A number of studies of the metabolism of enflurane have been carried out in efforts to evaluate the possibility that reactive intermediates may be formed that can initiate liver injury. One metabolic pathway for enflurane resulting in the formation of methoxydifluoroacetic acid suggests that enflurane may form a reactive acyl chloride (110). An enflurane-microsomal protein adduct can be detected in the livers of enflurane-exposed rats (111). The quantity of adduct is increased with cytochrome P450 induction by phenobarbital. As noted, anti-TFA antibodies will cross-react with enflurane metabolism-dependent antigens, so that there is a possibility of cross-sensitization between the two anesthetics.

Isoflurane

Isoflurane has been the subject of some controversy regarding its ability to cause hepatotoxicity in humans. Very few suspected cases have been reported, and of those, even fewer can be considered positive on close scrutiny. Although isoflurane in theory may form a reactive intermediate on its oxidative metabolism, parallel mechanisms to those of halothane oxidation are unlikely due to very low rates of isoflurane metabolism. Isoflurane does not produce hepatotoxicity in the hypoxic rat model used for halothane. It will, as discussed, produce hepatotoxicity if the rats are fasted and exposed to very low concentrations of oxygen.

Desflurane and Sevoflurane

Based on the extremely low rates of desflurane defluorination (112) and assuming that anesthetic liver damage is dependent on anesthetic metabolism, it may be predicted that desflurane has a low potential for liver toxicity. Investigations of its toxicity in guinea pig liver slices showed that desflurane minimally affects the cellular viability parameters of potassium (K^+) content and protein secretion (113).

Sevoflurane, an anesthetic undergoing clinical trials in the United States, appears to have low hepatotoxic potential. It is metabolized at slower rates than halothane, although faster than isoflurane and enflurane, and has not been shown to form reactive metabolites.

SUMMARY

Hepatotoxicity associated with the volatile halogenated anesthetics is a syndrome that continues to be difficult to study. The two animal models that have been developed have clear inadequacies and simply may demonstrate that the syndrome can be caused by multiple processes. The mechanism by which halothane is toxic in the hypoxic rat model may not be the mechanism by which it is toxic in the guinea pig or in humans under normoxic conditions. Of the fluorinated anesthetics, fluroxene appears to be the only predictable hepatotoxin that is toxic via metabolism to directly toxic intermediates.

The evidence that halothane hepatitis involves an immune response is substantial, but an immunopathologic mechanism for halothane needs to be confirmed. Research in this area may be promising because it may also provide a means for predicting the occurrence of anesthetic-induced liver toxicity in humans and identifying patients who should not be further exposed to halothane (88). Positive blood screens of patients for anti-TFA antibodies will indicate that the patient should not be exposed to halothane, or even enflurane, because both anesthetics form antigens that crossreact with halothane anti-TFA antibodies.

Even though most halogenated anesthetics have been assessed for liver toxicity in the context of the major proposed mechanisms in the animal models, it is of interest that the National Halothane Study (8) found diethyl ether to be as toxic or more so than halothane in humans. Diethyl ether contains no halogen and is not metabolized to reactive intermediates, but it is highly soluble in biologic media. For the most part, the solubility of the saturated halogenated anesthetics correlates roughly with their degree of metabolism, so nonspecific effects due to anesthetic solubility and retention in the cell are difficult to differentiate from metabolism. The low or nonexistent toxicity of desflurane and sevoflurane, for example, may be due not only to their resistance to metabolism but also to their lower solubilities in biologic tissues. Thus, they have less ability to disrupt cellular homeostasis.

REFERENCES

1. Defalque R J. The first delayed chloroform poisoning. *Anesth Analg* 1968;47:374–377.

2. Ravdin I S, Vars H M, Goldschmidt S, Klingensmith LE. Anesthesia and liver damage II. The effect of anesthesia on the blood sugar, the liver glycogen, and liver fat. *J Pharmacol Exp Ther* 1938;64:111–129.

3. Wells H G. Delayed chloroform poisoning, allied conditions: a note on the cause of the anatomic and clinical changes observed. *JAMA* 1906;46:341–343.

4. Dykes M H M. Anesthesia and the liver: history and epidemiology. *Can Anaesth Soc J* 1973;20:34–47.

5. Struck H C, Plattner E B. A study of the pharmacological properties of certain saturated fluorocarbons. *J Pharmacol Exp Ther* 1940;68:217–219.

6. Harrison G G, Smith J S. Massive lethal hepatic necrosis in rats anesthetized with fluroxene, after microsomal enzyme induction. *Anesthesiology* 1973;39:619–625.

7. Neuberger J, Williams R. Halothane hepatitis. *Digest Dis* 1988;6:52–64.

8. Subcommittee on the national halothane study of the committee on anesthesia, National Academy of Sciences–National Research Council. Summary of the national halothane study: possible association between halothane anesthesia and postoperative hepatic necrosis. *JAMA* 1966;197:775–788.

9. Zimmerman H J. *Hepatotoxicity: the adverse effects of drugs and other chemicals on the liver.* New York: Appleton-Century-Crofts; 1978;370–394.

10. Raventos J. The action of fluothane—a new volatile anesthetic. *Br J Pharmacol* 1956;11:394–409.

11. Bunker J P, Blumenfeld C M. Liver necrosis after halothane anesthesia. Cause or coincidence? *N Engl J Med* 1963;268:531–534.

12. Lindenbaum J, Leifer E. Hepatic necrosis associated with halothane anesthesia. *N Engl J Med* 1963;268:525–530.

13. Klion F M, Schaffner F, Popper H. Hepatitis after exposure to halothane. *Ann Intern Med* 1969;71:467–477.

14. Trey C, Lipworth L, Chalmers T C, et al. Fulminant hepatic failure: presumable contributions of halothane. *N Engl J Med* 1968;279:798–801.

15. Allan L G, Hussey A J, Howie J, et al. Hepatic glutathione-S-transferase release after halothane anaesthesia: open randomized comparison with isoflurane. *Lancet* 1987;i:771–774.

16. Hussey A J, Aldridge L M, Paul D, Ray D C, Beckett G J, Allan L G. Plasma glutathione-S-transferase concentration as a measure of hepatocellular integrity following a single general anaesthetic with halothane, enflurane or isoflurane. *Br J Anaesth* 1988;60:130.

17. Fee J P H, Black G W, Dundee J W, et al. A prospective study of liver enzyme and other changes following repeat administration of halothane and enflurane. *Br J Anaesth* 1979;51:1133–1141.

18. Kenna J G, Neuberger J M, Williams R. Specific antibodies to halothane-induced liver an-

tigens in halothane hepatitis. *Br J Anaesth* 1987;59:1286–1290.

19. Inman W H W, Mushin W W. Jaundice after repeat exposure to halothane: a further analysis of reports to the Committee on Safety of Medicines. *Br Med J* 1978;2:1455–1456.

20. Carney F M T, Van Dyke R A. Halothane hepatitis: a critical review. *Anesth Analg* 1972;51:135–160.

21. Davidson C S, Barbior B, Popper H. Concerning the hepatotoxicity of halothane. *N Engl J Med* 1966;275:1497.

22. Bottinger L E, Dalen E, Hallen B. Halothane-induced liver damage: an analysis of the material reported to the Swedish Adverse Drug Reaction Committee, 1966–1973. *Acta Anesth Scand* 1976;20:40–46.

23. Sipes I G, Brown B R Jr. An animal model of hepatotoxicity associated with halothane anesthesia. *Anesthesiology* 1976;45:622–628.

24. McLain G E, Sipes I G, Brown B R Jr. An animal model of halothane hepatotoxicity: roles of enzyme induction and hypoxia. *Anesthesiology* 1979;51:321–326.

25. Ross W T, Daggy B P, Cardell R A. Hepatic necrosis caused by halothane and hypoxia in phenobarbital-treated rats. *Anesthesiology* 1979;51:327–333.

26. Cousins M J, Sharp J H, Gourlay G K, Adams J F, Haynes W D, Whitehead R. Hepatotoxicity and halothane metabolism in an animal model with application to human toxicity. *Anaesth Intensive Care* 1979;7:9–24.

27. Van Dyke R, Chenoweth M, Poznak A V. Metabolism of volatile anesthetics—I. Conversion *in vivo* of several anesthetics to $^{14}CO_2$ and chloride. *Biochem Pharmacol* 1964;13:1239–1247.

28. Stier A. Trifluoroacetic acid as a metabolite of halothane. *Biochem Pharmacol* 1964;13:1544.

29. Rehder K, Forbes H, Alter H, et al. Halothane biotransformation in man: a quantitative study. *Anesthesiology* 1967;28:711–715.

30. Ahr H J, King L J, Nastainczyk W, Ullrich V. The mechanism of reductive dehalogenation of halothane by liver cytochrome P-450. *Biochem Pharmacol* 1982;31:383–390.

31. Jee R C, Sipes I G, Gandolfi A J, Brown B R Jr. Factors influencing halothane hepatotoxicity in the rat hypoxic model. *Toxicol Appl Pharmacol* 1980;52:267–277.

32. Van Dyke R A. Hepatic centrilobular necrosis in rats after exposure to halothane, enflurane, or isoflurane. *Anesth Analg* 1982;61:812–819.

33. Widger L A, Gandolfi A J, Van Dyke R A. Hypoxia and halothane metabolism in vivo. *Anesthesiology* 1976;44:197–201.

34. Mukai S, Morio M, Fujii K, Hanaki C. Volatile metabolites of halothane in the rabbit. *Anesthesiology* 1977;47:248–251.

35. Brown B R Jr, Sipes I G, Baker R K. Halothane hepatotoxicity and the reduced derivative, 1,1,1-trifluoro-2-chloroethane. *Environ Health Perspect* 1977;21:185–188.

36. Maiorino R M, Sipes I G, Gandolfi A J, Brown B R Jr, Lind R C. Factors affecting the forma-

tion of chlorotrifluoroethane and chlorodifluoroethylene from halothane. *Anesthesiology* 1981;54:383–389.

37. Van Dyke R A, Gandolfi A J. Anaerobic release of fluoride from halothane. Relationship to the binding of halothane metabolites to hepatic cellular constitutents. *Drug Metab Disp* 1976;4:40–44.

38. Trudell J R, Bosterling B, Trevor A J. Reductive metabolism of halothane by human and rabbit cytochrome P450. Binding of 1-chloro-2,2,2-trifluoroethyl radical to phospholipids. *Mol Pharmacol* 1982;21:710–717.

39. Glende E A Jr, Hruszkewycz A M, Recknagel R O. Critical role of lipid peroxidation in carbon tetrachloride-induced loss of aminopyrine demethylase, cytochrome P450 and glucose 6-phosphatase. *Biochem Pharmacol* 1976;25:2163–2170.

40. Wood C L, Gandolfi A J, Van Dyke R A. Lipid binding of a halothane metabolite: relationship to lipid peroxidation *in vitro*. *Drug Metab Disp* 1976;4:305–313.

41. Gorsky B H, Cascorbi H F. Halothane hepatotoxicity and fluoride production in mice and rats. *Anesthesiology* 1979;50:123–125.

42. Baker M T, Van Dyke R A. Metabolism-dependent binding of the chlorinated insecticide DDT and its metabolite, DDD, to microsomal proteins and lipids. *Biochem Pharmacol* 1984;33:255–260.

43. Krieter P A, Van Dyke R A. Cytochrome P450 and halothane metabolism. Decrease in rat liver microsomal P450 *in vitro*. *Chem Biol Interact* 1983;44:219–235.

44. Maiorino R M, Gandolfi A J, Brendel K, MacDonald J R, Sipes I G. Chromatographic resolution of amino acid adducts of aliphatic halides. *Chem Biol Interact* 1982;38:175–188.

45. Rice S A, Maze M, Smith C M, Kosek J C, Mazze R I. Halothane hepatotoxicity in Fisher 344 rats pretreated with isoniazid. *Toxicol Appl Pharmacol* 1987;87:411–419.

46. Mitchell J R, Zimmerman H J, Ishak K G, Nelson S D. Isoniazid liver injury: clinical spectrum, pathology, and probable pathogenesis. *Ann Intern Med* 1976;84:181–192.

47. Lind R C, Gandolfi A J, Hall P M. Isoniazid potentiation of a guinea pig model of halothane-associated hepatotoxicity. *J Appl Toxicol* 1990;10:161–165.

48. Hughes H C, Lang C M. Hepatic necrosis produced by repeated administration of halothane to guinea pigs. *Anesthesiology* 1972;36:466–471.

49. Lunam C A, Cousins M J, Hall P M. Guinea-pig model of halothane-associated hepatotoxicity in the absence of enzyme induction and hypoxia. *J Pharmacol Exp Ther* 1985;232:802–809.

50. Lunam C A, Hall P M, Cousins M J. The pathology of halothane hepatotoxicity in a guinea-pig model: a comparison with human halothane hepatitis. *Br J Exp Pathol* 1989;70:533–541.

51. Lind R C, Gandolfi A J, Brown B R, Hall P M.

Halothane hepatotoxicity in guinea pigs. *Anesth Analg* 1987;66:222–228.

52. Stock J G L, Strunin L. Unexplained hepatitis following halothane. *Anesthesiology* 1985;63:424–439.

53. Cohen P J. Effect of anesthetics on mitochondrial function. *Anesthesiology* 1973;39:153–164.

54. Van Dyke R A. Effect of fasting on anesthetic-associated liver toxicity. *Anesthesiology* 1981;55:A181.

55. Shingu K, Eger EI II, Johnson B H. Hypoxia may be more important than reductive metabolism in halothane-induced hepatic injury. *Anesth Analg* 1982;61:824–827.

56. Uetrecht J, Wood A J, Phythyon J M, Wood M. Contrasting effects on halothane hepatotoxicity in the phenobarbital-hypoxic and triiodothyronine model: mechanistic implications. *Anesthesiology* 1983;59:196–201.

57. Berman M L, Kuhnert L, Phythyon J M, Holaday D A. Isoflurane and enflurane-induced hepatic necrosis in triiodothyronine-pretreated rats. *Anesthesiology* 1983;58:1–5.

58. Smith A C, Roberts S M, Berman L M, Harbison R D, James R C. Effects of piperonyl butoxide on halothane hepatotoxicity and metabolism in the hyperthyroid rat. *Toxicology* 1988;50:95–105.

59. Gelman S. Halothane hepatotoxicity—again? *Anesth Analg* 1986;65:831–834.

60. Shingu K, Eger E I II, Johnson B H, et al. Hepatic injury induced by anesthetic agents in rat. *Anesth Analg* 1983;62:140–145.

61. Gelman S, Rimerman V, Fowler K, Bishop S, Bradley E L. The effect of halothane, isoflurane, and blood loss on hepatotoxicity and hepatic oxygen availability in phenobarbital-pretreated hypoxic rats. *Anesth Analg* 1984;63:965–972.

62. Gelman S I. The effect of enteral oxygen administration on the hepatic circulation during halothane anaesthesia: experimental investigations. *Br J Anaesth* 1975;47:1253–1259.

63. Becker G L, Miletich D J, Albrecht R F. Halogenated anesthetics increase oxygen consumption in isolated hepatocytes from phenobarbital-treated rats. *Anesthesiology* 1987;67:185–190.

64. White R E, Coon M J. Oxygen activation by cytochrome P450. *Annu Rev Biochem* 1980;49:315–356.

65. Wang Y, Baker M T. NADPH and oxygen consumption in isoflurane-facilitated 2-chloro-1,1-difluoroethene metabolism in rabbit liver microsomes. *Drug Metab Disp* 1993;21:299–304.

66. Steward A, Allott P R, Cowles A L, Mapelson W W. Solubility coefficients for inhaled anaesthetics for water, oil, and biological media. *Br J Anaesth* 1973;45:282–293.

67. Plummer J L, Wanwimolruk S, Jenner M A, Hall P M, Cousins M J. Effects of cimetidine and rantidine on halothane metabolism and hepatotoxicity in an animal model. *Drug Metab Disp* 1984;12:106–110.

68. Joyce J T, Roizen M F, Gerson J I, Grobecker H, Eger E I II, Forbes R A. Induction of

anesthesia with halothane increases plasma norepinephrine concentrations. *Anesthesiology* 1982;56:286–290.

69. White K A, Marletta M A. Nitric oxide synthase is a cytochrome P450 hemoprotein. *Biochemistry* 1992;31:6627–6631.

70. Ignarro L J. Signal transduction mechanisms involving nitric oxide. *Biochem Pharmacol* 1991;41:485–490.

71. Baker M T, Nelson R M, Van Dyke R A. The release of inorganic fluoride from halothane and halothane metabolites by cytochrome P450, hemin, and hemoglobin. *Drug Metab Disp* 1983;11:308–311.

72. Nicotera P, Bellomo G, Orrenius S. The role of Ca^{2+} in cell killing. *Chem Res Toxicol* 1990;3:484–494.

73. Gill D L, Grollman E F, Kohn L D. Calcium transport mechanisms in membrane vesicles from guinea pig brain synaptosomes. *J Biol Chem* 1981;256:184–192.

74. Gill D L. Sodium channel, sodium pump, and sodium-exchange activities in synaptosomal plasma membrane vesicles. *J Biol Chem* 1982;257:10986–10990.

75. Recknagel R O. A new direction in the study of CCl_4 hepatotoxicity. *Life Sci* 1983;33:401–408.

76. Farber J L. Calcium and the mechanisms of liver necrosis. *Prog Liver Dis* 1982;7:347–360.

77. Moore L. Inhibition of liver microsome calcium pump by *in vivo* administration of CCl_4, $CHCl_3$ and 1,1-dichloroethylene (vinylidene chloride). *Biochem Pharmacol* 1980;29:2505–2511.

78. Brattin W J, Pencil S D, Waller R L, Glende E A Jr, Recknagel R O. Assessment of the role of calcium ion in halocarbon hepatotoxicity. *Environ Health Perspect* 1984;57:321–323.

79. Agarwal A K, Mehendale H M. Perturbation of calcium homeostasis by CCl_4 in rats pretreated with chlordecone and phenobarbital. *Environ Health Perspect* 1984;57:289–291.

80. Iaizzo P A, Seewald M J, Powis G, Van Dyke R A. The effects of volatile anesthetics on Ca^{++} mobilization in rat hepatocytes. *Anesthesiology* 1990;72:504–509.

81. Iaizzo P A, Olsen R A, Seewald MJ, Powis G, Stier A, Van Dyke R A. Transient increases of intracellular CA^{++} induced by volatile anesthetics in rat hepatocytes. *Cell Calcium* 1990;11:515–524.

82. Farrell G C, Mahoney J, Bilous M, Frost L. Altered hepatic calcium homeostasis in guinea pigs with halothane-induced hepatotoxicity. *J Pharmacol Exp Ther* 1988;247:751–756.

83. Chien K R, Abrams J, Serroni A, Martin J T, Faber J L. Accelerated phospholipid degradation and associated membrane dysfunction in irreversible, ischemic liver cell injury. *J Biol Chem* 1978;253:4809–4917.

84. Vergani D, Mieli-Vergani G, Alberti A, et al. Antibiotics to the surface altered rabbit hepatocytes in patients with severe halothane-associated hepatitis. *N Engl J Med* 1980;303:66–71.

85. Vergani D, Tsantoulas D, Eddleston A L W F, Davis M, Williams R. Sensitization to halothane-altered liver components in severe he-

patic necrosis after halothane anaesthesia. *Lancet* 1978;ii:801–803.

86. Neuberger J, Mieli-Vergani G, Tredger J M, Davis M, Williams R. Oxidative metabolism of halothane in the production of altered hepatocyte membrane antigens in acute halothane-induced hepatic necrosis. *Gut* 1981;22:669–672.

87. Kenna J G, Neuberger J, Williams R. An enzyme-linked immunosorbent assay for detection of antibodies against halothane-altered hepatocyte antigens. *J Immunol Meth* 1984;75:3–14.

88. Martin J L, Kenna J G, Pohl L R. Antibody assays for the detection of patients sensitized to halothane. *Anesth Analg* 1990;70:154–159.

89. Sipes I G, Gandolfi A J, Pohl L R, Krishna G, Brown B R Jr. Comparison of the biotransformation and hepatotoxicity of halothane and deuterated halothane. *J Pharmacol Exp Ther* 1980;214:716–720.

90. Satoh H, Fukuda Y, Anderson D K, Ferrans V J, Gillette J R, Pohl L R. Immunological studies on the mechanism of halothane-induced hepatotoxicity: immunohistochemical evidence of trifluoroacetylated hepatocytes. *J Pharmacol Exp Ther* 1985;233:857–862.

91. Kenna J G, Neuberger J, Williams R. Identification by immunoblotting of three halothane-induced liver microsomal polypeptide antigens recognized by antibodies in sera from patients with halothane-associated hepatitis. *J Pharmacol Exp Ther* 1987;242:733–740.

92. Kenna J G, Satoh H, Christ D D, Pohl L R. Metabolic basis for a drug hypersensitivity: antibodies in sera from patients with halothane hepatitis recognize liver neoantigens that contain the trifluoroacetyl group derived from halothane. *J Pharmacol Exp Ther* 1988;245:1103–1109.

93. Satoh H, Martin B M, Schulick A H, Christ D D, Kenna J G, Pohl L R. Human antiendoplasmic reticulum antibodies in sera of patients with haothane-induced hepatitis are directed against a trifluoroacetylated carboxylesterase. *Proc Natl Acad Sci USA* 1989;86:322–326.

94. Martin J L, Pumford N R, LaRossa A C, et al. A metabolite of halothane covalently binds to an endoplasmic reticulum protein that is highly homologous to phosphatylinositol-specific phospholipase C-alpha but has no activity. *Biochem Biophys Res Commun* 1991;178:679–685.

95. Butler L E, Thomassen D, Martin J L, Martin B M, Kenna J G, Pohl L R. The calcium-binding protein calreticulin is covalently modified in rat liver by a reactive metabolite of the inhalation anesthetic halothane. *Chem Res Toxicol* 1992;5:406–410.

96. Kenna J G, Martin J L, Pohl L R. Purification of trifluoroacetylated protein antigens from livers of halothane-treated rats. *Eur J Pharmacol* 1990;183:1139–1140.

97. Martin T D, Martin B M, Pumford J L, Pohl L R. The role of a stress protein in the development of a drug-induced allergic response. *Eur J Pharmacol* 1990;183:1138–1139.

98. Kenna J G, Martin J L, Pohl L R. The topography of trifluoroacetylated protein antigens in liver microsomal fractions from halothane treated rats. *Biochem Pharmacol* 1992;44:621–629.

99. Martin J L, Dubbink D A, Plevak D J, et al. Halothane hepatitis 28 years after primary exposure. *Anesth Analg* 1992;74:605–608.

100. Siadat-Pajouh M, Hubbard A K, Roth T P, Gandolfi A J. Generation of halothane-induced immune response in a guinea pig model of halothane hepatitis. *Anesth Analg* 1987;66:1209–1214.

101. Hubbard A K, Roth T P, Schuman R S, Gandolfi A J. Localization of halothane-induced antigen *in situ* by specific anti-halothane metabolite antibodies. *Clin Exp Immunol* 1989;76:422–427.

102. Brown A P, Hastings K L, Gandolfi A J. Generation and detection of neoantigens in guinea pig liver slices incubated with halothane. *Int J Immunopharmacol* 1991;13:429–435.

103. Brown A P, Hasings K L, Gandolfi A J, Liebler D C, Brendel K. Formation and identification of protein adducts to cytosolic proteins in guinea pig liver slices exposed to halothane. *Toxicology* 1992;73:281–295.

104. Christen U R S, Burgen M, Gut J. Halothane metabolism: immunochemical evidence for molecular mimicry of trifluoroacetylated liver protein adducts by constitutive polypeptides. *Mol Pharmacol* 1991;40:390–400.

105. Welch W J. Mammalian stress response: cell physiology, structure/function of stress proteins, and implications for medicine and disease. *Physiol Rev* 1992;72:1063–1081.

106. Van Dyke R A, Mostofapour S, Marsh H M, Li Y, Chopp M. Immunocytochemical detection of the 72-kDa heat-shock protein in halothane-induced hepatotoxicity in rats. *Life Sci* 1992;50:PL41–PL45.

107. Joshi P H, Conn H O. The syndrome of methoxyflurane-associated hepatitis. *Ann Intern Med* 1974;80:395–401.

108. Baker M T, Van Dyke R A. Biochemical and toxicological aspects of the volatile anesthetic. In: Barash P G, Cullen B R, Stoelting R K, eds. *Clinical anesthesia,* 2nd ed. Philadelphia: JB Lippincott Co, 1992;467–480.

109. Lewis J H, Zimmerman H J, Ishak K G, Mullick F G. Enflurane hepatotoxicity, a clinicopathologic study of 24 cases. *Ann Intern Med* 1983;98:984–992.

110. Burke T R Jr, Branchflower R V, Lees D E, Pohl L R. Mechanism of defluorination of enflurane. Identification of an organic metabolite in rat and man. *Drug Metab Disp* 1981;9:19–24.

111. Christ D D, Satoh H, Kenna J G, Pohl L R. Potential metabolic basis for enflurane hepatitis and the apparent cross-sensitization between enflurane and halothane. *Drug Metab Disp* 1988;16:135–140.

112. Koblin D D, Eger E I II, Johnson B H, Konopka K, Waskell L. I-653 resists degradation in rats. *Anesth Analg* 1988;67:534–538.

113. Ghantous H N, Fernando J, Gandolfi A J, Brendel K. Minimal biotransformation and toxicity of desflurane in guinea pig liver slices. *Anesth Analg* 1991;72:796–800.

Anesthetic Toxicity, edited by
Susan A. Rice and Kevin J. Fish.
Raven Press, Ltd., New York © 1994.

6

Nephrotoxicity of Volatile Anesthetic Agents

Kevin J. Fish

*Department of Anesthesia, Stanford University School of Medicine,
Stanford, California 94305, and Department of Anesthesia, Veterans Affairs
Medical Center, Palo Alto, California 94304*

Until the early 1960s, it was thought that the volatile anesthetic agents were not metabolized to a significant degree by humans. The recognition that some patients who received methoxyflurane as an anesthetic agent developed postoperative renal dysfunction and that the renal dysfunction might be related to a metabolite of methoxyflurane was a major stimulus to an intensive study of the metabolism of methoxyflurane. This culminated in the recognition that the etiology of the methoxyflurane-induced renal dysfunction was due to metabolism of methoxyflurane and the release of inorganic fluoride (F^-), a known nephrotoxin. Recognition of the importance of metabolism to anesthesia-induced toxicity was the stimulus to a major and continuing research effort into the metabolism and toxicity of all the volatile anesthetic agents.

This chapter reviews the history of F^- nephrotoxicity and anesthetic metabolism to F^-. The factors that have been shown to enhance this toxicity are reviewed, and the significance of these factors to both current and future anesthetic agents and anesthetic practice is discussed.

INORGANIC FLUORIDE

The physiologic concentration of F^- in the blood is approximately 1 μM and is maintained by the balance between oral intake and elimination from the blood. Deposition in bone (about 55%) and urinary excretion (about 45%) are the two major mechanisms for elimination of an F^- load and control of serum F^- concentration. Only insignificant amounts are excreted in sweat and feces. Inorganic fluoride has a marked affinity for calcified tissues and accumulates in them by replacing ions and groups normally associated with hydroxyapatite crystals (1). Autoradiographic studies have demonstrated ^{18}F in the skeleton of rats only 2 minutes after i.v. injection (2). Once incorporated into skeletal tissue, the half-life of ^{18}F is 9 years, indicating that calcified tissues avidly retain F^- (3). The other major route of F^- elimination from blood is renal excretion. It has been demonstrated that over a range of urinary flow rates from 0.1 ml/minute to 6 ml/minute, there is a positive correlation between renal clearance of ^{18}F and urinary flow (4,5), with the maximum rate of clearance about one-half the glomerular filtration rate (GFR). Tubular reabsorption of F^- occurs by nonionic diffusion, apparently as hydrogen fluoride, and is inversely related to tubular fluid pH (6).

TOXICITY OF FLUORIDE-CONTAINING COMPOUNDS

The toxic effects of compounds containing organic fluoride have been known for years because of their common use as household pesticides. They became notorious as poisons because of the many human fatalities that occurred after accidental ingestion. Although organic fluorides may be poisonous, the toxicity is related to the organic compound unless there is metabolism and release of F^- from the parent compound. The toxicity of inorganic fluorides is related to the fluoride ion itself. An example is sodium fluoride, a highly soluble and easily absorbed compound, of which ingestion of as little as 5 to 10 g is lethal. Symptoms of acute sodium fluoride toxicity include intense salivation, vomiting, diarrhea, abdominal pain, convulsions, labored respiration, hypotension, hyperkalemia, and hemorrhage (7,8). Acute F^- toxicity is related to the blood F^- concentration and probably is due to the inhibition of several enzyme systems, such as enolases, phosphatases, and dehydrogenases (9). The systemic effects and treatment of acute F^- toxicity have been reviewed recently and are not discussed further here (8).

NEPHROTOXICITY OF INORGANIC FLUORIDE

The nephrotoxic effects of F^- in humans were first reported by Goldemberg (10) in 1930. He treated patients with thyrotoxicosis with sodium fluoride i.v. but had to discontinue these efforts when several patients developed a polyuric syndrome that he called *diabetes insipidus fluorique*. In 1961, Taylor et al. (11) documented the renal effects of the i.v. administration of near lethal doses of sodium fluoride. They noted increased urinary output and protein excretion and observed a decrease in urinary specific gravity. These findings persisted for several days after the administration of the sodium fluoride. Additionally, they observed that the kidneys were one of the first organs to show changes in function following acute exposure to high doses of

F^-. However, it is likely that these early changes are not due to increased renal sensitivity to the toxic effects of F^- but rather to the high renal F^- concentrations that are established during urine formation (12). Alkalinization of the urine enhances renal excretion of F^- and increases the ability of the patient to tolerate a given serum F^- concentration (13). In patients who have acute F^- toxicity, alkalinization of the urine enhances F^- excretion and can be used as a treatment to increase urinary excretion of F^- and to minimize the systemic toxicity (8).

MECHANISMS OF INORGANIC FLUORIDE NEPHROTOXICITY

The precise way in which F^- produces its toxic effect on the kidneys is not clear, although several possible mechanisms have been suggested. Roman et al. (14) examined the tubular site of action of F^- in Fischer 344 rats using clearance techniques. They found that during sodium fluoride infusion, free water clearance (i.e., tubular reabsorption of water) was markedly reduced, whereas sodium excretion was increased. Their conclusions were that F^- inhibits tubular reabsorption of water, primarily in the medullary portion of the ascending limb of the loop of Henle, and they suggested that this occurred by inhibition of the active chloride pump located in this portion of the nephron segment. They were unable to exclude the collecting duct as a site of F^- action.

Wallin and Kaplan (15) studied two different strains of rats, the hereditary hypothalamic diabetes insipidus rat and the Sprague-Dawley rat. They found that free water clearance was unaltered during sodium fluoride infusion and thought that it was unlikely that significant alteration of chloride reabsorption occurred. They pointed out that at lower F^- dosages, urinary osmolality increased and volume decreased with administration of exogenous vasopressin. This response was lost at higher F⁻ dosages, suggesting that there was a defect in the ability of the collecting tubule to respond to vasopressin. To support this view, they examined cAMP and vasopressin excretion rates in urine in response to sodium fluoride administration. Vasopressin excretion was increased, but cAMP excretion rate was decreased. Urinary excretion of vasopressin was increased by the administration of exogenous vasopressin, indicating access of the hormone to the end-organ. They suggested three possible explanations for their findings. First, they suggested that F⁻ may disrupt the ATP-generating system through its effect on intermediary metabolism. Second, there might be defective binding of vasopressin to its receptor sites. Finally, qualitative defects in adenylcyclase or increased phosphodiesterase activity could be present.

In another study, Whitford and Stringer (16) showed in Fischer 344 rats that during a 2-hour i.v. infusion of sodium fluoride, urinary flow rates increased moderately, whereas inner medullary sodium and chloride concentrations, GFR, and the excretion rates of sodium, chloride, and potassium decreased. Changes were proportional to the dose of sodium fluoride. Although plasma F⁻ concentrations decreased rapidly from their peak values at the end of the infusion, this decline was not accompanied by recovery of urinary osmolality or medullary sodium and chloride concentrations. Instead, these variables showed only a gradual return toward control values over 40 hours. Glomerular filtration rate continued to fall throughout the first day after stopping the infusion of sodium fluoride. They suggested that increased vasa recta blood flow with subsequent medullary solute washout was the underlying mechanism for the initial effects of F⁻ that they observed. The precise mechanism by which F⁻ depresses glomerular filtration remains unknown and may be due to alterations in either the permeability characteristics of glomeruli or the internal distribution of intrarenal blood flow.

The histologic appearance of the rat kidney following i.p. injection of nephrotoxic but not lethal doses of F⁻ was described by Mazze et al. (17). Employing light microscopy, glomeruli appeared to be normal, but there was dilatation of proximal convoluted tubules and marked reduction in the height of littoral cells. There were also many foci of hypereosinophilia, nuclear pyknosis, and karyorrhexis, and intraluminal slough of necrotic proximal tubular epithelial cells. Electron microscopy showed swelling and occasional rupture of mitochondria, most notably in proximal convoluted tubules. Seven days after exposure to F⁻, evidence of tubular regeneration was demonstrable.

In summary, the answer to the question regarding the precise mechanism and site of action of F⁻ in the kidney remains unclear. There are at least three possibilities.

1. Inorganic fluoride produces proximal tubular damage that interferes with iso-osmotic reabsorption of proximal tubular fluid. The excessive fluid load presented to the distal nephron prevents development of maximum medullary hyperosmolality, which leads to decreased reabsorption of water from the collecting ducts. Large volumes of dilute urine are formed despite the presence of antidiuretic hormone.

2. Inorganic fluoride inhibits Na^+ and K^+ ATPase and other enzymes that are involved in ion transport in the ascending limb of the loop of Henle. This leads to decreased renal medullary hyperosmolality and polyuric renal insufficiency.

3. Inorganic fluoride is a potent vasodilator. Vasodilation of the vasa recta leads to increased medullary solute washout and an inability to concentrate urine.

NEPHROTOXICITY OF METHOXYFLURANE

The commonly used inhalation anesthetic agents are either halogenated ethanes or ethers. Halogenation of hydrocarbons decreases their volatility and inflammability.

Halogenation of ethers also decreases their water solubility and in some cases increases their lipid solubility. Following the introduction of halothane into clinical practice in 1956, an intensive search was conducted for other fluorinated hydrocarbons with similar anesthetic properties. This led to the introduction of methoxyflurane into clinical practice in 1960. In 1966, Crandell et al. (18) reported the development of high-output renal insufficiency in 16 of 94 patients anesthetized with methoxyflurane. Polyuria was associated with a negative fluid balance, elevations of serum sodium, osmolality, and urea nitrogen concentrations, and a fixed urinary osmolality close to that of serum. Patients were unable to concentrate urine despite fluid deprivation and vasopressin administration. Renal impairment lasted from 10 to 20 days in most cases, but in three patients, abnormalities persisted for longer than 1 year. They concluded that methoxyflurane was in some way responsible for the renal abnormalities observed in their patients, but they were unable to define the precise connection.

In 1970, Taves et al. (19) suggested that accumulation of excessive concentrations of nephrotoxic metabolites might be the cause of the polyuric renal failure associated with methoxyflurane administration. They implicated F^- as the toxic metabolite, noting that oxalate, another potentially nephrotoxic metabolite of methoxyflurane, is associated with oliguric rather than polyuric renal failure. They postulated that several factors would be of importance in determining whether high-output renal failure would develop following methoxyflurane anesthesia. These included the duration of anesthesia, the amount of anesthetic retained (especially in the obese patient), the rate of metabolism, and the rate of clearance of F^- and organic fluoride from the body.

Mazze et al. (20) subsequently reported increased blood concentrations of F^- in all patients anesthetized with methoxyflurane and showed that the highest serum F^- concentrations occurred in the patients with the greatest degree of renal impairment. The demonstration by Mazze et al. (21) of strain differences in rats in both methoxyflurane defluorination and susceptibility to the nephrotoxic effects of F^- was an important step in establishing the cause–effect relationship between F^- and anesthetic nephrotoxicity. Among the five rat strains they studied, only Fischer 344 rats exhibited both a high rate of methoxyflurane defluorination and susceptibility to the nephrotoxic effects of F^-. Using this strain as an animal model, they were able to show that renal functional and morphologic changes were proportional to the dose of methoxyflurane (17) and that strikingly similar renal changes occurred following either methoxyflurane administration or i.p. injection of sodium fluoride. Furthermore, polyuria after both treatments was resistant to antidiuretic hormone, as had been reported in patients with methoxyflurane-induced toxicity (18).

An additional refinement of the animal studies, which has enhanced our understanding of the metabolism of methoxyflurane and other volatile anesthetic agents and the factors that affect this process, was the application of *in vitro* techniques to studies of hepatic drug metabolism. Like many drugs, volatile anesthetic agents primarily undergo oxidative metabolism by the hepatic microsomal cytochrome P450 system. Rat liver microsomal preparations isolated by ultracentrifugation contains this enzyme system and, under suitable conditions, can be used to determine rates of defluorination and other factors that might affect the cytochrome P450 enzyme system, such as enzyme induction and enzyme inhibition (22) (see chapter by Waskell).

FLUORIDE RELEASE FROM ANESTHETIC AGENTS

Dehalogenation of anesthetics follows enzymatic oxidation of the carbon atom that carries the halogen atom(s) rather than direct attack on the carbon–halogen bond. This occurs predominantly in the liver. Oxidation results in an unstable molecule, leading to loss of all halogen atoms on that carbon. The carbon–fluorine bond is the most stable of the carbon–halogen bonds, with chlorine, bromine, and iodine following fluorine in decreasing order of carbon bond strength. Thus, halothane is resistant to oxidative defluorination, although it is debrominated and dechlorinated (Fig. 1). Methoxyflurane is extensively dehalogenated, probably because it has two sites for enzymatic attack, one at the dichlorocarbon and the other at the ether linkage. From the structure of enflurane, one would expect that it would be metabolized relatively easily by liver enzymes. In fact, this is not the case. The ether linkage appears to be stabilized by the presence of four fluorine atoms, two on either side of the ether linkage. Defluorination occurs slowly and probably only at the terminal carbon atom of the ethyl moiety. Isoflurane has a terminal trifluorocarbon atom and an ether linkage surrounded by three halogen atoms. It is even more stable than enflurane. Desflurane is the most stable fluorinated volatile anesthetic. In contrast, sevoflurane is susceptible to defluorination, probably because it has a low halogen density around its ether linkage.

Substrate availability is an important factor governing anesthetic defluorination. Substrate availability is primarily related to anesthetic solubility, with the duration of administration particularly important for the highly fat-soluble agents that are slowly released into the blood for a prolonged period of time following anesthesia. For example, methoxyflurane is highly fat soluble (oil/gas partition coefficient = 930). Following an anesthetic of 3 to 4 hours' duration, it may be present at concentrations that permit maximum rates of defluorination for hours or even days (23). Cousins and Mazze (24) demonstrated the relationship between duration of exposure to methoxyflurane, F^- production and nephrotoxicity in both Fischer 344 rats (17) and patients. They showed that hypernatremia, serum hyperosmolality, and elevated blood urea nitrogen and serum F^- concentrations were dose-related effects and that peak serum F^- concentrations occurred as late as 24 to 72 hours following termination of methoxyflurane anesthesia. By contrast, the blood concentrations of less soluble agents, such as isoflurane and enflurane (oil/gas partition coefficient = 98) or sevoflurane (oil/gas partition coefficient = 55), fall relatively quickly after anesthesia due to more rapid pulmonary excretion. Thus, in humans exposed to enflurane for periods as long as 9 hours, peak serum F^- concentration is usually observed within 4 to 6 hours after the end of anesthesia (25).

Another aspect of anesthetic solubility is the role it plays in determining the access of anesthetic agents to the enzymatic site. Enflurane, for example, is five times less soluble in microsomes than is methoxyflurane (26). The affinity of anesthetics for enzymatic site, however, is not known. The state of anesthesia itself may affect the ex-

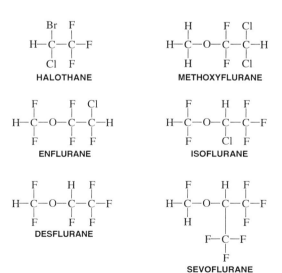

FIG. 1. Structural formulae of six fluorinated anesthetic agents.

tent of anesthetic biotransformation. This may happen by inhibition of mitochondrial respiration during anesthesia, which leads to depletion of NADPH, an essential cofactor for anesthetic metabolism. Hence, cofactor availability could limit the rate of defluorination of anesthetic agents, so that maximum rates of anesthetic metabolism might not occur during surgical anesthesia (26).

A number of *in vivo* and *in vitro* studies in animal and humans have demonstrated that other concurrently administered agents also might affect the metabolism of volatile anesthetic agents (27–31). For example, halothane has been shown to inhibit the metabolism of enflurane in rats and humans (28,29). Propylene glycol is the solvent for etomidate, an i.v. anesthetic agent, and propylene glycol also has been shown to inhibit the metabolism of enflurane (30). Aune et al. (32) demonstrated that enflurane and halothane could inhibit antipyrine oxidation and paracetamol conjugation in isolated rat hepatocytes. In another animal study, Hanna et al. (33) showed that pretreatment with paracetamol decreased metabolism of enflurane. The volatile anesthetic agents themselves have been shown to induce hepatic microsomal enzymes (34,35).

Considerable variation in hepatocellular activity may occur both among individuals and within an individual. Interindividual variations in rates of metabolism are due to differences in genetic composition, concurrent drug therapy, and environmental exposure to chemical substances. Intraindividual differences are due to the latter two factors because metabolism of a particular compound by a given individual is remarkably constant in the presence of a stable environment (see chapter by Wood).

ROLE OF ENZYME INDUCTION

The cytochrome P450 system consists of a profile of similar enzymes, all considered mixed-function oxidases. They are induci-

ble to different degrees by different compounds. For example, cytochrome P450 is induced by the administration of phenobarbital, whereas cytochrome P448 is induced by polycyclic hydrocarbons, such as 3-methylcholanthrene. The anesthetic agents themselves are weak inducing agents (34,35). Of more concern to anesthesiologists is the large group of compounds that patients may be chronically medicated with or exposed to in their environment. These chemicals could influence the metabolism of anesthetic agents by inducing or inhibiting their biotransformation.

A number of studies have examined the interaction between administration of enzyme-inducing agents and the metabolism of the volatile anesthetic agents. Prior administration of phenobarbital consistently enhanced the defluorination of methoxyflurane (36), isoflurane (37), and sevoflurane (38) *in vitro* but did not increase defluorination of enflurane (or did so only marginally). Similar results have been observed *in vivo* in Fischer 344 rats (39). Churchill et al. (40) reported the case of a patient who received secobarbital for 1 month before a 2.5 hour exposure to minimal concentrations of methoxyflurane. The patient's peak serum F^- concentration was 114 μM, a value three times higher than expected after a methoxyflurane exposure of this duration. The most likely explanation for this high F^- concentration was enhanced defluorination as a consequence of enzyme induction.

The effects of administration of enzyme-inducing drugs on enflurane metabolism were studied by Maduska (41), who also studied patients having more than one exposure to enflurane or treated with pentobarbital before anesthesia. They concluded that increased F^- production was unlikely to follow enflurane anesthesia among patients treated with enzyme-inducing drugs or having had a previous recent exposure to enflurane. Similar conclusions were reached by Dooley et al. (42). They measured serum F^- concentration in 102 surgical patients anesthetized with enflurane and chronically treated with a wide variety of drugs ranging from known enzyme-inducing agents, such as phenobarbital and phenytoin, to weak inducing agents, such as ethanol. They were unable to show that any of these drugs were associated with unusually high peak serum F^- concentrations. Additionally, 5 of their patients had two exposures to enflurane over a period of several weeks to months. The second exposure did not result in increased serum F^- concentrations above those that occurred after the initial exposure.

There are exceptions to the finding that enflurane defluorination is not inducible. Cousins et al. (43) reported the case of a patient receiving isoniazid who had a peak serum F^- concentration of 106 μM following 5 hours of enflurane anesthesia. This concentration was three times higher than expected and was within the nephrotoxic range. The patient was a heavy smoker, had a history of heavy alcohol intake, and was receiving treatment with chlorpromazine, diazepam, and isoniazid. Although it certainly was possible that this isolated high serum F^- concentration was due to individual variation, a number of subsequent studies strongly suggest that this very high peak serum F^- concentration was due to enzyme induction by isoniazid and not to the other drugs.

In a series of *in vitro* and *in vivo* experiments, isoniazid and its metabolites were shown to enhance the defluorination of methoxyflurane, isoflurane, sevoflurane, and enflurane (44,45). The extent of defluorination was only slightly less than that seen after phenobarbital pretreatment for the first three anesthetics and well beyond that reported for enflurane. These studies also reported that isoniazid and other drugs containing the hydrazine linkage are potent inducing agents of cytochrome P451, a variant of cytochrome P450. A subsequent study (46) demonstrated that the ethanol-inducible cytochrome P450-3A was responsible for enflurane defluorination in the rabbit and showed that this enzyme may be enhanced by a number of agents, including ethanol, isoniazid, imidazole, acetone, diabetes, and prolonged fasting.

In a follow-up study of patients receiving isoniazid and enflurane anesthesia, Mazze et al. (47) demonstrated that approximately half of the patients receiving isoniazid had very elevated serum F^- concentrations following anesthesia. The results were suggestive that this phenomenon could be related to the bimodal distribution of isoniazid metabolism into fast and slow acetylators of the drug. It may be that rapid acetylators develop high concentrations of hydrazine-containing metabolites of isoniazid that induce enflurane defluorination. There is recent evidence to suggest that the metabolism of isoflurane is also inducible by isoniazid in humans and that there also may be the same bimodal distribution of fast and slow metabolizers of isoflurane in patients receiving isoniazid (48). It would be advisable to avoid the use of enflurane (or other fluorinated volatile anesthetic agents that are metabolized to a significant degree) in patients taking isoniazid or other drugs that contain the hydrazine moiety.

ROLE OF OBESITY

Unusually high serum F^- concentrations have been reported in morbidly obese patients exposed to enflurane anesthesia. Cousins et al. (43) reported a peak serum F^- concentration of 52 μM after 5 hours of exposure to enflurane in an obese patient weighing 130 kg. They attributed this concentration, which was about twice that expected, either to individual variation in enflurane metabolism or to prolonged postoperative release and metabolism of enflurane due to the patient's unusually large storage capacity for fat-soluble drugs. Bentley et al. (49) measured peak serum F^- concentrations and the rate of rise in serum F^- concentration in 24 morbidly obese and 7 nonobese patients (127.6 $\pm$ 6.0 vs 67.3 $\pm$ 1.2 kg) receiving enflurane anesthesia. Peak serum F^- concentrations in obese patients were higher (28.0 ± 1.9 vs 17.3 ± 1.3 μM) when compared with the control group. Twenty-four hours after anesthesia, F^- concentrations remained significantly higher in the obese patients (18.8 ± 2.3 vs 10.7 ± 3.1 μM). There was a linear increase in serum F^- concentration with time in both groups, but the rate of rise in obese patients was more than twice that in nonobese counterparts. Whether subclinical renal dysfunction occurred was not determined. However, peak serum F^- concentrations and the duration of elevated F^- concentrations were similar to those reported to cause impairment of the urine-concentrating mechanism (25).

Rice and Fish (50) investigated the nephrotoxic potential of prolonged anesthesia with enflurane or isoflurane in obesity using an animal model and found that exposure to enflurane for 4 hours resulted in significantly elevated peak serum F^- concentrations in obese compared with nonobese animals (62 ± 11 vs 27 ± 6 μM). In the obese animals there were clinical signs of nephrotoxicity, including polyuria and decreased urea nitrogen and creatinine clearance. Exposure to isoflurane also produced significantly elevated mean peak serum F^- concentrations in obese compared with nonobese animals (27 ± 8 vs 9 ± 0.4 μM). In the obese animals receiving isoflurane, there was subclinical nephrotoxicity manifested by significantly decreased urea and creatinine clearances, but there was no polyuria. It would appear that there is potential for developing subclinical F^--induced nephrotoxicity in obese patients following even isoflurane anesthesia.

The higher mean peak serum F^- concentrations and the increased rate of rise of serum F^- concentrations seen in these animal and human studies support the premise that increased biotransformation of at least some of the volatile anesthetics occurs in markedly obese patients. There are several possible explanations for these results. There could be differences in hepatic delivery or extraction of volatile anesthetics, altered hepatic microsomal enzyme activity, or differences in F^- kinetics. Excessive adipose tissue can act as an increased depot for storage of highly fat-soluble volatile anesthetics, such as methoxyflurane, with prolonged release and hepatic delivery in the postoperative period. A recent study of the metabolism of sevoflurane in obese patients failed to demonstrate that there was any difference in peak serum F^- concentration between obese and nonobese patients exposed to sevoflurane (51). Sevoflurane has very low solubility and is rapidly eliminated from the body following anesthesia. Thus, although it is metabolized during anesthesia, the serum F^- concentration falls rapidly even in obese patients following anesthesia. In this respect, sevoflurane is very different from methoxyflurane and even enflurane. Whether F^- kinetics are different in obese patients is not known.

Increased hepatic lipid could lead to increased uptake of lipid-soluble anesthetics by the liver. Fatty infiltration of the liver occurs in more than 80% of obese patients, and increases in hepatic lipid content were seen in an animal model of obesity (52). The increased hepatic lipid content could lead to increased uptake of enflurane by the liver and, hence, to increased biotransformation. Increased anesthetic biotransformation is not limited to those agents that undergo defluorination but has been observed also in obese animals receiving halothane anesthesia (53).

In humans, important factors that affect microsomal activity include age, gender, diet, concurrent drug administration, and smoking habits. In an animal model that controlled for these factors, Rice et al. (52) studied the effect of chronic ingestion of a high-fat diet on hepatic enzyme content and activity. They found that the hepatic microsomal contents of cytochromes P450 and b_5 were not different from control animals and that the rates of hepatic microsomal defluorination of methoxyflurane, enflurane, and isoflurane were not different between dietary groups. Thus the enhanced *in vivo* anesthetic metabolism does not appear to

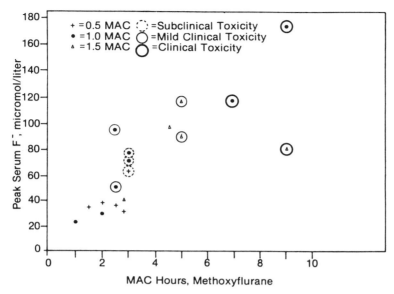

FIG. 2. Peak serum F⁻ concentration and degree of nephrotoxicity are shown at increasing doses of methoxyflurane (MAC-hours). Methoxyflurane dose correlated with both peak serum inorganic fluoride concentration and degree of nephrotoxicity. (From Cousins M J, Mazze R I. Methoxyflurane nephrotoxicity: a study of dose–response in man. *JAMA* 1973;225:1611–1616.) Copyright 1973, American Medical Association.

be the result of an increase in specific activity of anesthetic-metabolizing enzymes.

Redistribution of cardiac output with increased splanchnic blood flow is also a feature of obesity, possibly presenting a greater fraction of administered enflurane to the liver and increasing the amount of F⁻ released into the circulation. Miller et al. (54) demonstrated that in obese patients, arterial enflurane reached maximal concentrations three times faster than in nonobese patients and that the blood/gas partition coefficient for enflurane in obese patients was 30% lower than that in nonobese patients. This may explain the differences they observed in enflurane uptake between obese and nonobese patients.

RENAL THRESHOLD OF F⁻ NEPHROTOXICITY

What serum F⁻ concentration will produce renal impairment? The generally accepted and often quoted serum F⁻ concen-

tration that will reliably produce clinically apparent renal dysfunction following anesthesia is 50 μM, suggested by observations in surgical patients by Cousins and Mazze (24). They correlated the serum F⁻ concentrations seen after methoxyflurane anesthesia with the degree of postsurgical renal dysfunction (Fig. 2). Patients who received 2.0 MAC-hours[1] of methoxyflurane or less had peak serum F⁻ concentrations below 40 μM, which were not apparently associated with nephrotoxicity. The threshold of toxicity occurred at a dosage of 2.5 to 3.0 MAC-hours and occurred at peak serum F⁻ concentrations ranging from 50 to 80 μM. These patients had a delayed return to maximum preoperative urinary osmolality and

---

[1] MAC, minimum alveolar concentration of an anesthetic at steady state that inhibits movement in response to a noxious stimulus in 50% of subjects. MAC-hour, The integral of end-tidal concentration expressed as a fraction of MAC multiplied by the time of exposure. For example, an end-tidal concentration of 0.5 MAC (0.4%) of halothane maintained for 1 hour is a 0.5 MAC-hour of exposure.

unresponsiveness to antidiuretic hormone administration. Overt clinical toxicity occurred at a dosage of 5.0 MAC-hours (serum F^- concentrations ranging from 90 to 120 μM), as evidenced by serum hyperosmolality, hypernatremia, polyuria, and low urinary osmolality. Overt and serious clinical toxicity was associated with methoxyflurane dosages greater than 7.0 MAC-hours (serum F^- concentrations ranging from 80 to 175 μM). Patients demonstrated marked serum and urinary electrolyte abnormalities, daily weight loss of almost 1 kg, and significant dehydration. Urinary output was increased in all subjects and in one patient exceeded more than 9 L in 1 day.

However, there is considerable evidence from both laboratory studies in animals and clinical studies in humans that the threshold for subclinical F^--induced renal toxicity is lower than 50 μM. Whitford and Taves (12) demonstrated significant reductions of inner medullary sodium concentration and increases in urine flow rate in rats when the serum F^- concentration was only 32 μM. Roman et al. (14) measured changes in renal tubular function at serum F^- concentrations of only 18.6 $\pm$ 7.2 μM. In obese Fischer 344 rats that received 4 hours of isoflurane anesthesia, Rice and Fish (50) reported that mean peak serum F^- concentrations were 27 $\pm$ 8 μM. Polyuria was not evident, but there was a decrease in creatinine clearance of approximately 66% that was still present 72 hours after anesthesia. In these animals, there was no significant change in serum creatinine. In the same study, obese Fischer 344 rats receiving enflurane showed polyuria and a similar decrease in creatinine clearance. Again, in these animals with obvious F^- nephrotoxicity, serum creatinine did not increase significantly, and serum creatinine alone would appear to be a poor marker of acute F^- nephrotoxicity.

Evidence of subclinical nephrotoxicity has been observed in humans by Mazze et al. (25) at peak serum F^- concentrations less than 50 μM. In this study, healthy volunteers were exposed to 9.6 $\pm$ 0.1 MAC-hours of enflurane, and their response to vasopressin was examined. After this exposure, mean peak serum F^- concentrations of 33.6 $\pm$ 2.8 μM were seen 6 hours after anesthesia. Mean peak urinary osmolality was approximately 800 mOsm/kg, a 26% reduction in maximum urinary concentrating ability. By day 5, concentrating ability had returned to preanesthetic values. Other than during anesthesia, there were no changes in serum creatinine or creatinine clearance associated with this reduction in urinary concentrating ability. In another study of patients receiving isoflurane for sedation in an ICU, serum F^- concentrations rose to a mean peak of 25 μM. There were no changes in serum creatinine concentration or creatinine clearance (55). There were no changes observed in urinary osmolality, but not surprisingly in this group of patients, no vasopressin-urine-concentration tests were administered.

What is apparent is that elevations of serum F^- concentration that are considerably lower than 50 μM are associated with measurable renal dysfunction. The important distinction between methoxyflurane and the volatile anesthetics currently used clinically is that following methoxyflurane administration, F^- concentrations peak 24 to 72 hours after anesthesia is discontinued and fall only slowly thereafter. Under normal circumstances, the elevations of serum F^- concentration following anesthesia with enflurane or sevoflurane usually are not maintained for long enough to produce clinically significant renal dysfunction. Isoflurane and desflurane are even less susceptible to metabolism and less likely to produce significant amounts of F^-.

PATIENTS WITH PREEXISTING RENAL DYSFUNCTION

In patients undergoing surgery, other factors that might be expected to contribute to the development of renal insufficiency in the perioperative period include the effect of preexisting renal dysfunction, the administration of other nephrotoxic agents, and finally the superimposition of other acute renal injury, such as hypotension, hypoxemia, renal vascular spasm, or sepsis. Patients undergoing anesthesia who have preexisting renal dysfunction present a clinical dilemma to the anesthesiologist. Might even a small degree of additional renal impairment secondary to F^- exposure in such patients be clinically significant? This is an appropriate question because in the presence of reduced renal function, there is potential for impaired excretion of F^- and serum F^- concentrations after anesthesia might reach higher levels and remain elevated for longer periods of time. Also, it is possible that the nephrotoxic threshold for F^- nephrotoxicity might be lower in patients with preexisting renal impairment.

There have only been three reported occurrences of significant postoperative renal impairment in patients with preexisting renal dysfunction that could possibly be attributed to F^- from metabolism of a volatile anesthetic other than methoxyflurane. In these cases, the circumstances implicating enflurane and suggesting F^--induced nephropathy as the cause of postoperative renal failure were equivocal. Hartnett et al. (56) described the case of a 42-year-old woman with a low preoperative creatinine clearance (55 ml/min) who developed non-oliguric renal insufficiency after a 3-hour exposure to enflurane. Serum F^- concentrations were not documented. She had a period of mild intraoperative hypotension and was treated during and after operation with several potentially nephrotoxic antibiotics. Loehning and Mazze (57) reported the case of a patient in whom enflurane anesthesia may have been a factor in the deterioration of function of a transplanted kidney. In this case, renal insufficiency probably was exacerbated by inadequate perioperative fluid replacement. Peak serum F^- concentration was only 16 μM.

Eichhorn et al. (58) reported the third case, that of a patient with renal failure after a 6-hour exposure to enflurane for creation of an ileal loop urinary diversion. The postoperative course in this patient was complicated by anuria, which is not typical of F^- nephrotoxicity. Also, the serum F^- concentration measured on the second postoperative day was 96 μM, a very high concentration following enflurane anesthesia, and it did not return to normal until 2 weeks later. The anuria, the high F^- concentration, and the unusual pattern of fall of serum F^- concentrations after enflurane anesthesia make this case difficult to explain.

Carter et al. (5) studied F^- kinetics in healthy and anephric patients and in patients with poor renal function. No clinically or statistically significant differences could be demonstrated among the three groups with respect to maximum serum F^- concentration or the rate of fall of serum F^- concentrations after anesthesia. Inorganic fluoride concentrations were below 50 μM in all patients. In a subsequent animal study, Sievenpiper et al. (59) demonstrated that there were no differences in the renal response to either enflurane or halothane anesthesia in Fischer 344 rats with surgically induced chronic renal insufficiency. They reported that after the first 12 hours, serum F^- concentrations were similar in rats with normal renal function and those with chronic renal failure. Also, there was no evidence in this study of a lowered threshold for nephrotoxicity in kidneys that had preexisting dysfunction.

It is likely that following anesthesia with any of the volatile anesthetics in current clinical practice, the reduction in the ability of the kidney to excrete a normal F^- load is compensated for by uptake into the calcified tissues of the body. Hence, preexisting renal impairment does not result in significant abnormalities of F^- kinetics in patients with abnormal renal function, and renal impairment is not likely to be aggravated by F^-. In the presence of other predisposing factors or therapy with drugs known to have nephrotoxicity as a side effect of treatment, this may not be true.

CONCURRENT ADMINISTRATION OF OTHER NEPHROTOXINS

Concurrent exposure of patients to more than one nephrotoxic agent may have unexpectedly severe adverse effects on renal function. Kuzucu (60) reported a toxic interaction between tetracycline and methoxyflurane. Mazze and Cousins (61) described a patient with methoxyflurane-induced F^- nephropathy in whom postoperative administration of gentamicin led to permanent impairment of renal function. Barr et al. (62) confirmed the interaction between methoxyflurane and gentamicin in Fischer 344 rats, demonstrating that rats exposed to both gentamicin and methoxyflurane had greater renal insufficiency than rats treated with either drug alone. Several possible explanations were postulated for this interaction. A reduction in renal F^- excretion might increase both the peak serum F^- concentration and the duration of exposure to high serum F^- concentrations. Uptake into bone appears to compensate for reduced renal excretion at the lower serum F^- concentrations common after enflurane anesthesia. However, it is unlikely that this pathway can accommodate the larger F^- load that results from methoxyflurane biotransformation. Thus, an initially appropriate dose of gentamicin will become toxic as GFR is reduced due to the combined effects of the two nephrotoxins. This hypothesis may not explain the results fully. It may well be that the toxic interaction is more involved and is due to a combination of gentamicin, F^-, and oxalic acid interaction.

Is there any potential for interaction between other volatile anesthetic agents and gentamicin? Fish et al. (63) investigated the possibility that there may be interaction between enflurane and gentamicin, using the same chronic renal failure animal model employed by Sievenpiper et al. (59). In this experiment, rats with chronic renal failure were treated with gentamicin and exposed to 2 MAC-hours of enflurane or halothane anesthesia. Serum gentamicin concentrations were in the upper therapeutic range, and mild rises in serum creatinine concentration and urinary volume attributable to gentamicin therapy were observed. Peak serum F^- concentrations, 23 μM, were the same in the gentamicin-enflurane and saline-enflurane treatment groups. No interaction between gentamicin and enflurane or halothane anesthesia was demonstrable. The investigators concluded that concurrent therapy with gentamicin was not a contraindication to the use of enflurane.

One other drug that has been investigated for its potential to interact with F^- is cyclosporine A. It is a widely used immunosuppressive agent and is currently the most successful agent in prolonging homograft transplantation survival (64). Unfortunately, its use is limited by serious side effects, the most important of which is nephrotoxicity, a frequent result of treatment with adequate immunosuppressive doses of cyclosporine A. Complicating the management of cyclosporine A therapy, interactions between many different drugs and cyclosporine A have been demonstrated, leading to unexpected increases in nephrotoxicity (65–67). Fish et al. (68) investigated the potential for interaction of cyclosporine A with F^- in an animal model. This study examined the effects on renal function in male Fischer 344 rats of pretreatment with a 10-day course of cyclosporine A, followed by enflurane anesthesia. They were unable to identify any interaction between cyclosporine A and F^- produced from metabolism of enflurane. Thus, it appears that interaction between the nephrotoxicity of cyclosporine A and the low serum F^- concentrations produced from metabolism of currently used volatile anesthetic agents is not likely to occur.

DESFLURANE

Desflurane recently has been introduced into clinical practice in the United States. It has two characteristics that make it attractive to anesthesiologists. It has a blood/gas partition coefficient of 0.42, which is essentially the same as that of nitrous oxide and far less than that of other clinically available volatile anesthetic agents. This confers on desflurane the property of rapid induction and emergence from anesthesia, which may be particularly advantageous for patients having surgery as outpatients. Desflurane is also an extremely stable molecule, resistant to degradation both by soda lime and by drug-metabolizing enzymes of the body. The disadvantages of desflurane are that it has a boiling point of 23.5°C, which necessitates the use of a heated vaporizer for its safe clinical use, and it has a somewhat pungent and irritating odor.

With the combination of stability and low solubility that the desflurane molecule possesses, one would predict that biotransformation should be minimal. This is indeed the case. In healthy volunteers receiving 7.35 ± 0.81 MAC-hours of desflurane, Sutton et al. (69) were unable to measure any alterations of serum F^- concentration in these volunteers, nor was there any increase of urinary excretion of F^- or organic fluoride following anesthesia. Trifluoroacetic acid appeared in the serum of volunteers exposed to desflurane and remained elevated 6 days after anesthesia. These concentrations of trifluoroacetic acid were approximately 10-fold less than concentrations seen after exposure to isoflurane. These results in humans were consistent with results from earlier animal studies (70,71). In two human studies of hepatic and renal function in volunteers exposed to desflurane (72,73), there were no clinical or biochemical indications of hepatic or renal dysfunction.

The low concentrations of metabolites, especially the virtual absence of metabolism to F^-, would seem to indicate that desflurane is devoid of potential for producing nephrotoxicity.

SEVOFLURANE

Sevoflurane was first synthesized in the early 1970s and, in common with desflurane, has very low blood solubility. Its physical characteristics are similar to those of the other common volatile anesthetic agents. It has a boiling point of 58.5°C and, unlike desflurane, can be delivered using standard vaporization techniques. Its advantages are that with a blood/gas partition coefficient of 0.60, uptake and elimination are almost as fast as desflurane, and, therefore, it too will produce a rapid induction and emergence from anesthesia. In addition, it has a very nonirritating odor and is, therefore, particularly suited to use as an induction agent in children.

It has two major disadvantages compared to desflurane and isoflurane. First, in the presence of soda lime or Baralyme, sevoflurane undergoes significant degradation to a number of potentially toxic compounds (74), of which the most important are $CF_2{=}C(CF_3)OCH_2F$ (compound A) and $CH_3OCF_2CH(CF_3)OCH_2F$ (compound B). The rate of degradation increases as the temperature of the soda lime is raised. Neither compound has been shown to be nephrotoxic at low concentrations. At lethal concentrations (LC_{50} was calculated as 1090 ppm in male rats and 1050 ppm in female rats, with exposure for 1 hour) of compound A, however, degeneration and necrosis of renal tubules were seen histologically (74). Because these animals were exposed only to compound A or B and not to the parent compound sevoflurane, the possibility of *in vivo* interaction between compound A and F^- released from hepatic metabolism of sevoflurane could not be assessed.

Frink et al. (75) quantified the production of compounds A and B during closed circuit anesthesia in humans. After 4 hours of anesthesia, the mean peak circuit concentration of compound A was 8.2 ± 2.7 ppm when soda lime was used as the CO_2 absorbent and 20.3 ± 8.6 ppm when Baralyme was used as the CO_2 absorbent. These concentrations are low and would presumably have been even lower if the fresh gas flow rate into the circuit had been higher. There was no clinical evidence in the patients of any toxicity associated with the inhalation of these low concentrations of degradation products. There have been more than 1 million clinical anesthetics administered to patients in Japan without any evidence of toxicity related to these compounds, and there have been a number of clinical studies here in the United States with similar observations. It should be remembered that sevoflurane is not the only anesthetic to be degraded by soda lime to toxic compounds. Under similar conditions, halothane is broken down to considerably more toxic compounds (76). However, it has been suggested by Mazze that this issue has not been resolved completely (77).

The second disadvantage of sevoflurane is that it is metabolized by the liver to hexafluoroisopropanol and to F^-. Of these, F^- is probably the more important product of metabolism because hexafluoroisopropanol is rapidly conjugated to form the nontoxic glucuronide. Cook et al. (78) administered sevoflurane to Fischer 344 rats and found that urinary excretion of F^- was a third to a fourth that associated with methoxyflurane administration. However, using hepatic microsomes, they observed that sevoflurane and methoxyflurane were metabolized *in vitro* at approximately the same rate. They attributed the discrepancy between the *in vivo* and *in vitro* results to the difference in solubility between the two drugs. There were no functional renal or morphologic defects following sevoflurane administration. Comparison of data with a previous *in vivo*

study with enflurane revealed similar peak serum F^- concentrations and serum F^- concentration decay curves.

In humans, a similar picture has been observed. In all the studies reported, during clinical anesthesia, serum F^- concentrations rose rapidly and peaked at 1 to 2 hours following anesthesia. Frink et al. (79) studied 50 patients receiving sevoflurane for up to 7 MAC-hours and observed a mean peak serum F^- concentration of 29.3 μM (Fig. 3). By 8 hours, serum F^- concentration had fallen to 18 μM. However, 5 of their patients who had prolonged anesthesia with sevoflurane had peak serum F^- concentrations greater than 50 μM. This study did not evaluate discrete abnormalities in renal concentrating ability, although no abnormalities in serum electrolytes, blood urea nitrogen, or creatinine concentration occurred in any of these patients (80). Similar results were seen in a second study (81). In this study, exposure to sevoflurane was greater (13.5 ± 1.7 MAC-hours) and the mean peak serum F^- concentration was higher (42.5 ± 4.5 μM). Five of the ten patients they studied had peak serum F^- concentrations higher than 50 μM and remained above 40 μM for more than 6 hours. Twenty-four hours after anesthesia, the mean serum F^- concentrations were less than 30 μM. Biochemical data were suggestive that there were no adverse effects on the kidneys or other organs. However, again there were no studies of renal concentrating ability following anesthesia.

Until these questions have been resolved, the future of sevoflurane as a clinically useful agent remains unclear. It seems likely that it could fulfill a clinical need for a rapidly acting inhalation induction agent in pediatric practice. It is also likely that it could find a role in anesthesia for patients who are having surgery on an outpatient basis, where surgical times usually are short and rapid emergence and recovery are desirable. The potential for nephrotoxicity would seem to preclude the use of sevoflurane in prolonged anesthesia.

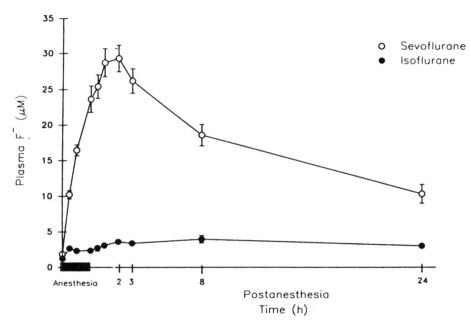

FIG. 3. Mean plasma F⁻ concentration during and after isoflurane or sevoflurane anesthesia. Data points shown are mean ± SEM. (From Frink E J, Ghantous H, Malan T P, et al. Plasma inorganic fluoride with sevoflurane anesthesia: correlation with indices of hepatic and renal function. *Anesth Analg* 1992;74:231–235.) Copyright 1992, International Anesthesia Research Society.

PROLONGED ANESTHESIA WITH ISOFLURANE

Surgical anesthesia with the inhalation anesthetics is usually of relatively short duration, and the cumulative dosage of these agents absorbed by the body is low. Thus, peak serum F⁻ concentration seen with isoflurane anesthesia is usually low, even in the obese patient (82). There have been a number of reports of the use of isoflurane for prolonged sedation in the ICU (83,84), where cumulative doses of up to 107 MAC-hours have been administered. In adults exposed to isoflurane who received a mean of 8.7 MAC-hours of isoflurane, the mean peak serum F⁻ concentration was 25.3 μM. However, one patient who received more than 30 MAC-hours of isoflurane sedation had a peak serum F⁻ concentration higher than 90 μM. It must be remembered that

these were critically ill patients in an intensive care unit and that these patients received low concentrations for long periods of time. In a study of pediatric patients who received isoflurane sedation for a mean duration of 131 MAC-hours (range 13 to 497 MAC-hours), Truog and Rice (84) found that mean peak serum F⁻ concentration was only 11 μM, and the highest F⁻ concentration was 26.1 μM after 441 MAC-hours. In contrast, in a group of adult patients having prolonged surgical anesthesia with isoflurane, Murray and Trinick (85) found that following a mean exposure of only 19.2 MAC-hours, mean peak serum F⁻ concentration was 43.2 μM. Forty percent of the patients had a peak plasma F⁻ concentration of more than 50 μM. Despite these concentrations, there were no changes in biochemical markers of renal function, nor was polyuria present.

CONCLUSIONS

The studies of methoxyflurane metabolism and the recognition of the role of its metabolite in toxicity triggered a considerable research effort into the metabolism of other anesthetic agents and the role that their metabolites might play in anesthetic toxicity. Reflecting the concern over toxicity resulting from metabolism of volatile anesthetics, isoflurane supplanted enflurane as the most popular anesthetic agent for the last 15 years in the United States. Desflurane recently was released commercially in the United States and is probably the least metabolized of any of the volatile anesthetic agents. Sevoflurane has been in clinical trials in the United States and Europe. These trials will have to resolve a number of questions regarding the toxicity of its metabolites before it is likely to receive regulatory approval. It is noteworthy that it has been released for clinical use in Japan. However, the increased awareness of the importance of anesthetic biotransformation that has resulted from the history of F^- nephrotoxicity makes it unlikely that nephrotoxicity will occur with fluorinated inhalation anesthetic agents in current clinical usage or introduced in the future.

ACKNOWLEDGMENT

The author would like to acknowledge the assistance of Dr. R. I. Mazze with the preparation of the early drafts of this manuscript.

REFERENCES

1. Armstrong, W D, Cedalia I, Singer L, Weatherel J A, Weidmann S M. Distribution of fluorides. In: *Fluorides and human health*. Geneva: WHO Monograph Series 1970;59:93–139.
2. Ericsson Y, Ulberg S. Autoradiographic investigations of the distribution of ^{18}F in mice and rats. *Acta Odontol Scand* 1958;16:362–374.
3. Carlsson C H, Armstrong W D, Singer L. Distribution and excretion of radiofluoride in the human. *Proc Soc Exp Biol Med* 1960;104:235–239.
4. Hosking D J, Chamberlain M J. Studies in man with ^{18}F. *Clin Sci* 1972;42:153–161.
5. Carter R, Heerdt M, Acchiardo S. Fluoride kinetics after enflurane anesthesia in healthy and anephric patients and in patients with poor renal function. *Clin Pharmacol Ther* 1976;20:565–570.
6. Whitford G M, Pashley D H, Stringer G I. Fluoride renal clearance: a pH-dependent event. *Am J Physiol* 1976;230:527–532.
7. Caruso S F, Maynard E A, DiStefano V. Pharmacology of sodium fluoride. In: Smith F, ed. *Handbook of experimental pharmacology*, vol XX, Part 2. New York: Springer-Verlag, 1970: 144–165.
8. McIvor M E. Acute fluoride toxicity: pathophysiology and management. *Drug Safety* 1990; 5:79–85.
9. Wiseman A. Effect of inorganic fluoride on enzymes. In: Smith F, ed. *Handbook of experimental pharmacology*, vol XX, Part 2. New York: Springer-Verlag, 1970:48–97.
10. Goldemberg L. Treatement de la maladie de Basedow et de l'hyperthyroidisme par le fluor. *Presse Med* 1930;102:1751–1754.
11. Taylor J M, Scott J K, Maynard E A, Smith F A, Hodge H C. Toxic effects of fluoride on the rat kidney. *Toxicol Appl Pharmacol* 1961;3:278–289.
12. Whitford G M, Taves D R. Fluoride-induced diuresis. *Anesthesiology* 1973;39:416–427.
13. Whitford G M, Reynolds K E, Pashley D H. Acute fluoride toxicity: influence of metabolic alkalosis. *Toxicol Appl Pharmacol* 1979;50:31–39.
14. Roman R J, Carter J R, North W C, Kanker M J. Renal tubular site of action of fluoride in Fisher 344 rats. *Anesthesiology* 1977;46:260–264.
15. Wallin J D, Kaplan R A. Effect of sodium fluoride on concentrating and diluting ability in the rat. *Am J Physiol* 1977;232:F335–F340.
16. Whitford G M, Stringer G I. Duration of the fluoride-induced urinary concentrating defect in rats (39987). *Proc Soc Exp Biol Med* 1978;157: 44–49.
17. Mazze R I, Cousins M J, Kosek J C. Dose-related methoxyflurane nephrotoxicity in rats: a biochemical and pathologic correlation. *Anesthesiology* 1972;36:571–587.
18. Crandell W B, Pappas S G, Macdonald A. Nephrotoxicity associated with methoxyflurane anesthesia. *Anesthesiology* 1966;27:591–607.
19. Taves D R, Fry B W, Freeman R B, Gillies A J. Toxicity following methoxyflurane anesthesia. II. Fluoride concentrations in nephrotoxicity. *JAMA* 1970;214:91–95.
20. Mazze R I, Trudell J R, Cousins M J. Methoxyflurane metabolism and renal dysfunction. *Anesthesiology* 1971;35:247–252.
21. Mazze R I, Cousins M J, Kosek J C. Strain differences in metabolism and susceptibility to the nephrotoxic effects of methoxyflurane in rats. *J Pharmacol Exp Ther* 1973;184:481–488.
22. Peck C, Temple R, Collins J M. Understanding consequences of concurrent therapies. *JAMA* 1993;269:1550–1552.

23. Mazze R I, Hitt B A. Methoxyflurane metabolism. *Anesthesiology* 1976;44:369–371.
24. Cousins M J, Mazze R I. Methoxyflurane nephrotoxicity: a study of dose–response in man. *JAMA* 1973;225:1611–1616.
25. Mazze R I, Calverley R, Smith N. Inorganic fluoride nephrotoxicity: prolonged enflurane and halothane anesthesia in volunteers. *Anesthesiology* 1977;46:265–271.
26. Cohen P J. Effect of anesthetics on mitochondrial function. *Anesthesiology* 1973;39:153–164.
27. Fiserova-Bergerova V. Inhibitory effect of isoflurane upon oxidative metabolism of halothane. *Anesth Analg* 1984;63:399–404.
28. Fish K J, Rice S A. Halothane inhibits metabolis of enflurane in Fischer 344 rats. *Anesthesiology* 1983;59:417–420.
29. Fish K J, Rice S A, Weissman D B. Halothane inhibits metabolism of enflurane in surgical patients. *Anesthesiology* 1984;61:A268.
30. Fish K J, Rice S A, Margary J. Contrasting effects of etomidate and propylene glycol upon enflurane metabolism and adrenal steroidogenesis in Fischer 344 rats. *Anesthesiology* 1988;68:189–193.
31. Oikkonen M P. Isoflurane inhibits enflurane metabolism in man. *Anaesthesia* 1989;44:763–764.
32. Aune J, Bessesen A, Olsen H, Morland J. Acute effects of halothane and enflurane on drug metabolism and protein synthesis in isolated rat hepatocytes. *Acta Pharmacol Toxicol* 1983;53:363–368.
33. Hanna A N, McDonald J S, Miller C H, Couri D. Pretreatment with paracetamol inhibits metabolism of enflurane in rats. *Br J Anaesth* 1989;62:429–433.
34. Brown B R, Sagalyn A M. Hepatic microsomal enzyme induction by inhalation anesthetics: mechanism in the rat. *Anesthesiology* 1974;40:152–161.
35. Berman M L, Green O C, Calverley R K, Smith N T, Eger E I. Enzyme induction by enflurane in man. *Anesthesiology* 1976;44:496–500.
36. Mazze R I, Hitt B A, Cousins M J. Effect of enzyme induction with phenobarbital on the *in vivo* and *in vitro* defluorination of isoflurane and methoxyflurane. *J Pharmacol Exp Ther* 1974;190:523–529.
37. Greenstein L R, Hitt B A, Mazze R I. Metabolism *in vitro* of enflurane, isoflurane and methoxyflurane. *Anesthesiology* 1975;42:420–424.
38. Cook T L, Beppu W J, Hitt B A, Kosek J C, Mazze R I. A comparison of renal effects and metabolism of sevoflurane and methoxyflurane in enzyme-induced rats. *Anesth Analg* 1975;54:829–834.
39. Barr G A, Cousins M J, Mazze R I, Hitt B A, Kosek J C. A comparison of the renal effects and metabolism of enflurane and methoxyflurane in Fischer rats. *J Pharmacol Exp Ther* 1974;188:257–264.
40. Churchill D, Yacoub J M, Symes A, Gault M H. Toxic nephropathy after low-dose methoxyflurane anesthesia: drug interaction with secobarbital. *Can Med Assoc J* 1976;114:326–329.
41. Maduska A L. Serum inorganic fluoride levels in patients receiving enflurane anesthesia. *Anesth Analg* 1974;53:351–353.
42. Dooley J R, Mazze R I, Rice S A, Borel J D. Is enflurane defluorination inducible in man? *Anesthesiology* 1979;50:213–217.
43. Cousins M J, Greenstein L R, Hitt B A, Mazze R I. Metabolism and renal effects of enflurane in man. *Anesthesiology* 1976;44:44–53.
44. Rice S A, Talcott R E. Effects of isoniazid treatment on selected hepatic mixed function oxidases. *Drug Metab Disp* 1979;7:260–262.
45. Fish M P, Rice S A. Effects of isoniazid metabolites on the rate of hepatic microsomal defluorination of volatile fluorinated ether anesthetics. In: Coon M J, Conney A H, Westabrook R, eds. *Microsomes, drug oxidations and chemical carcinogenesis.* New York: Academic Press, 1980;2:885–888.
46. Hoffman J, Konopka K, Buckhorn C, Koop R, Waskell L. Ethanol-inducible cytochrome P450 in rabbits metabolizes enflurane. *Br J Anaesth* 1989;63:103–108.
47. Mazze R I, Woodruff R E, Heerdt M E. Isoniazid-induced enflurane defluorination in humans. *Anesthesiology* 1982;57:5–8.
48. Gauntlett I S, Koblin D D, Fahey M R, et al. Metabolism of isoflurane in patients receiving isoniazid. *Anesth Analg* 1989;69:245–249.
49. Bentley J B, Vaughan R W, Miller M S, Calkins JM, Gandolfi AJ. Serum inorganic fluoride levels in obese patients during and after enflurane exposure. *Anesth Analg* 1979;58:409–412.
50. Rice S A, Fish K J. Anesthetic metabolism and renal function in obese and nonobese Fischer 344 rats following enflurane or isoflurane anesthesia. *Anesthesiology* 1986;65:28–34.
51. Frink E J, Malan T P, Brown E A, Morgan S E, Brown B R. Plasma inorganic fluoride levels with sevoflurane anesthesia in morbidly obese and nonobese patients. *Anesth Analg* 1993;76:1333–1337.
52. Rice S A, Fish K J, Hoover-Plow J, Jawaharlal K. *In vitro* hepatic drug and anesthetic metabolism of rats with dietary-induced obesity. *Arch Int Pharmacodyna Ther* 1989;299:286–293.
53. Bierman J S, Rice S A, Fish K J, Serra M T. Metabolism of halothane in obese Fischer 344 rats. *Anesthesiology* 1989;71:431–437.
54. Miller M S, Gandolfi A J, Vaughan R W, Bentley J B. Disposition of enflurane in obese patients. *J Pharmacol Exp Ther* 1980;215:292–296.
55. Spencer E M, Willats S M, Prys-Roberts C. Plasma inorganic fluoride concentrations during and after prolonged isoflurane sedation: effect on renal function. *Anesth Analg* 1991;73:731–737.
56. Hartnett M N, Lane W, Bennett W M. Nonoliguric renal failure and enflurane. *Ann Intern Med* 1974;81:560.
57. Loehning R, Mazze R I. Possible nephrotoxicity from enflurane in a patient with severe renal disease. *Anesthesiology* 1974;40:203–205.
58. Eichhorn J H, Hedley-Whyte J, Steinman T I, Kaufmann J M, Laasberg L H. Renal failure following enflurane anesthesia. *Anesthesiology* 1976;45:557–560.

59. Sievenpiper T S, Rice S A, McClendon F, Kosek J C, Mazze R I. Renal effects of enflurane anesthesia in Fischer 344 rats with pre-existing renal insufficiency. *J Pharmacol Exp Ther* 1979; 211:36–41.

60. Kuzucu E Y. Methoxyflurane, tetracycline, and renal failure. *JAMA* 1970;211:1162–1164.

61. Mazze R I, Cousins M J. Combined nephrotoxicity of gentamicin and methoxyflurane anesthesia in man. *Br J Anaesth* 1973;45:394–398.

62. Barr G A, Mazze R I, Cousins M J, Kosek J C. An animal model for combined methoxyflurane and gentamicin nephrotoxicity. *Br J Anaesth* 1973;45:306–312.

63. Fish K J, Sievenpiper T J, Rice S A, Wharton R S, Mazze R I. Renal function in Fischer 344 rats with chronic renal impairment after administration of enflurane and gentamicin. *Anesthesiology* 1980;53:481–488.

64. Kahan B. Cyclosporine. *N Engl J Med* 1989; 321:1725–1738.

65. Murray B M, Edwards L, Morse G D, Kohli R R, Venuto R C. Clinically important interaction of cyclosporine and erythromycin. *Transplantation* 1987;43:602–604.

66. Daneshmend T K. Ketoconazole–cyclosporine interaction. *Lancet* 1982;2:1342–1343.

67. Whiting P H, Simpson J G. The enhancement of cyclosporine A-induced nephrotoxicity by gentamicin. *Biochem Pharmacol* 1983;82:2025–2028.

68. Fish K J, Rice S A, Peterson K L. Renal function following cyclosporine and enflurane. *Anesthesiology* 1990;73:A361.

69. Sutton T S, Koblin D D, Gruenke L D, et al. Fluoride metabolites after prolonged exposure of volunteers and patients to desflurane. *Anesth Analg* 1991;73:180–185.

70. Koblin D D, Eger E I, Johnson B H, et al. I-653 resists degradation in rats. *Anesth Analg* 1988; 67:534–538.

71. Koblin D D, Weiskopf R B, Holmes M A, et al. Metabolism of I-653 and isoflurane in swine. *Anesth Analg* 1989;68:147–149.

72. Jones R M, Koblin D D, Cashman J N, Eger E I, Johnson B H, Damask M C. Biotransformation and hepatorenal function in volunteers after exposure to desflurane. *Br J Anesth* 1990; 64:482–487.

73. Weiskopf R B, Eger E I, Ionescu P, et al. Desflurane does not produce hepatic or renal injury in human volunteers. *Anesth Analg* 1992;74: 570–574.

74. Morio M M, Fujii K, Satoh N, et al. Reaction of sevoflurane and its degradation products with soda lime: toxicity of the byproducts. *Anesthesiology* 1992;77:1155–1164.

75. Frink E J, Malan T P, Morgan S E, Brown E A, Malcomson M, Brown B R. Quantification of the degradation products of sevoflurane in two CO_2 absorbants during low-flow anesthesia in surgical patients. *Anesthesiology* 1992;77:1064–1069.

76. Brown B R, Frink E J. Whatever happened to sevoflurane? *Can J Anaesth* 1992;39:207–209.

77. Mazze R I. The safety of sevoflurane in humans. *Anesthesiology* 1992;77:1062–1063.

78. Cook T L, Beppu W J, Hitt B A, Kosek J C, Mazze R I. Renal effects and metabolism of sevoflurane in Fischer 344 rats: an *in vivo* and *in vitro* comparison with methoxyflurane. *Anesthesiology* 1975;43:70–77.

79. Frink E J, Ghantous H, Malan T P, et al. Plasma inorganic fluoride with sevoflurane anesthesia: correlation with indices of hepatic and renal function. *Anesth Analg* 1992;74:231–235.

80. Frink E J, Malan T P, Atlas M, Dominguez L M, DiNardo J A, Brown B R. Clinical comparison of sevoflurane and isoflurane in healthy patients. *Anesth Analg* 1992;74:241–245.

81. Kobayashi Y, Ochiai R, Takeda J, Sekiguchi H, Fukushima K. Serum and urinary inorganic fluoride concentrations after prolonged inhalation of sevoflurane in humans. *Anesth Analg* 1992;74:753–757.

82. Strube P J, Hulands G H, Halsey M J. Serum fluoride levels in morbidly obese patients: enflurane compared with isoflurane. *Anaesthesia* 1988;42:685–689.

83. Arnold J H, Truog R D, Rice S A. Prolonged administration of isoflurane to pediatric patients during mechanical ventilation. *Anesth Analg* 1993;76:520–526.

84. Truog R D, Rice S A. Inorganic fluoride and prolonged isoflurane anesthesia in the intensive care unit. *Anesth Analg* 1989;69:843–845.

85. Murray J M, Trinick T R. Plasma fluoride concentrations during and after prolonged anesthesia: a comparison of halothane and isoflurane. *Anesth Analg* 1992;74:236–240.

Anesthetic Toxicity, edited by
Susan A. Rice and Kevin J. Fish.
Raven Press, Ltd., New York © 1994.

7

Toxicity of Local Anesthetic Agents

Hal S. Feldman

*Department of Anesthesia Research Laboratories, Brigham and Women's Hospital,
Harvard Medical School, Boston, Massachusetts 02115*

This chapter examines the toxicity associated with the use of local anesthetic agents. Some historical background on the development of local anesthetics and their toxicity is provided, with particular attention to the early use of cocaine and its associated toxicity and addiction liability. In order to understand the systemic toxicity of this class of drug, information on the various factors that influence its toxic action are discussed. Systemic toxic reaction involving the central nervous system (CNS) and cardiovascular system (CVS) are addressed, as well as local neurotoxicity and allergic reactions. A discussion of prevention and treatment of systemic toxic reaction involving local anesthetic agents is provided.

HISTORY

Early History

Around 1553, Francisco Pizarro found the Incas chewing the leaves of the coca plant (in combination with lime or ash) as a stimulant. Additionally, it was noted that during the surgical procedure of trephination, the surgeon would allow saliva containing the extract from the chewed coca leaves to drip on the surgical incision, producing local anesthesia (1). In 1848, James Young Simpson published some of the results of his experiments on the topical application of several different liquids. Unfortunately, his studies were not successful, but his concept of local anesthesia and its importance was explicit: "if we could by any means endure a local anesthesia without that temporary absence of consciousness, which is found in the state of general anesthesia, many would regard it as a still greater improvement in this branch of practice" (2). In 1858, Benjamin Ward Richardson published his studies using an apparatus that sprayed ether topically and froze the peripheral nerves by evaporation (2).

Introduction of Cocaine

The use of leaves from the coca plant (*Erythroxylon coca*) by the native Indians of the South American Andes was known since the time of the Spanish conquest of that area. Very little scientific research was performed relative to this plant, partly because the leaves decomposed considerably on the long journey back to Europe (3). In 1857, Mantegazza was the first to describe in some detail its systemic effects and "declared coca leaves to be a new and exciting weapon against disease" (1). In 1860, a purified substance was isolated from the coca leaf that produced numbness of the tongue and was termed *cocaine* (2).

Over the next 20 years, several other reports of the pharmacologic properties of cocaine appeared in the literature. In 1868, the first report of cocaine-induced seizures in animals was cited by Moreno y Maiz. Maiz also reported cutaneous anesthesia and queried as to whether this agent could be used as a local anesthetic (4). In 1874, Bennett reported seizures and respiratory arrest as well as local anesthetic properties in animals and numbness of the tongue (5). In 1880, von Anrep published an extensive evaluation of the pharmacology of cocaine, including its toxicity and ability to numb the skin if applied subcutaneously. Von Anrep concluded that the drug possessed qualities that would make it medically important (3). In 1855, Alexander Wood was the first to present the concept of blocking a nerve by the direct application of a drug (2).

Sigmund Freud was intrigued by the reports of cocaine and in 1884 published his extensive review of the drug, "Über Coca" (6). Freud and Karl Koller began work on the systemic effects of cocaine. Koller, an intern in opthalmology, was determined to find an agent that could be used as a local anesthetic in the eye. He was familiar with the ability of cocaine to produce local anesthesia but did not make the important connection between its effects and his search for some time. He did finally realize cocaine's potential and performed experiments on animals, on his colleagues, and on himself. On September 11, 1884, he performed an operation for glaucoma using cocaine as a topical anesthetic (7). The news of Koller's success reached the United States, and by the end of November 1884, a report appeared in US literature of over 150 successful cases of corneal and conjunctival anesthesia (8).

In 1884, Hall reported his results of successfully blocking his own ulnar nerve with cocaine and the success of his colleague, Halstead, in removing a small cystic tumor after injecting cocaine locally and into the supraorbital notch. Hall also reported that Nash, a dental surgeon, operated on his upper incisor tooth after injecting cocaine into the infraorbital nerve (9). The procedure

was painless, and the introduction of cocaine local anesthesia in dentistry had been made. This was done at some cost, as Halstead and Hall had become addicted to cocaine as a result of their experiments (7).

In 1885, Corning reported the results of what he termed spinal anesthesia. Using cocaine, he injected a dog between the vertebral spinous processes, which resulted in anesthesia and paralysis of the hind limbs. He then repeated the procedure in a patient (10). Before long, the use of cocaine in medicine was widespread, and there soon appeared reports of toxic reactions associated with its use. In 1891, Mattison published his work entitled "Cocaine Poisoning" (11), citing more than 125 cases of toxic reactions to cocaine, including 7 deaths. In 1919, Eggleston and Hatcher presented experimental data on acute toxic reactions as well as recommendations for the prevention and treatment of such reactions (12).

Cocaine had certain drawbacks. Particularly, its propensity to cause addiction and its acute systemic toxicity made it less desirable than originally thought. The search for a synthetic substitute was undertaken by Einhorn. Early efforts resulted in a series of synthetics that were of little use clinically (13). Around 1905, however, the group produced procaine (an ester-type agent like cocaine). Dibucaine (the first clinically successful amide type local anesthetic) was synthesized in 1929, and in 1931, tetracaine (another ester-type agent) was synthesized. In 1948, Löfgren reported his success in synthesizing and testing lidocaine (14), perhaps the most extensively used clinical local anesthetic agent in history. There followed a period of chemical synthesis that produced hundreds of agents, most of which had little clinical use. Several, however, remain in clinical use today: chloroprocaine (1955), mepivacaine (1957), prilocaine (1960), bupivacaine (1963), etidocaine (1972), and recently, ropivacaine (which began clinical trials late in 1984) (15,16).

The early use of cocaine and the development of local or regional anesthesia was a huge step forward for the practice of medicine. As seemingly safer agents were introduced and techniques were refined, reporting of adverse events became less frequent. It is unclear whether it was because of a reduced incidence or a desire for anonymity in relation to such events (17).

Toxicity of Local Anesthetic Agents

Local anesthetic agents are potentially toxic if sufficiently high doses are given or if they are administered into the incorrect anatomic site. Their mechanism of action is by blocking impulse conduction in nerves. Similar effects are seen in other organs that are impulse conductors, for example, the heart and brain. They can have profound effects on the central CNS and the CVS. The most frequent clinical toxic reaction to local anesthetics involves the CNS. Early signs of CNS irritation may be followed by overt seizures, respiratory arrest and myocardial depression, and even death.

The synthetic local anesthetics solved the addiction problem associated with cocaine and also provided a wider range of clinical usefulness in duration of action and potency. Toxicity, however, remained a problem. In 1970, Löfström accurately noted that fatal cases had been reported from every country where local anesthetic techniques were practiced. Many could be explained by massive overdoses, but some were in conjunction with small doses, as in the practice of dentistry. His review of clinical and experimental reports of the 1960s led him to suggest that the whole concept of toxicity of local anesthetics should be reexamined (18). The preclinical requirements of governmental regulatory agencies at that time were not as stringent as they are today. Thus, the pharmacologic and toxicologic data on these compounds may have been lacking in certain areas. The last decade has witnessed vast changes in the manner in which preclinical testing of new local anesthetic agents is conducted and presented. Additionally, more detailed research has been conducted on several of the older agents that were already in clinical use.

Recent History: Bupivacaine and Etidocaine

In 1977, Edde and Deutsch presented a clinical report of cardiac arrest following the injection of 100 mg bupivacaine for interscalene brachial plexus block (19). This was followed by a report of cardiac arrest after the injection of 250 mg of etidocaine for caudal anesthesia (20). In 1979, Albright published his editorial that detailed several cases of cardiovascular consequences, including ventricular arrhythmias, cardiovascular collapse, and death (21). Albright implied a relationship between these toxic events and the long-acting, highly lipid-soluble, highly protein-bound agents, bupivacaine and etidocaine. Subsequently, Heath (22) and Rosenberg et al. (23) presented clinical reports of toxic reactions and fatalities associated with the use of bupivacaine for i.v. regional anesthesia (Bier blocks).

In 1983, a special meeting of the United States Food and Drug Commission, Anesthetic and Life Support Drugs Advisory Committee examined these issues (24). At this meeting, Albright presented 49 cases of cardiac arrest involving bupivacaine, of which there were 21 deaths (43%). Of the 21 deaths associated with bupivacaine, 16 were obstetric cases (76%). Albright later reported 52 deaths following bupivacaine administration (25). Of these, there were 31 maternal deaths (60%), and 5 were infants (9%). Subsequently, the FDA recommended that 0.75% bupivacaine should not be employed in obstetric use and declared its use in i.v. regional anesthesia contraindicated.

In 1985, there were no reports of severe local anesthetic-related cardiotoxicity (25). This apparently amazing reduction in the incidence of cardiotoxicity was not due solely to the restrictions and recommendation of the FDA. The importance of the use of a test dose, often containing epinephrine to help identify an intravascular injection, was stressed (26). Administering the local anesthetic in increments and at a slower rate of injection helped to avoid massive overdoses. Equipment and medication for the rapid treatment of toxic events were kept within easy reach of the procedure areas. Perhaps most importantly, those using local anesthetics in clinical practice developed a new and well-deserved respect for these agents.

The occurrence of sudden cardiovascular collapse, ventricular arrhythmias, difficult resuscitation, and death associated with doses that were considered clinically acceptable was still unexplained. It appeared that bupivacaine and possibly etidocaine are different from the other clinically used agents with respect to cardiotoxicity.

Factors Influencing Local Anesthetic Toxicity

Local anesthetic toxicity generally results when blood levels of drug reach sufficiently high concentrations that toxic reactions take place. This can occur as a result of accidental i.v. injection during a regional anesthetic procedure if excessive doses are used or if drug is administered into the incorrect anatomic site.

Local anesthetic toxicity is the result of a complex interaction of several factors. The rate and route of administration, preexisting medical conditions, pregnancy, acid-base balance, age, weight, and other physical and medical factors can influence the toxicity of local anesthetic agents. Physicochemical properties, such as lipid solubility, pKa, rate, and route of metabolism are also contributing factors.

Chemical Structure

Local anesthetic agents in current clinical use fall into two structural groups, amino amides and amino esters (Fig. 1). The molecule is made up of three parts, the aromatic ring, the intermediate chain, and the amino group. Bonding between the ar-

omatic ring and the intermediate chain is with either an ester or an amide link.

The amine portion of the molecule can be a tertiary amine or secondary amine, such as in lidocaine and procaine. Within the amino amide group of anesthetics, there exists a subgroup, consisting of mepivacaine, bupivacaine, and ropivacaine, that possess a piperidine ring. Prilocaine, etidocaine, mepivacaine, bupivacaine, and ropivacaine possess an asymmetric carbon atom and, therefore, the existence of stereoisomerism. These chiral agents are supplied for clinical use in the racemic form, except ropivacaine, which is an S-isomer. Some experimental evidence indicates that specific isomers may possess different therapeutic and toxic potencies. A recent study in rats that examined the D- and L-enantiomers of bupivacaine found that the D-enantiomer was more cardiotoxic than the L-enantiomer (27). No well-controlled studies to evaluate the local anesthetic profile of the enantiomers exist, however.

Chemical structure also influences the site and rate of metabolism or degradation of these compounds. The amino ester agents are hydrolyzed rapidly by cholinesterases in the blood. As a result, toxicity associated with these agents is generally of short duration. The amino amide agents are for the most part metabolized by the liver. This process of biotransformation in humans takes a relatively longer time compared with the degradation of ester agents. Terminal elimination half-lives and mean body residence times are between 1.5 and 3 hours for these agents (28). The result is that toxic reactions caused by amino amides can be expected to last longer than those induced by amino esters.

Potency

Relative anesthetic potency of local anesthetics is based on the amount of drug necessary to produce an equivalent neural blockade. An agent that has a relative an-

AGENT	CHEMICAL STRUCTURE			MOLECULAR WEIGHT (base)	RELATIVE ANESTHETIC POTENCY	PERCENT PROTEIN BINDING	LIPID SOLUBILITY (25°C)*	pKa (25°C)*
	Aromatic	Intermediate Chain	Amine					
ESTERS Procaine	H_2N-⟨ring⟩	$COOCH_2CH_2$	$-N(C_2H_5)(C_2H_5)$	236	1	5.8	1.7	9.1
Chloro-procaine	H_2N-⟨ring, Cl⟩	$COOCH_2CH_2$	$-N(C_2H_5)(C_2H_5)$	271	1	—	9.0	9.3
Tetracaine	$H_9C_4N(H)-$⟨ring⟩	$COOCH_2CH_2$	$-N(CH_3)(CH_3)$	264	8	76	221	8.6
AMIDES Prilocaine	⟨ring, CH_3⟩	$NHCOCH(CH_3)$	$-N(H)(C_3H_7)$	220	2	55	25	8.0
Lidocaine	⟨ring, CH_3, CH_3⟩	$NHCOCH_2$	$-N(C_2H_5)(C_2H_5)$	234	2	64	43	8.2
Mepivacaine	⟨ring, CH_3, CH_3⟩	$NHCO$	⟨N-CH_3 ring⟩	246	2	78	21	7.9
Etidocaine	⟨ring, CH_3, CH_3⟩	$NHCOCH(C_2H_5)$	$-N(C_2H_5)(C_3H_7)$	276	6	94	800	8.1
Ropivacaine	⟨ring, CH_3, CH_3⟩	$NHCO$	⟨N-C_3H_7 ring⟩	274	7	95	115	8.2
Bupivacaine	⟨ring, CH_3, CH_3⟩	$NHCO$	⟨N-C_4H_9 ring⟩	288	8	96	346	8.2

FIG. 1. Chemical structure, molecular weight, and some physicochemical properties of clinically used local anesthetic agents. *Lipid solubility determined by octanol:buffer partitioning; pKa determined by spectrophotometric method. *Lipid solubility and pKa data from Strichartz G R, Sanchez V, Arthur G R, Chafetz R, Martin D. Fundamental properties of local anesthetics. II. Measured octanol:buffer partition coefficients and pKa values of clinically used drugs. *Anesth Analg* 1990;71:158–170.)

esthetic potency of 2 requires half as much drug to produce neural blockade as an agent with a potency of 1. Procaine, being the weakest local anesthetic agent in terms of local anesthetic potency, has a grade of 1. A more potent agent, e.g., bupivacaine, has a potency of 8. Other agents lie intermediate to these (Fig. 1).

A parallel relationship exists between relative anesthetic potency and systemic toxicity. In 1938, Schaumann concluded that a close relationship existed between conduction anesthesia and systemic toxicity (29), and in 1942, Beutner and Calesnick found parallel relationships between corneal anesthetic potency and convulsant effects of a series of local anesthetics (30). The amount of drug required to cause toxicity tends to parallel the local anesthetic potency. For example, the convulsive dose of procaine in cats was reported to be 33 mg/kg, and that for bupivacaine was 3.5 mg/kg (31). Other agents studied had convulsive doses that were intermediate (lidocaine 15 mg/kg, mepivacaine 17 mg/kg, and prilocaine 22 mg/kg). The agents' CNS toxicity potencies parallel their local anesthetic potencies. In a more recent study in dogs receiving i.v. bolus injections, the convulsive dose for lidocaine was about 22 mg/kg compared to 8 mg/kg for etidocaine, 5 mg/kg for bupivacaine, and 4 mg/kg for tetracaine, thus yielding a CNS toxicity ratio of 4:2:1:1, respectively, for these four agents in the dog (32). Convulsive dose data from studies using monkeys yielded similar results (33–35). Table 1 presents comparative toxicity data for several local anesthetic agents.

Parallelism also occurs when cardiovascular toxicity is considered. Studies using isolated guinea pig atria demonstrate that procaine was the least potent agent and bupivacaine the most potent in terms of negative inotropy (36). Similar correlations have been reported for cardiac depression in isolated guinea pig and rabbit hearts (37,38). Stewart et al. studied the changes in myocardial contractile force caused by i.v. injection of procaine, chloroprocaine, lidocaine, hexylcaine, cocaine, and tetracaine in dogs. The agents studied had relative toxicity ratios that paralleled their anesthetic potency (39) (Fig. 1). Another study in anesthetized, ventilated dogs showed a similar relationship for reduction in cardiac output (40). These relationships suggest that the more potent agents may produce CNS and CVS toxicity at lower doses and blood levels than less potent agents.

pKa, Lipid Solubility, and Protein Binding

The pKa of an agent is the pH at which there are equal amounts of the ionized and the nonionized form of the drug. The nonionized form of the drug penetrates the nerve and other biologic membranes more easily and is, therefore, a primary contributor to the onset of action.

Lipid solubility is an expression of the relative ability of a chemical to penetrate lipids (Fig. 1). Because nerve membranes are essentially a lipoprotein matrix, consisting of approximately 90% lipids and 10% proteins, lipid solubility is probably the primary determinant of anesthetic potency. Therefore, agents that are highly lipid soluble penetrate nerve membranes more easily than those with lower lipid solubility (41). In effect, to produce blockade of a nerve, relatively fewer molecules of a highly lipid-soluble agent are required, resulting in a lower total dose and a high relative anesthetic potency.

The possible relationship of lipid solubility and acute systemic toxicity is speculative. It is possible that the more highly lipid-soluble agents penetrate cells of the brain and heart more readily than less lipid-soluble agents. Experiments in awake dogs have shown that agents of low lipid solubility (lidocaine, mepivacaine, ropivacaine, and tetracaine) are less toxic than agents of high lipid solubility (etidocaine and bupivacaine) (32,40,42). However, no definitive correlation exists between the degree of lipid solubility and the occurrence of deaths due to ventricular fibrillation in the dog (39,43).

Protein binding is an agent's ability to bind with protein in the body, either in the blood or in the nerve or tissue membrane. Protein binding is reported to be related to duration of anesthetic blockade. Agents with high protein-binding capabilities are thought to bind strongly with receptors in the sodium channels of nerves that are primarily protein in nature. Thus, they will tend to remain longer than those that are less firmly bound, resulting in longer blockade of the nerves (44). Studies in laboratory animals have not shown a precise correlation between CNS or cardiovascular toxicity and the extent of protein binding. In general, the results indicate that agents that are highly protein bound are more toxic than agents that are less protein bound. However, bupivacaine, ropivacaine, and etidocaine are equally protein bound, and etidocaine is less toxic than ropivacaine, which is less toxic than bupivacaine (Fig. 1).

Acid-Base Balance and Oxygenation

Acid-base status and oxygenation can have profound effects on the sensitivity of the CNS to toxicity associated with local anesthetic agents. After the onset of seizures, acidosis may develop rapidly as a result of the increase in lactic acid produced secondary to increased muscle activity and increased oxygen demand. Additionally, hypoxia may occur secondary to inadequate respiration (45–48).

Changes in arterial blood pH and Pco_2 can alter the dose of local anesthetic required to produce convulsions. Studies in laboratory cats demonstrated an inverse relationship between the convulsive dose and $Paco_2$. When $Paco_2$ was elevated from about 40 mm Hg to about 90 mm Hg, the convulsant doses of procaine, mepivacaine, prilocaine, lidocaine, and bupivacaine were reduced 45% to 50% (31,49,50). A direct relationship exists for arterial pH. As the pH is lowered (as a result of an increase in Pco_2), the convulsive dose is also lowered (49).

There are several possible explanations as to why increased $Paco_2$ and decreased pH enhance local anesthetic CNS toxicity. Increases in $Paco_2$ tend to increase cerebral blood flow, thus delivering more drug per unit time to the brain (49). In addition, acidosis and hypercarbia decrease the protein-binding capability of local anesthetics and result in more unbound drug in the blood and thus available to the tissues (50,51). Increases in $Paco_2$ have been shown to cause excitability of various regions of the brain (50). A decrease in pH associated with an increase in $Paco_2$ will cause dissociation of local anesthetics, with a resulting reduction in the concentration of the base form, reducing the amount of drug that can easily pass the blood–brain barrier and raising the dose necessary to cause seizures. However, lowering of the intracellular pH would convert intracellular drug to the cationic form and thereby entrap it within the cells

of the brain or heart. The cationic form of these agents has been shown to be the active form (52). This ion trapping may result in enhanced and prolonged activity. Studies performed in monkeys with lidocaine-induced seizures show a significant prolongation of seizure activity when severe metabolic acidosis (base defict = 15.9 ± 6.8 mEq/L of blood) occurred (53).

Changes in acid-base balance also have effects on the cardiovascular toxicity of local anesthetics. Studies in sheep and pigs have demonstrated an increase in cardiac toxicity of bupivacaine in the presence of hypoxia and acidosis (54,55). Intact isolated human atria exposed to mepivacaine or acidosis show a reduction in contractility. In the presence of combined acidosis and mepivacaine, the effects were additive (56). Studies in fetal baboons subjected to asphyxia also demonstrated an increased toxicity to lidocaine (57). Studies in spontaneously beating isolated guinea pig atria showed that hypoxia and simulated respiratory or metabolic acidosis had no exacerbating effect on lidocaine as compared with the depression seen with these agents under normal acid-base conditions and oxygenation. In contrast, the combination of acidosis and hypoxia significantly increases the depressant effects of bupivacaine on spontaneous rate and contractile force (58).

Animals tend to hyperventilate during periods of seizure activity (59–61). Studies in dogs have shown that local anesthetic-induced seizures are not accompanied by acidosis or hypoxia, but there were several instances of sudden ventricular fibrillation and death. Therefore, it appears that acidosis or hypoxia or both are not prerequisites for ventricular fibrillation. However, a recent study by Heavner et al. indicates that severe hypoxia (Pao_2 < 40 mm Hg) but not borderline moderate hypoxia (Pao_2 40 to 62 mm Hg) may increase the likelihood that bupivacaine will induce arrhythmias before seizures (62).

TABLE 1. The intravenous convulsive and lethal dose with blood concentrations of several local anesthetic agents in various unanesthetized animal species and humans

Drug	Relative anesthetic potency	Species	Route[a]	Toxicity[b]	Dose (mg/kg)	Concentration[c] (µg/ml)	Reference
Procaine	1	Human	i.v.-inf	MTD	19.2 ± 1.7	—	17
			i.v.	CD	22.8	38.3(w)	103
		Mouse	i.v.-inf	LD$_{50}$	58.6 ± 5.4	—	176
			i.v.	LD$_{50}$	57.0 ± 1.0		177
			i.v.	LD$_{50}$	52 ± 1.7		178
Chloroprocaine	2	Human	i.v.-inf	MTD	22.8 ± 1.3	—	17
Prilocaine	2	Monkey	i.v.-inf	CD	18.1 ± 3.2	20.5 ± 5.2(p)	33
Cocaine		Mouse	i.v.	LD$_{50}$	19.0 ± 1.0	—	178
Lidocaine	2	Human	i.v.	CD	7.33	—	103
		Monkey	i.v.-inf	MTD	6.4 ± 0.5	5.3 ± 0.6(p)	17
			i.v.-inf	CD	19.3 ± 3.5	13.7 ± 0.6(p)	79
			i.v.-inf	CD	22.7 ± 2.8	26.1 ± 1.8(p)	34
			i.v.-inf	CD	22.5 ± 4.4	18.2 ± 1.5(p)	35
			i.v.-inf	CD	14.2 ± 3.2	24.5 ± 4.5(p)	33
			i.v.-bolus	CD	15.1 ± 1.5		79
			i.v.-inf	CD	13.8 ± 3.0	24.5 ± 4.5(p)	53
		Dog	i.v.-bolus	CD	20.8 ± 4.0	47.2 ± 5.4(p)	42
			i.v.-inf	CD	11.0 ± 1.0		179
		Cat	i.v.-bolus	CD	10–12.5		111
	2	Sheep	i.v.-bolus	CD	≈2.4	40(w)	181
			i.v.-inf	CD	5.6 ± 0.9	17(w)	120
			i.v.-inf	CD	5.8 ± 1.8	11.7 ± 2.0(w)	71
			i.v.-inf	CD	6.8 ± 0.8	54 ± 19(w)	180
			i.v.-inf	LD	30.8 ± 5.8		180
			i.v.-inf	LD	36.7 ± 3.3	41.2 ± 6.7(w)	71
		Rabbit	i.v.-bolus	CD	5–6		111
		Mouse	i.v.	LD$_{50}$	25.6 ± 1.0		176
			i.v.	LD$_{50}$	20.0 ± 2.0		178
			i.v.	LD$_{50}$	23.0 ± 2.0		177
			i.v.-inf	LD$_{50}$	30.3 ± 1.7		176
Mepivacaine	2	Human	i.v.-inf	MTD	9.8 ± 0.5		96
		Monkey	i.v.-inf	CD	18.8 ± 6.3	22.4 ± 4.2(p)	33
		Dog	i.v.-bolus	CD	13.0 ± 1.2		180
		Sheep	i.v.-inf	CD	7.5 ± 1.0	17.4 ± 1.7(p)	70
			i.v.-inf	LD	51.7 ± 5.3	41.6 ± 2.4(p)	70
		Rabbit	i.v.	LD$_{50}$	22 ± 2		177
			i.v.	LD$_{50}$	27.8 ± 1.0		176
		Guinea pig	i.v.	LD$_{50}$	20.0 ± 1.4		177

Drug	No.	Species	Route	Measure	Value	Conc.	Ref.
	2	Mouse	i.v.	LD$_{50}$	32.0 ± 2.0		177
			i.v.-inf	LD$_{50}$	40.3 ± 3.2		176
			i.v.	LD$_{50}$	40		97
Etidocaine	6	Human	i.v.-inf (20/mg/min)	MTD	≈2.3	2.27 ± 0.2(p)	77
			i.v.-inf (10/mg/min)	MTD	≈3.4		77
		Monkey	i.v.-bolus	CD	3.0 ± 0.5	3.8 ± 0.5(p)	79
			i.v.-inf	CD	5.3 ± 1.3	4.3 ± 1.4(p)	79
			i.v.-inf	CD	5.4 ± 1.2		35
		Dog	i.v.-serial	CD	3.0–4.3	5.0(p)	98
			i.v.-bolus	CD	4.6 ± 0.4		179
			i.v.-serial	LD	≈10		98
		Sheep	i.v.-inf	CD	2.2 ± 0.2	3.0 ± 0.4(w)	94
			i.v.-inf	LD	9.4 ± 1.4	6.6 ± 0.9(w)	94
Ropivacaine	7	Human	i.v.-inf	MTD	≈1.7 ± 0.5	1.70 ± 0.5(p)	102
		Dog	i.v.-inf	CD	4.9 ± 0.5	11.4 ± 0.9(p)	42
		Sheep	i.v.-bolus	CD	1.31	20	181
			i.v.-inf	CD	3.5 ± 0.5	17.1 ± 5.9	180
			i.v.-inf	CD	6.1 ± 0.6	4.2 ± 0.5(p)	69
			i.v.-inf	LD	7.3 ± 1.0		180
			i.v.-inf	LD	11.3 ± 1.1	7.3 ± 0.3(p)	69
Tetracaine	8	Human	i.v.-inf	MTD	2.5 ± 0.2		17
		Monkey	i.v.-bolus	CD	3.4 ± 0.7		79
		Dog	i.v.-bolus	CD	3.0 ± 0.0		179
		Mouse	i.v.	LD$_{50}$	7.3 ± 0.3		178
			i.v.	LD$_{50}$	8.0 ± 1.0		180
Bupivacaine	8	Human	i.v.-inf	MTD	≈1.4 ± 0.4	1.2 ± 0.4(p)	102
			i.v.-inf	MTD	≈1.6	2.2 ± 0.5(p)	77
		Monkey	i.v.-inf	CD	4.3 ± 0.8	5.5 ± 1.8(p)	34
			i.v.-inf	CD	4.4 ± 1.2	4.5 ± 1.7(p)	35
		Dog	i.v.-inf	CD	4.3 ± 0.4	18 ± 2.7	42
			i.v.-bolus	CD	3.4 ± 0.4		179
		Pig	i.v.-inf	LD	8.4 ± 1.2	25.7 ± 4.5(p)	84
		Sheep	i.v.-bolus	CD	1.0	14(w)	181
			i.v.-inf	CD	1.4 ± 0.1	11(w)	120
			i.v.-inf	CD	1.6 ± 0.2	10.1 ± 4.3(w)	180
			i.v.-inf	CD	2.7 ± 0.4	5.2 ± 0.9(p)	68
			i.v.-inf	LD	3.7 ± 1.1		180
			i.v.-inf	LD	8.9 ± 0.9	8.0 ± 0.9(p)	68
		Mouse	i.v.	LD$_{50}$	7.8 ± 0.4		182
			i.v.	LD$_{50}$	8		97

[a] i.v.-inf, intravenous infusion; i.v.-bolus, intravenous bolus; i.v., intravenous.
[b] MTD, maximum tolerated dose; CD, dose to cause convulsion; LD, dose to cause death; LD$_{50}$, dose to cause death in 50% of population.
[c] p, plasma; w, whole blood.

Preexisting Conditions

Preexisting conditions can influence the systemic toxicity of local anesthetic agents. For example, patients with impaired hepatic function may not be able to metabolize amide agents at a normal rate, resulting in elevated blood concentrations for prolonged periods of time (see section on drug interaction). During periods of local anesthetic toxicity, the ability to metabolize these agents may be of critical importance. Similarly, conditions that reduce the amount of circulating cholinesterases would reduce the ability to hydrolyze amino ester agents.

Renal failure may result in hyperkalemia, which has been shown to reduce heart rate and prolong the P-R interval of the electrocardiogram *in vitro* (63). A clinical report implicates hyperkalemia and acidosis in a patient with chronic renal failure as a major contributing factor in a toxic reaction to bupivacaine (64). Anemia may produce hypoxia of cardiac or cerebral tissue and enhance local anesthetic toxicity. Edde and Deutsch report that a patient with hyperkalemia resulting from renal failure and a hematocrit of 12% developed sudden ventricular fibrillation without preceding convulsions (19).

Several conditions involving the CVS may pose potential problems in conjunction with local anesthetics. Heart failure may result in reduced blood flow to the liver and interfere with metabolic degradation of local anesthetic agents. Conditions that involve the intracardiac conduction system, such as heart block, may be exacerbated in the presence of high concentrations of amide local anesthetic (65). There is some evidence that prior myocardial damage, such as infarction, may exacerbate local anesthetic cardiotoxicity (43,66,67).

The effects of pregnancy on local anesthetic toxicity have been examined in several studies in sheep. Morishima et al. (68) and Santos et al. (69) demonstrated that pregnant ewes were more susceptible to the toxic effect of bupivacaine than were nonpregnant ewes. In contrast, they also showed that no difference existed in the systemic toxicity of lidocaine, mepivacaine, or ropivacaine between pregnant and nonpregnant ewes (68–70). Thus, in general, it appears that pregnancy *per se* does not alter the systemic toxicity of local anesthetic agents. Bupivacaine, however, appears to be more toxic during pregnancy than does lidocaine, mepivacaine, or ropivacaine.

Several animal studies indicate that age affects local anesthetic toxicity. Morishima et al. studied the toxicity of lidocaine in adult, newborn, and fetal sheep. The dose required to produce seizures was 5.8 ± 1.8 mg/kg in adults, 18.4 ± 2.2 in newborns, and 41.9 ± 6.0 in fetuses (71). A study in anesthetized pigs showed that 2-day-old pigs are more resistant to the toxic effects of bupivacaine than are 2-week-old and 2-month-old pigs (72). These age differences in the relative toxicity of local anesthetic agents may be due to differences in species, protein binding, metabolism, or distribution of local anesthetic. Additionally, Badgwell et al. suggest that the immaturity of the CNS and CVS in young animals may play a role in the relative resistance to local anesthetic toxicity (72).

This is not always the case. Liu et al. demonstrated that the doses of etidocaine, bupivacaine, lidocaine, and chloroprocaine at which 50% of mice convulse (CD_{50}) and 50% die (LD_{50}) were consistently lower in immature mice as compared with adults (73). Additionally, the CD_{50} and LD_{50} for etidocaine and bupivacaine in adult mice was lower than in elderly mice. In elderly mice, less lidocaine and chloroprocaine are required than in adult mice (73).

The clinical experience varies as much as the experimental animal data. McIlvaine et al. present evidence that suggests that children may have a higher threshold for bupivacaine toxicity than adults (74). McCloskey et al. present three cases of toxic reactions to bupivacaine in children occurring with continuous caudal epidural infusion (75). These clinical reports involve continuous infusion for anesthesia and analgesia and may present a scenario more related to pharmacokinetic differences that may not play an important role in the case of an accidental i.v. injection of a large amount of drug.

Technical Aspects

Technical aspects of regional anesthesia can influence systemic toxicity of local anesthetics. The site of injection will influence the rate at which drug enters the bloodstream. Direct i.v. injection will result in the most rapid and highest peak blood level of drug for a given dose and is potentially the most toxic. Injections into anatomic sites of high vascularity also will result in rapid absorption into the bloodstream. Intercostal injections produce the highest peak blood concentration of the extravascular sites (15). Injections into less vascular regions produce lower peak blood levels at a slower rate (15,76).

Local anesthetics are, in general, vasodilators, and as a result, absorption into the bloodstream after injection is enhanced. This results in shorter duration of anesthetic action and faster rise to peak blood concentrations. To counteract the intrinsic vasodilator action of local anesthetics and thus retard absorption and removal of drug from the site of action, vasoconstrictor agents often are added to the local anesthetic solution.

The rate of injection has a profound influence on systemic toxicity. Scott studied the threshold dose for CNS toxicity of etidocaine in healthy volunteers (77). When etidocaine was infused i.v. at a rate of 20 mg/minute, a mean dose of 161 mg was required for threshold CNS symptoms as compared with administration at 10 mg/minute with a mean threshold dose of 236 mg. In awake dogs, the convulsive dose administered as a bolus injection was 3.4 mg/kg for bupivacaine and 3.0 mg/kg for ropivacaine. The same doses were administered

by i.v. infusion over 15 minutes, with no seizure activity (78). Other studies in animals and humans support these findings (16,79).

The combination of two local anesthetic agents is not an uncommon clinical practice. Mixtures of either amide–amide or amide–ester local anesthetics show no evidence of synergism or antagonism (80,81). de Jong and Bonin noted that mixing increased the margin between convulsant and lethal doses (80). Mixtures containing bupivacaine appear to exhibit a greater benefit in regard to toxic reactions (80,82).

Drug Interaction

The two primary target organ systems of local anesthetic toxicity are the CNS and the CVS. Therefore, other drugs that affect these systems may interact with local anesthetic effects and result in increased susceptibility to toxicity. It has been shown that premedication with some CNS depressant agents can increase the dose of local anesthetic necessary to produce seizures. Intramuscular diazepam (0.25 mg/kg) increased the convulsive dose of lidocaine 100% in cats (83). Premedication with benzodiazepine lowered the incidence of bupivacaine-induced seizures in pigs but did not alter the dose or blood levels necessary to cause cardiovascular collapse (84). General anesthesia also has been shown to increase the dose necessary for the production of seizures by local anesthetics. However, a caveat is in order. The suppression of the CNS may eclipse the toxic signs of local anesthetic overdosage. The initial undetected signs of CNS toxicity may result in massive overdosage of local anesthetic. Under these conditions, the CVS toxicity associated with massive local anesthetic overdosage may be the first sign of toxicity observed (85).

Regional anesthesia often is employed for postoperative pain relief following thoracotomy. Patients often are treated with cardiodepressant drugs, such as β-adrenergic blockers or calcium channel blockers. These agents and others that inhibit cardiac impulse propagation may create an additive effect when combined with local anesthetic agents, in particular, bupivacaine. Increased susceptibility to bupivacaine cardiotoxicity in the presence of calcium channel blockers, β-adrenergic blockers, and cardiac glycosides has been reported in animals (86–88).

Recently, Roitman et al. presented a case report that supports these experimental findings (89). A patient pretreated with digoxin and metoprolol received an intercostal block with 100 mg bupivacaine and demonstrated bradycardia, A-V block, and asystole without CNS toxicity. The authors speculated that the combination of the three drugs, all of which slow intracardiac conduction, acted to produce cardiotoxicity at a lower bupivacaine blood concentration than would normally be expected to cause such cardiac effects. Interestingly, on a subsequent day, the patient was given another intercostal block with the same amount of bupivacaine, but with lower digoxin levels, without any adverse effects.

Another concern is the possible effect of β-blockers on clearance of local anesthetic. Propranolol reduces hepatic blood flow and inhibits the metabolism and clearance of lidocaine and bupivacaine (90). Other drugs that reduce hepatic blood flow may reduce clearance of amide local anesthetic agents. Cimetidine, an H_2 receptor antagonist, has been implicated in reducing hepatic blood flow and inhibiting hepatic enzyme activity (91). Kim and Tasch found a significant decrease in the convulsive dose of lidocaine in mice after cimetidine pretreatment but not after ranitidine (92). However, these investigators also found a significant reduction in the convulsive dose of 2-chloroprocaine with a cimetidine concentration that caused no change in the convulsive dose of lidocaine. Therefore, they concluded that the mechanism may not be wholly related to hepatic blood flow or hepatic enzyme activity.

Effects on the Central Nervous System

The CNS is the primary target organ for local anesthetic toxicity. The CVS is generally more resistant to the toxic effects of local anesthetics in animals and humans (16,17,31,33,35,49,54,69,71,72,93–103).

A general pattern of symptoms and signs of increasing CNS toxicity resulting from the i.v. administration of local anesthetics has been described by Scott (104):

1. Numbness of the tongue, or circumoral numbness. (This is not a CNS effect but a result of drug leaving the vascular space and affecting the sensory nerve endings in the extravascular space.)
2. Lightheadedness
3. Tinnitus
4. Visual disturbances
5. Slurring of speech
6. Muscular twitching
7. Irrational conversation
8. Unconsciousness
9. Grand mal convulsions
10. Coma
11. Apnea

These progressive symptoms are more related to a slow i.v. infusion than to a rapid i.v. bolus injection, when the signs and symptoms change rapidly and convulsions may be the first symptom observed (104).

It appears that local anesthetics exert a dose-dependent and blood concentration-dependent action on the CNS. First, there is a sedative or suppressive state at very low doses, followed by an excitatory state at higher doses (seizures), and finally a state of complete depression (coma) (33,35, 104,105). Although it may appear that local anesthetics are CNS stimulants, as evidenced by seizure activity, the experimental and clinical findings indicate that these effects are probably based on their CNS depressant action. At very critical, low concentrations, local anesthetics are effective anticonvulsant agents (15,106–110). The mechanism is believed to be depression of hyperexcitable cortical neurons (15). The dose and blood concentration necessary for anticonvulsant activity are very low compared to the dose necessary for seizure activity. However, some animal researchers report that animals are asleep or nonresponsive before the onset of seizures (33,35). Lightheadedness, drowsiness, and euphoria have been reported in some patients before the onset of seizures (15), and these symptoms may reflect a similar condition. Because of the availability of other, more effective anticonvulsants, local anesthetics are rarely employed in the treatment of seizures.

The convulsive action of local anesthetic agents also is believed to be related to their depressive action. Although CNS stimulation is clinically observed in the form of seizures, it is probably due to the suppression or blockade of inhibitory cortical synapses or inhibitory cortical neurons. This suppression or blockade of inhibitory pathways allows facilitatory neurons to function unopposed, leading to an increase in excitation of the CNS, finally manifested as convulsions (15). As the dose and brain concentrations continue to increase, the facilitatory pathways also become blocked, leading to a state of overall CNS depression, as evidenced by coma and flat line electroencephalograph (EEG) recordings.

Several investigators have studied the EEG changes associated with local anesthetic administration. Attempts to identify specific foci of seizure production have been inconclusive. In animals, the amygdala appears to play an important role (33,105,111). Studies have shown a dose-dependent change in EEG patterns recorded from this region. At low subconvulsive doses, Wagman et al. describe the pattern as rhythmic spindling (111). As the blood and brain concentrations increase, the EEG shows slow high-voltage cortical activity. With the occurrence of tonic/clonic convulsion, a pattern of amygdaloid spiking occurs. Bilateral ablation of the amygdala in rats prevented the development of cocaine-induced seizures (113).

In humans, however, the EEG has not consistently demonstrated the occurrence of prodromal signs. Usubiaga et al. infused healthy volunteers with procaine or lidocaine until seizures occurred (103). Low doses of both drugs caused no EEG changes even though there were clinical signs of dizziness, facial warmth, and tachycardia. Some reduction in alpha waves was reported in connection with slightly higher doses and clinical signs of sedation. Seizure activity was associated with EEG tracings consistent with seizures. A postictal state of no electrical activity also was recorded. There was no correlation between EEG and symptomatic preconvulsive signs, but the muscular contractions did correlate with EEG seizure activity (103). In healthy volunteers receiving an i.v. infusion of bupivacaine, etidocaine, or lidocaine, no specific EEG changes were noted even during severe muscle twitching (77). Munson et al. reported preconvulsive changes in the EEG of monkeys receiving lidocaine but not in those receiving infusions of prilocaine or etidocaine (33–35). The variable results reported in laboratory animal studies and the inability to predict seizures in human studies make surface EEG recordings not useful as a routine clinical procedure for predicting the onset of seizure activity.

In summary, local anesthetics are CNS depressants. At critical, low dosages, their depressant effects can be therapeutic in the prevention or abolition of certain types of seizures. At higher concentrations, the suppression of inhibitory pathways results in facilitatory pathways functioning unopposed, resulting in seizures. At very high doses, the facilitatory pathways also are blocked, resulting in complete suppression of the CNS. This condition is associated with coma and depression of respiratory and circulatory centers ultimately leading to death. Surface EEG recordings in the clinical settings are generally of little use in predicting an impending convulsion.

Effects on the Cardiovascular System

The CVS tends to be more resistant to the toxic effects of local anesthetic than does the CNS. CVS toxicity also appears to parallel local anesthetic potency.

Just as local anesthetics possess anticonvulsant activity at certain doses, they also act as antiarrhythmic agents at certain doses. The ability to block sodium channels and thereby retard or block impulse conductors is responsible for this antiarrhythmic action. Lidocaine has been used as an antiarrhythmic for three decades and is probably the most effective and widely used local anesthetic/antiarrhythmic agent (114). Procaine was used clinically before the introduction of procainamide (115). Other agents have proven effective in the treatment or prevention of a variety of experimentally induced arrhythmias (116–119).

In general, local anesthetics have a suppressant effect on the heart, reducing myocardial contractile force and prolonging or blocking intracardiac conduction. They also may be vasodilators. High doses of local anesthetics cause a reduction in heart rate and blood pressure, cardiac conduction defects, and arrhythmias, including ventricular tachycardia and fibrillation. There is, for the most part, a separation between the dose and blood concentration required to cause CNS toxicity and CVS toxicity. Studies in dogs that compared the dose to cause seizures in awake animals (32) and the dose to cause CVS collapse in anesthetized animals (40,85) indicated that lidocaine, etidocaine, tetracaine, and bupivacaine had ratios between 3.5 and 6.7. Similar relationships have been reported in sheep (71).

Sudden cardiovascular collapse, ventricular arrhythmias, ventricular fibrillation, and death have been reported in humans (19–25, 46) and laboratory animals (39,42,43,101,120–128) following the administration of some local anesthetics. The majority of these findings occurred with the potent, highly lipid-soluble, highly protein-bound agents, such as bupivacaine and etidocaine. However, other agents, such as procaine and tetracaine, also have been associated with the occurrence of ventricular fibrillation (43). Cocaine has been the causative factor in numerous reports of sudden death, ventricular fibrillation, and even myocardial infarction, mostly related to its recreational abuse (129).

Cardiac Electrophysiology and Arrhythmogenicity

Studies of local anesthetic effects on cardiac electrophysiology have been performed for many agents. The findings generally indicate a depressant effect on cellular electrophysiology and intracardiac conduction. The amount of depression and concentration of drug required vary depending on the agent but tend to parallel the potency of the local anesthetic.

Clarkson and Hondeghem demonstrated that both lidocaine and bupivacaine depress the maximal rate of rise (V_{max}) of the cardiac action potential. This depression was rate and dose dependent. Bupivacaine was approximately 15 times more depressant than lidocaine in the physiologic heart rate range (130). Recovery from bupivacaine was slower than from lidocaine. The V_{max} is indicative of the rapid inward flow of sodium through the sodium channel. It, therefore, would appear that bupivacaine is more strongly bound to the receptor site within the channel than is lidocaine.

Arlock studied lidocaine, bupivacaine, and ropivacaine in the isolated guinea pig papillary muscle (131). He reported depression of V_{max} and recovery from block that was similar to earlier reports (132). Arlock found that lidocaine was the least potent and bupivacaine the most potent, whereas ropivacaine was intermediate. These results support the fast in–slow out theory of bupivacaine blockade and binding to sodium channels as well as the fast in–fast out description for lidocaine (132), with ropivacaine being fast in–relatively fast out (131).

Studies in rabbit Purkinje fiber–ventricular muscle preparation also showed bupivacaine to be the most depressant agent, lidocaine the least, and ropivacaine intermediate. These studies also described a peculiar characteristic in relation to bupivacaine, that of electrical alternans (alternating amplitude of the action potential). The combined depressant effects of bupivacaine resulted in the conclusion that reentrant type arrhythmias are more likely in the presence of bupivacaine (133). Recently, De La Coussaye et al. demonstrated reentrant arrhythmias associated with bupivacaine in an isolated rabbit heart model (134).

The effects of local anesthetics on intracardiac conduction have been examined by several investigators. Block and Covino studied intracardiac conduction in an isolated rabbit heart preparation. They demonstrated a dose-related decrease in conduction through the intracardiac conduction system and correlated anesthetic potency and depression of intracardiac conduction. Bupivacaine, etidocaine, and tetracaine produced depressant effects at lower concentrations than did lidocaine, mepivacaine, or prilocaine (38). In the isolated rabbit heart, Pitkanen et al. found that bupivacaine was more cardiodepressant and arrhythmogenic than ropivacaine or lidocaine (135). Tanz et al. also studied lidocaine and bupivacaine in a similar preparation and reported rhythm disturbances with bupivacaine, as well as sinoatrial (SA) blockade (37). In an isolated canine cardiac preparation, Wheeler et al. reported SA blockade also and noted that bupivacaine was 15 times more potent than lidocaine (136).

In anesthetized ventilated dogs, Hotvedt et al. noted that bupivacaine increased intraatrial, atrioventricular (A-V) nodal, and His-Purkinje impulse conduction velocity (137). Similar results have been reported for cocaine in awake dogs (138). In other studies, no prolongation of P-R interval was noted after lidocaine or ropivacaine infusion, but significant prolongation was observed after bupivacaine infusion (42,126). Other laboratory studies have demonstrated prolongation of cardiac conduction with bu-

pivacaine with little or no change observed for other agents. Many of these studies indicate a dose-response relationship (39,101, 124,125,127).

The clinical reports that documented sudden, unexpected CVS collapse and death have been a primary focus for recent research investigations evaluating various local anesthetic agents for their relative arrhythmogenicity and their overall CVS toxicity. In addition, research efforts have been directed at elucidating the differential mechanisms responsible for (increased) arrhythmogenicity. The sudden development of ventricular arrhythmias, fibrillation, and cardiovascular collapse usually was associated with rapid i.v. injection of local anesthetics. At this time, experimental animal models mimicking this clinical scenario were not widely employed in the pharmacologic and toxicologic evaluation of local anesthetics. Most experimental studies were performed in anesthetized, sedated, or paralyzed animals, and the administration of drug was by slow i.v. infusion or increasing serial doses.

A number of studies mimicking the clinical situation of accidental intravascular injection of large doses of local anesthetics confirmed the clinical reports of sudden cardiovascular collapse. Of 7 awake, unsedated dogs receiving a rapid i.v. bolus injection, 2 dogs developed ventricular fibrillation at 57 and 65 seconds after the injection of 3.4 and 5.1 mg/kg bupivacaine, respectively, and died. Other animals receiving similar doses survived. Animals receiving lidocaine 11.0 to 16.5 mg/kg had no ventricular arrhythmias and all survived (124). Similar studies in awake dogs examined bupivacaine, lidocaine, and ropivacaine given as a bolus injection of twice the convulsive dose (60). Lidocaine (41.7 $\pm$ 8.0 mg/kg) was devoid of arrhythmogenicity. Bupivacaine (8.6 $\pm$ 0.7 mg/kg) showed the highest incidence of ventricular arrhythmias (83%), consisting of premature ventricular contractions, atrioventricular dissociation, ventricular tachycardia, and fibrillation, alone or in combination. Ventricular arrhythmias were seen in 2 of the 6 (33%) dogs treated with ropivacaine (9.75 ± 0.9 mg/kg).

A large amount of data subsequently appeared in the literature that clearly indicated that bupivacaine was the most toxic of the local anesthetics to the CVS. Bupivacaine's propensity to cause ventricular fibrillation, CVS collapse, and death is well illustrated in a series of pooled data from a single research laboratory (139). Figure 2 illustrates the results in dogs receiving rapid i.v. bolus injections of several local anesthetics. Bupivacaine was the only drug to cause death at the convulsive dose. At two times the convulsive dose, bupivacaine still caused the greatest percentage of deaths and the highest incidence of ventricular fibrillation, followed by etidocaine. It is clear from these combined data and data of other investigators that bupivacaine is more cardiotoxic than etidocaine, ropivacaine, lidocaine, or mepivacaine. Lethality parallels anesthetic potency for the most part.

There are at least three possible mechanisms responsible for the arrhythmias produced by local anesthetics: direct action on the CNS or specific areas of the brain, direct effects on the myocardium or the conduction system, or a combination of these effects.

Certain specific regions of the brain have been identified as sources for arrhythmia production after local anesthetic administration. Heavner injected several local anesthetic agents into the lateral cerebral ventricle of the cat (140). Bupivacaine resulted in all animals developing arrhythmias. A high percentage experienced arrhythmias with procaine (71%). Conversely, lidocaine resulted in only one of six animals developing arrhythmias. In rats receiving equimolar doses of bupivacaine or lidocaine injected into the nucleus tractus solitarius, ventricular arrhythmias were produced in about 50% of the animals. Lidocaine-induced arrhythmias spontaneously reverted to normal sinus rhythm, whereas only half of the bupivacaine-treated animals reverted back to sinus rhythm. Death occurred in the remaining rats (141).

Although the brain may play a role in local anesthetic-induced arrhythmias, it does not appear to be the sole contributing fac-

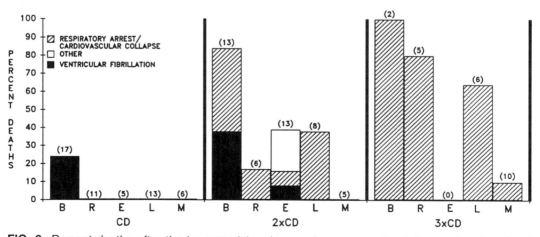

FIG. 2. Percent deaths after the i.v. convulsive dose and supraconvulsant doses of various local anesthetic agents in the unanesthetized dog. Presented are pooled data from a single research laboratory. Parenthetical numbers are sample size (*n*). B, bupivacaine; R, ropivacaine; E, etidocaine; L, lidocaine; M, mepivacaine; CD, convulsive dose; 2 × CD, 2 times the convulsive dose; 3 × CD, 3 times the convulsive dose. (From Feldman HS. The relative acute systemic toxicity of selected local anesthetic agents. ACTA Universitatis Upsaliensis Comprehensive Summaries of Uppsala Dissertations from the Faculty of Medicine, No. 226, 1989.)

tor. Several studies have shown the occurrence of ventricular arrhythmias and ventricular fibrillation in animals receiving i.v. local anesthetic agents under general anesthesia (43, 101, 125–127). In these studies, the CNS was depressed by general anesthesia and was somewhat protected from the toxic effects of high doses of local anesthetics. However, neuronal innervation and feedback mechanisms to the CVS remained functional, and the CNS could not be completely ruled out as a contributing factor in the formation of ventricular arrhythmias.

Several studies were designed to isolate cardiac tissue *in situ*. Nath et al. injected local anesthetics directly into the coronary circulation of pigs at doses not toxic if injected into the general circulation (125). Both bupivacaine and lidocaine produced ventricular arrhythmias, but bupivacaine was more cardiotoxic. Other studies using denervated hearts or completely isolated hearts have demonstrated the ability of these agents to produce arrhythmias in cardiac tissue (134, 135).

In general, the cardiac electrophysiologic effects of local anesthetics do not differ greatly, but their relative potency for toxicity does. At certain dosages, bupivacaine produces effects that are different from those of other local anesthetics. There is considerable experimental evidence to support the contention that bupivacaine exerts a strong direct effect on the myocardium. The degree to which the brain, the CNS in general, and direct myocardial effects contribute to the overall cardiotoxic profile of local anesthetic agents has not been determined.

Effects on Myocardial Contractility, Heart Rate, and Blood Pressure

The chronotropic and inotropic effects of local anesthetics have been studied extensively. Studies in anesthetized, ventilated dogs given increasing serial bolus injections of procaine, chloroprocaine, mepivacaine, lidocaine, prilocaine, etidocaine, tetracaine, and bupivacaine have clearly demonstrated that these agents are capable of causing profound depression of heart rate, cardiac output, and mean arterial pressure (40, 85). The relative cardiovascular toxicity of these agents correlated well with their relative anesthetic potencies. Death in these animals was due to progressive hypotension and cardiovascular collapse. Bupivacaine had the lowest lethal dose, followed closely by tetracaine and etidocaine. Procaine required the highest dose to cause death.

At blood concentrations in the clinically acceptable range, local anesthetics have very little effect on cardiac rate, contractility, or blood pressure (18). Studies in isolated cardiac tissues and in intact animals and humans, however, have shown negative inotropic and chronotropic effects of local anesthetics that paralleled their local anesthetic potency (36–38).

The mechanism involved in local anesthetic myocardial depression is not clearly understood. It is possible that local anesthetic agents decrease contractility in the myocardium by the blockade of sodium channels, thus inactivating or reducing activation of myocardial cells. Kuperman et al. demonstrated that procaine and tetracaine can increase calcium release from isolated skeletal muscle, and their ability to do this was proportional to their local anesthetic potency (142). This led Covino to speculate that perhaps local anesthetic agents increase the release of calcium from the myocardium and thus reduce contractility. Other studies support this or report a depression of calcium entry (143–145).

Eledjam et al. have shown that in isolated rabbit right atrium, a calcium-enriched bathing solution did not completely counteract the negative inotropic effect of bupivacaine (146). However, the combination of calcium and adenosine triphosphate significantly decreased the negative inotropic effects of bupivacaine, indicating some possible relationship to energy metabolism. More recently, De La Coussaye et al. reported that the depressant effect of bupivacaine may be due to the amount of drug that enters the myocardial cell and, further, that the action may be on the sarcoplasmic reticulum or energy metabolism or both, in addition to effects on myocardial sodium channels (147). They studied the effects of 0.5 μg/ml bupivacaine and lidocaine on rabbit right atrium. Bupivacaine caused a 68% decrease in contractility as compared to 6% with lidocaine. To enhance entry of lidocaine into the cell, a membrane-permeant lipophilic anion, tetraphenylboron, was added to the lidocaine-containing bath solution. This resulted in depression equal to that of 0.5 μg/ml bupivacaine. This implies that perhaps bupivacaine's greater negative inotropic action is related to the amount of drug entering the cell. If equal amounts of other local anesthetics were to enter the cells, a similar degree of depression could result.

Treatment of Toxicity

The best treatment for local anesthetic toxicity is prevention. Respect for the potency of the local anesthetic in use and careful attention to dosage and route of administration are required. Local anesthetics should be injected only after negative aspiration to exclude i.v. injection. A test dose should be administered slowly, with careful attention to the patient and vital signs. Sufficient time should be allowed before additional drug is administered slowly in divided doses.

The use of epinephrine (1:200,000) as an additive to the local anesthetic solutions has been advocated (26,148). This provides a marker for i.v. injections because epinephrine will cause an increase in heart rate. Additionally, it is thought that the epinephrine will help counteract myocardial depression in the event of a toxic reaction. However, this is a controversial issue, and other investigators cite epinephrine as re-

sponsible for a reduction in the dose of bupivacaine to cause cardiac arrhythmias in pigs (149). Other attempts at decreasing the possibility of toxic local anesthetic reactions have included encapsulation in liposomes. Boogaerts et al. found that significantly higher doses of liposome-encapsulated bupivacaine than of plain bupivacaine were required to cause seizure and ventricular tachycardia in the rabbit (150).

The vast majority of clinically encountered toxic reactions to local anesthetic involve the CNS. These are a result of excessive dosage, administration into the incorrect anatomic site, or some combination of factors that allow large amounts of drug into the central circulation. Cardiovascular complications are seldom encountered. When they are present, however, they pose a potentially life-threatening situation. The treatment of both CNS and CVS complications remains controversial, and no definitive regimen for treatment has been defined.

The treatment of CNS complications is directed primarily at maintaining an open airway, providing proper ventilation, and controlling seizure activity. Barbiturates may be used to prevent or arrest seizures induced by local anesthetics in animals and humans (40,42,128). Currently, the use of small doses of short-acting barbiturates, such as thiopental, has been suggested as an effective means of controlling seizures (112). Diazepam also has been used to terminate local anesthetic-induced seizures in humans (46). In laboratory cats and pigs, diazepam was effective in decreasing the incidence of CNS toxicity, although in pigs it did not alter the dose of bupivacaine required to cause CVS collapse (84). In cats, cardiac arrhythmias were fewer in diazepam-pretreated animals (151). Gregg et al. studied diazepam in bupivacaine-toxic rats and found a higher incidence of severe arrhythmias after pretreatment with diazepam (127).

The primary reason to control overt seizure activity is to facilitate ventilation and avoid hypoxemia. Eggleston and Hatcher in 1919 noted some success is preventing cocaine-induced death in cats with the use of artificial respiration and epinephrine, but they noted that artificial respiration alone was not sufficient (12). Moore and Bridenbaugh reported clinical success in terminating local anesthetic-induced seizure in 84 of 93 patients with oxygen administrated by bag and mask (152).

More complicated systemic toxic reactions involve CVS manifestations of toxicity, such as hypotension, atrioventricular block, electromechanical dissociation, ventricular tachycardia, and fibrillation. The treatment of cardiovascular complications is controversial. The use of epinephrine in the treatment of hypotension associated with local anesthetics has received much attention. Moore and Scurlock indicated that the use of epinephrine as an additive in conjunction with administration of the local anesthetic reduces the incidence of toxic manifestations (153). However, a study in pigs revealed no difference in the dose to cause cardiovascular collapse between plain and epinephrine-containing solutions of bupivacaine (149). In addition, the group receiving epinephrine experienced arrhythmias and seizures at a lower total dose of bupivacaine. Epinephrine, added to the bupivacaine solution, did not protect against CVS collapse, nor did it render animals any easier to resuscitate after collapse.

Some laboratory studies have shown success in the use of epinephrine as part of a resuscitation protocol (100,122,154), whereas others have reported little or no success (11,128). Feldman et al. used epinephrine as part of their resuscitation protocol in dogs receiving bupivacaine or ropivacaine, but with little success (128). One animal developed ventricular tachycardia and hypertension immediately after the injection of epinephrine. They suggested that another vasopressor agent with less direct cardiac effects, such as phenylephrine, may be beneficial. Recently, a study in pigs found some success with the use of amrinone, a bipyridine compound. Amrinone's action in increasing cardiac output is nonadrenergic

and may have some advantage in decreasing the possibility of inducing arrhythmias while providing some treatment for depression of contractility (155).

The treatment of ventricular arrhythmias associated with local anesthetic overdosage has been addressed experimentally. Bretylium was used successfully as part of a resuscitation protocol in bupivacaine-intoxicated sheep (156) but was found not to be of value in dogs (128). de Jong and Davis reported successful use of lidocaine in the conversion of persistent arrhythmias induced by bupivacaine in cats (157). Scalabrini et al. demonstrated significant prevention against intraventricular conduction disturbances and ventricular arrhythmias with the use of 7.5% sodium chloride pretreatment in dogs intoxicated with bupivacaine (158). Direct current cardioversion has met with mixed success in animal studies (128). There is some experimental evidence from *in vitro* studies suggesting that intracardiac pacing by means of an electrode catheter may be useful in difficult resuscitations (135). In extreme cases, the rapid use of cardiopulmonary bypass has been successful (159,160).

In summary, the treatment of systemic toxicity due to local anesthetics should be instituted rapidly and aggressively. Appropriate equipment and pharmacologic agents should be kept close at hand. Maintenance of an open airway and administration of oxygen appear important. Support of the circulation and control of arrhythmias are essential for maintaining adequate perfusion of the vital organs as well as assisting in the removal of local anesthetic from the tissue and detoxification. Persistence in the resuscitation process is essential, as some resuscitations may be difficult.

Local Neurotoxicity

Factors that may contribute to neurotoxicity include pH, additives or preservatives, and concentration of the local anesthetic agent. Virtually all clinically used agents have been associated with some type of neurologic deficit, and there does not seem to be any consistent relationship to the individual local anesthetic employed. Rosen et al. studied 2-chloroprocaine, bupivacaine, and lidocaine in clinically used concentrations in the sheep and monkey and found that none of the solutions were more neurotoxic than the others (161).

Clinically, neurotoxicity due to local anesthetics can occur after an accidental subarachnoid injection of an epidural dose of an agent. Relatively large volumes (10 to 30 ml) of anesthetic solution can be injected accidentally into the subarachnoid space. The pH of commercial preparations range between 3.13 and 6.38 (161). The cerebrospinal fluid (CSF) has poor buffering capabilities, and drugs are removed slowly from this space. The results can be prolonged sensory/motor deficit and, in some cases, permanent neurologic deficit. pH, however, has not been identified as the sole causative factor (162). The concentration of local anesthetic and the use of additives in the solutions also have been implicated as contributing factors. Some believe that this neurologic damage is a result of spinal cord ischemia either due to prolonged hypotension during surgery or as a consequence of arterial vasoconstriction resulting from the use of epinephrine in the local anesthetic solution (164). Others have implicated preservatives, such as sodium bisulfite, as the causative entity (165–167). This subject was reviewed by Kane in 1981 (168). He presented many data to support the fact that these neurologic deficits are very infrequent after epidural anesthesia.

There appears to be a relationship between concentration and neurotoxicity. Ready et al. studied the toxicity of several local anesthetic agents at varying concentrations, saline, and the preservative, sodium bisulfite, in a rabbit model (166). They found that high concentrations of lidocaine (up to 32%) and tetracaine (up to 8%) caused neural injury. The highest concentrations of bupivacaine (3.3%) and 2-chlo-roprocaine (4.0%) were not consistently associated with comparable neural damage. This study confirms early opinions (169) and Greene's statement that "histotoxicity being a function of concentration, prevention of neurological complications also includes strict limitations of the concentration of local anesthetic employed" (170).

Microbore Catheters and Neurotoxicity

Small-bore catheters for use in continuous spinal anesthesia (CSA) were introduced into clinical practice recently (171). These microbore catheters allowed a small puncture to be made in the dura for catheter insertion, reducing the incidence of postdural puncture headache from CSF leaking out of the subarachnoid space. For this reason, the new catheters were popular and rapidly came into frequent use. Within a short time, reports of cauda equina syndrome (CES) associated with the use of these small-bore catheters and CSA appeared in the literature. The cauda equina is the lower lumbar portion of the spinal cord and contains numerous small neural fibers that possibly are more susceptible to damage from ischemia, arachnoiditis (170), and local anesthetic solutions. On May 29, 1992, the FDA recalled the small-bore catheter from clinical use. The reasons given were that there are no drugs currently approved for continuous spinal anesthesia and that the microbore catheters do not seem to function in the same manner as larger-bore catheters.

Various investigators speculate that the combination of the small-bore catheter and local anesthetics is responsible for the apparent cauda equina cases associated with its use. They believe the catheter does not promote mixing of the local anesthetic in the CSF, and it is thought that high concentrations of hyperbaric solution (5% lidocaine in 7.5% dextrose) cause the solution to settle in the cauda equina and bathe it in a high concentration of drug, resulting in damage (172,173). It must be kept in mind that CES has occurred with large-bore catheters, after single injection through a needle, and with a variety of local anesthetics.

Allergic Reactions

Allergic reactions to local anesthetics are extremely rare. Amino ester local anesthetics, such as procaine, chloroprocaine, and tetracaine, are derivatives of para-aminobenzoic acid (PABA), a known allergen. Because PABA is a byproduct of the hydrolysis of amino ester local anesthetics, allergic reactions to it are more common than with the amino amide type agents that are not structurally related to PABA. Many of the reports of allergic reactions to local anesthetics were dermatologic in nature and associated with the use of amino ester agents in dentistry. Since the introduction of the amino amide agents, the incidence of allergic reactions has decreased.

Some commercial preparations of amino amide agents employ methylparaben as a preservative. Methylparaben is chemically related to PABA and also has been identified as an allergen (174). The rare occurrence of allergic reactions to amino amide agents is probably due to the preservative rather than to the amino amide local anesthetics *per se.* Aldrete and O'Higgins studied a group of patients who had some historical inclination toward allergic reactions to local anesthetics and a group with no such historical inclination (175). Both amino amide and amino ester type agents were studied, as was methylparaben. Using an intracutaneous testing technique, the investigators found no reactions to the amino amides in either patient population. Reactions to amino ester agents occurred in both groups, and methylparaben caused positive reactions in some of the nonallergic group.

In summary, allergic reactions to local anesthetic agents are extremely rare. Amino ester agents produce PABA as a metabolite,

and it is a known allergen. Methylparaben is also a known allergen, and it is used occasionally as a preservative in commercial preparations of some amino amide agents. Reactions are generally dermatologic in nature when they occur and rarely are systemic or anaphylactoid. Recommendations for screening suspect patients can be found in the literature and generally involve skin tests (174,175).

REFERENCES

1. Vandam L D. Some aspects of the history of local anesthesia. In: Strichartz G R, ed. *Local anesthetics.* New York: Springer-Verlag, 1987: 1–19.
2. Wildsmith J A W. The history and development of local anesthesia. In: Wildsmith J A W, Armitage E N, eds. *Principles and practice of regional anaesthesia.* New York: Churchill Livingstone, 1987:1–7.
3. Wildsmith J A W. Carl Koller (1857–1944) and the introduction of cocaine into anesthetic practice. *Reg Anesth* 1984;9:161–164.
4. Holmstedt B, Fredga A. Sundry episodes in the history of coca and cocaine. *J Ethnopharm* 1981;3:113–147.
5. Bennett A. The physiological action of coca. *Br Med J* 1874;1:510.
6. Freud S. Über Coca. *Zentralbl Ges Ther* 1884; 2:289–314.
7. Fink B R. History of neural blockade. In: Cousins M J, Bridenbaugh P O, eds. *Neural blockade in clinical anesthesia and management of pain.* Philadelphia: JB Lippincott Company, 1988:3–15.
8. Bull C S. The hydrochlorate of cocaine as a local anaesthetic in ophthalmic surgery. *N Y Med J* 1884;40:609–611.
9. Hall R J. Hydrochlorate of cocaine. *NY Med J* 1884;40:643–644.
10. Corning J L. Spinal anaesthesia and local medication of the cord. *NY Med J* 1885;42:483–485.
11. Mattison J B. Cocaine poisoning. *Med Surg Rep* 1891;LX:645–650.
12. Eggleston C, Hatcher R A. A further contribution to the pharmacology of the local anesthetics. *J Pharmacol Exp Ther* 1919;13:433–487.
13. Einhorn A. On the chemistry of local anesthetics. *MMW* 1889;46:1218–1220.
14. Löfgren N. Studies on local anesthetics. Xylocaine a new synthetic drug. Doctoral Dissertation, Faculty of Mathematics and Natural Sciences, University of Stockholm: Ivar Haeggströms, Stockholm, 1948.
15. Covino B G, Vassallo H G. *Local anesthetics. Mechanisms of action and clinical use.* New York: Grune & Stratton, 1976.

16. Rosenberg P H, Heinonen E. Differential sensitivity of a and c nerve fibres to long-acting amide local anaesthetics. *Br J Anaesth* 1983; 55:163–167.

17. Foldes F F, Molloy R, McNall P G, Koukal L R. Comparison of toxicity of intravenously given local anesthetic agents in man. *JAMA* 1960;172:1493–1498.

18. Löfström B. Aspects of the pharmacology of local anesthetic agents. *Br J Anaesth* 1970; 42:194–206.

19. Edde R R, Deutsch S. Cardiac arrest after interscalene brachial-plexus block. *Anesth Analg* 1977;56:446–447.

20. Prentiss J E. Cardiac arrest following caudal anesthesia. *Anesthesiology* 1979;50:51–53.

21. Albright G A. Cardiac arrest following regional anesthesia with etidocaine or bupivacaine. *Anesthesiology* 1979;51:285–287.

22. Heath M L. Deaths after intravenous regional anaesthesia. *Br Med J* 1982;285:913–914.

23. Rosenberg P H, Kalso E A, Tuominen M K, Lindén H B. Acute bupivacaine toxicity as a result of venous leakage under the tourniquet cuff during a bier block. *Anesthesiology* 1983; 58:95–98.

24. Department of Health and Human Services, Public Health Service, Food and Drug Administration. Minutes of fifth meeting, Anesthetic and Life Support Drugs Advisory Committee. Bethesda, MD, October 1983.

25. Reiz S, Nath S. Cardiotoxicity of local anaesthetic agents. *Br J Anaesth* 1986;58:736–746.

26. Moore D C, Batra M S. The components of an effective test dose prior to epidural block. *Anesthesiology* 1981;55:693–696.

27. Denson D D, Behbehani M M, Gregg R V. Enantiomer-specific effects of an intravenously administered arrhythmogenic dose of bupivacaine on neurons of the nucleus tractus solitarius and the cardiovascular system in the anesthetized rat. *Reg Anesth* 1992;17:311–316.

28. Tucker G T. Local anesthetic drugs—mode of action and pharmacokinetics. *Anaesthesia* 1989;2:983–1010.

29. Schaumann O. *Naunyn-Schmeidebergs Arch Exp Path Pharmacol* 1938;190:30.

30. Beutner R, Calesnick B. The essential characteristics of local anesthetic. *Anesthesiology* 1942;3:673–682.

31. Englesson S. The influence of acid-base changes on central nervous system toxicity of local anaesthetic agents I. *Acta Anaesth Scand* 1974;18:79–87.

32. Liu P L, Feldman H S, Giasi R, Patterson M K, Covino B G. Comparative CNS toxicity of lidocaine, etidocaine, bupivacaine and tetracaine in awake dogs following rapid intravenous administration. *Anesth Analg* 1983;62:375–379.

33. Munson E S, Gutnick M J, Wagman I H. Local anesthetic drug-induced seizures in rhesus monkeys. *Anesth Analg* 1970;49:986–997.

34. Munson E S, Martucci R W, Wagman I H. Bupivacaine and lignocaine-induced seizures in rhesus monkeys. *Br J Anaesth* 1972;44:1025–1028.

35. Munson E S, Tucker W K, Ausinsch B, Malagodi H. Etidocaine, bupivacaine, and lidocaine seizure thresholds in monkeys. *Anesthesiology* 1975;42:471–478.

36. Feldman H S, Covino B M, Sage D J. Direct chronotropic and inotropic effects of local anesthetic agents in isolated guinea pig atria. *Reg Anesth* 1982;7:149–156.

37. Tanz R D, Heskett T, Loehning R W, Fairfax C A. Comparative cardiotoxicity of bupivacaine and lidocaine in the isolated perfused mammalian heart. *Anesth Analg* 1984;63:549–556.

38. Block A, Covino B G. Effect of local anesthetic agents on cardiac conduction and contractility. *Reg Anesth* 1981;6:55–61.

39. Stewart D M, Rogers W P, Mahaffey J E, Witherspoon S, Woods E F. Effect of local anesthetics on the cardiovascular system of the dog. *Anesthesiology* 1963;24:620–624.

40. Liu P, Feldman H S, Covino B M, Giasi R, Covino B G. Acute cardiovascular toxicity of intravenous amide local anesthetics in anesthetized ventilated dogs. *Anesth Analg* 1982;61:317–322.

41. Covino B G. Pharmacology of local anaesthetic agents. *Br J Anaesth* 1986;58:701–716.

42. Feldman H S, Arthur G R, Covino B G. Comparative systemic toxicity of convulsant and supraconvulsant doses of intravenous ropivacaine, bupivacaine, and lidocaine in the conscious dog. *Anesth Analg* 1989;69:794–801.

43. Long J H, Oppenheimer M J, Wester M R, Durant T M. The effect of intravenous procaine on the heart. *Anesthesiology* 1949;10:406–415.

44. Covino B G. General considerations, toxicity and complications of local anaesthesia. *Anaesthesia* 1989;2:1011–1033.

45. Moore D C, Crawford R D, Scurlock J E. Severe hypoxia and acidosis following local anesthetic-induced convulsions. *Anesthesiology* 1980;53:259–260.

46. Davis N L, de Jong R H. Successful resuscitation following massive bupivacaine overdose. *Anesth Analg* 1982;61:62–64.

47. Mallampati S R, Liu P L, Knapp R M. Convulsions and ventricular tachycardia from bupivacaine with epinephrine: successful resuscitation. *Anesth Analg* 1984;63:856–859.

48. Moore D C, Thompson G E, Crawford R D. Long-acting local anesthetic drugs and convulsions with hypoxia and acidosis. *Anesthesiology* 1982;56:230–232.

49. Englesson S, Grevsten S. The influence of acid-base changes on central nervous system toxicity of local anaesthetic agents II. *Acta Anaesth Scand* 1974;18:88–103.

50. de Jong R H, Wagman T H, Prince D A. Effect of carbon dioxide on the cortical seizure threshold to lidocaine. *Exp Neurol* 1967;17:221–232.

51. Coyle D E, Denson D D, Thompson G A, Myers J A, Arthur G R, Bridenbaugh P O. The

influence of lactic acid on the serum protein binding of bupivacaine: species differences. *Anesthesiology* 1984;61:127–133.

52. Ritchie J M, Ritchie B, Greengard P. The active structure of local anesthetics. *J Pharmacol Exp Ther* 1965;150:152–159.
53. Munson E S, Wagman I H. Acid-base changes during lidocaine induced seizures in *Macaca mulatta. Arch Neurol* 1969;20:406–412.
54. Rosen M A, Thigpen J W, Shnider S M, Foutz S E, Levinson G, Koike M. Bupivacaine-induced cardiotoxicity in hypoxic and acidotic sheep. *Anesth Analg* 1985;64:1089–1096.
55. Heavner J E, Dryden C F, Sanghani V, Huemer G, Bessire A, Bagwell J M. Severe hypoxia enhances central nervous system and cardiovascular toxicity of bupivacaine in lightly anesthetized pigs. *Anesthesiology* 1992;77:142–147.
56. Andersson K E, Gennser G, Nilsson E. Influence of mepivacaine on isolated human foetal hearts at normal and low pH. *Acta Physiol Scand* 1970;80(suppl 353); 34–47.
57. Morishima H O, Covino B G. Toxicity and distribution of lidocaine in nonasphyxiated and asphyxiated baboon fetuses. *Anesthesiology* 1981; 54:182–186.
58. Sage D J, Feldman H S, Arthur G R, et al. Influence of lidocaine and bupivacaine on isolated guinea pig atria in the presence of acidosis and hypoxia. *Anesth Analg* 1984;63:1–7.
59. Jorfeldt L, Löfstrom B, Pernow B, Persson B, Wahren J, Widman B. The effect of local anaesthetics on the central circulation and respiration in man and dog. *Acta Anaesth Scand* 1968;12:153–169.
60. Feldman H S, Arthur G R, Covino B G. Comparative systemic toxicity of convulsant and supraconvulsant doses of intravenous ropivacaine, bupivacaine and lidocaine in the conscious dog. *Anesth Analg* 1989;69:1–8.
61. Rutten A J, Nancarrow C, Mather L E, Ilsley A H, Runciman W B, Upton R N. Hemodynamic and central nervous system effect of intravenous bolus doses of lidocaine, bupivacaine, and ropivacaine in sheep. *Anesth Analg* 1989;69:291–299.
62. Heavner J E, Dryden C F, Sanghani V, Huemer G, Bessire A, Badgwell J M. Severe hypoxia enhances central nervous system and cardiovascular toxicity of bupivacaine in lightly anesthetized pigs. *Anesthesiology* 1992;77:142–147.
63. Komai H, Rusy B F. Effects of bupivacaine and lidocaine on AV conduction in the isolated rat heart: modification by hyperkalemia. *Anesthesiology* 1981;55:281–285.
64. Gould D B, Aldrete J A. Bupivacaine cardiotoxicity in a patient with renal failure. *Acta Anaesth Scand* 1983;27:18–21.
65. Gupta P K, Lichstein E, Chadda K D. Lidocaine-induced heart block in patients with bundle branch block. *Am J Cardiol* 1974;33:487–492.
66. Widman B. Some circulatory and respiratory effects of intravenously infused local anes-
thetics. *Acta Anaesthesiol Scand* 1966;(Suppl 25):34–36.
67. Wojtczak J A, Pratilas V, Griffin R M, Kaplan J A. Cellular mechanisms of cardiac arrhythmias induced by bupivacaine. *Anesthesiology* 1984;61:A37.
68. Morishima H O, Pedersen H, Finster M, et al. Bupivacaine toxicity in pregnant and nonpregnant ewes. *Anesthesiology* 1985;63:134–139.
69. Santos A C, Arthur G R, Pedersen H, Morishima H O, Finster M, Covino B G. Systemic toxicity of ropivacaine during ovine pregnancy. *Anesthesiology* 1991;75:137–141.
70. Santos A C, Pederson H, Harmon T W, et al. Does pregnancy alter the systemic toxicity of local anesthetics? *Anesthesiology* 1989;70:991–995.
71. Morishima H O, Pedersen H, Finster M, et al. Toxicity of lidocaine in adult, newborn, and fetal sheep. *Anesthesiology* 1981;55:57–61.
72. Badgwell J M, Heavner J E, Kytta J. Bupivacaine toxicity in young pigs is age-dependent and is affected by volatile anesthetics. *Anesthesiology* 1990;73:297–303.
73. Liu P L, Covino B M, Feldman H S. Effect of age on local anesthetic central nervous system toxicity in mice. *Reg Anesth* 1983;8:57–60.
74. McIlvaine W B, Knox R F, Fennessey P V, Goldstein M. Continuous infusion of bupivacaine via intrapleural catheter for analgesia after thoracotomy in children. *Anesthesiology* 1988;69:261–264.
75. McCloskey J J, Haun S E, Deshpande J K. Bupivacaine toxicity secondary to continuous caudal epidural infusion in children. *Anesth Analg* 1992;75:287–290.
76. de Jong R H, Bonin J D. Local anesthetics: injection route alters relative toxicity of bupivacaine. *Anesth Analg* 1980;59:925–928.
77. Scott D B. Evaluation of the toxicity of local anaesthetic agents in man. *Br J Anaesth* 1975;47:56–61.
78. Arthur G R, Feldman H S, Covino B G. Comparative pharmacokinetics of bupivacaine and ropivacaine, a new amide local anesthetic. *Anesth Analg* 1988;67:1053–1058.
79. Munson E S, Paul W L, Embro W J. Central nervous system toxicity of local anesthetic mixtures in monkeys. *Anesthesiology* 1977;46:179–183.
80. de Jong R H, Bonin J D. Mixtures of local anesthetics are no more toxic than the parent drugs. *Anesthesiology* 1981;54:177–181.
81. Spiegel D A, Dexter F, Warner D S, Baker M T, Todd M M. Central nervous system toxicity of local anesthetic mixtures in the rat. *Anesth Analg* 1992;75:922–928.
82. de Jong R H, Bonin J D. Toxicity of local anesthetic mixtures. *Toxicol Appl Pharmacol* 1980;54:501–507.
83. de Jong R H, Heavner J E. Diazepam prevents local anesthetic convulsions. *Anesthesiology* 1971;34:523–531.
84. Bernards C M, Carpenter R L, Rupp S M, et

al. Effect of midazolam and diazepam premedication on central nervous system and cardiovascular toxicity of bupivacaine in pigs. *Anesthesiology* 1989;70:318–323.

85. Liu P L, Feldman H S, Covino B M, Giasi R, Covino B G. Acute cardiovascular toxicity of procaine, chloroprocaine, and tetracaine in anesthetized ventilated dogs. *Reg Anesth* 1982; 7:14–19.

86. Edouard A R, Berdeaux A, Ahmad R, Samii K. Cardiovascular interactions of local anesthetics and calcium entry blockers in conscious dogs. *Reg Anesth* 1991;16:95–100.

87. Timour Q, Freysz M, Couzon P, et al. Possible role of drug interactions in bupivacaine-induced problems related to intraventricular conduction disorders. *Reg Anesth* 1990;15:180–185.

88. De Kock M, Gautier P, Vandewalle F, Renotte M-T. Digoxin enhances bupivacaine toxicity in rats. *Reg Anesth* 1991;16:272–277.

89. Roitman K, Sprung J, Wallace M, Matjasko J. Enhancement of bupivacaine cardiotoxicity with cardiac glycosides and β-adrenergic blockers: a case report. *Anesth Analg* 1993;76:658–661.

90. Bowdle T A, Freund P R, Slattery J T. Propranolol reduces bupivacaine clearance. *Anesthesiology* 1987;66:36–38.

91. Henry D A, MacDonald I A, Kitchingman G, Bell G D, Langman M J S. Cimetidine and ranitidine: comparison of effects on hepatic drug metabolism. *Br Med J* 1980;281:775–777.

92. Kim K C, Tasch M D. Effects of cimetidine and ranitidine on local anesthetic central nervous system toxicity in mice. *Anesth Analg* 1986;65:840–842.

93. Steinhaus J E. Local anesthetic toxicity: a pharmacological re-evaluation. *Anesthesiology* 1957;18:275–281.

94. Morishima H O, Pedersen H, Finster M, Feldman H S, Covino B G. Etidocaine toxicity in the adult, newborn and fetal sheep. *Anesthesiology* 1983;58:342–346.

95. Morishima H O, Pedersen H, Finster M, et al. Is bupivacaine more cardiotoxic than lidocaine? *Anesthesiology* 1983;59:A409.

96. Foldes F F, Davidson G M, Duncalf D, Kuwabara S. The intravenous toxicity of local anesthetic agents in man. *Clin Pharmacol Ther* 1965;6:328–335.

97. Widman B. LAC-43 (Marcaine®)—a new local anaesthetic. *Acta Anaesthesiol Scand Suppl* 1966;(Suppl 25):59–66.

98. Eicholzer A W, Feldman H S. Acute toxicity of etidocaine following various routes of administration in the dog. *Toxicol Appl Pharmacol* 1976;37:13–21.

99. Morishima HO, Pedersen H, Finster M et al. Toxicity of lidocaine in the adult, newborn and fetal sheep. *Anesthesiology* 1981;55:57–61.

100. de Jong R H, Bonin J D. Deaths from local anesthetic-induced convulsions in mice. *Anesth Analg* 1980;59:401–405.

101. Chadwick H S. Toxicity and resuscitation in lidocaine- or bupivacaine-infused cats. *Anesthesiology* 1985;63:385–390.

102. Scott D B, Lee A, Fagan D, Bowler G M R, Bloomfield P, Lundh R. Acute toxicity of ropivacaine compared with that of bupivacaine. *Anesth Analg* 1989;69:563–569.

103. Usubiaga J E, Wikinski J, Ferrero R, Usubiaga L E, Winiski R. Local anesthetic-induced convulsions in man: an electroencephalographic study. *Anesth Analg* 1966;45:611–620.

104. Scott D B. Toxic effects of local anaesthetic agents on the central nervous system. *Br J Anaesth* 1986;58:732–735.

105. de Jong R H. In: *Local anesthetics,* Springfield, IL: Charles C Thomas, 1977.

106. Julian R M. Lidocaine in experimental epilepsy. *J Life Sci* 1973;4:27–30.

107. Bernhard C G, Bohm E. *Local anaesthetics as anticonvulsants: A study on experimental and clinical epilepsy.* Stockholm: Almqvist & Wiksell, 1965.

108. Krenis L J, Liu P L, Ngai S H. The effect of local anesthetics on the central nervous system toxicity of hyperbaric oxygen. *Neuropharmacology* 1971;10:637–641.

109. Lemmen L J, Klassen M, Duiser B. Intravenous lidocaine in the treatment of convulsions. *JAMA* 1978;239:2025.

110. Wikiniski J A, Usubiaga J E, Morales R L, Torrieri A, Usubiaga L E. Mechanism of convulsions elicited by local anesthetic agents. I. Local anesthetic depression of electrically induced seizures in man. *Anesth Analg* 1970; 49:504–510.

111. Wagman I H, de Jong R H, Prince D A. Effects of lidocaine on the central nervous system. *Anesthesiology* 1967;28:155–172.

112. Covino B G. Toxicity and systemic effects of local anesthetic agents. In: Strichartz G, ed. *Local anesthetics.* New York: Springer-Verlag, 1987:187–209.

113. Eidelberg E, Neer H M, Miller M K. Anticonvulsant properties of some benzodiazepine derivatives. Possible use against psychomotor seizures. *Neurology* 1965;15:223–230.

114. Weiss W A. Intravenous use of lidocaine for ventricular arrhythmias. *Anesth Analg* 1960;39:369–381.

115. Burnstein C. Treatment of acute arrhythmias during anesthesia by intravenous procaine. *Anesthesiology* 1946;7:113–121.

116. Dunbar R W, Boettner R B, Gatz R N, et al. The effect of mepivacaine, bupivacaine, and lidocaine on digitalis-induced ventricular arrhythmias. *Anesth Analg* 1970;49:761–766.

117. Boettner R B, Dunbar R W, Haley J V, Morrow DH. The comparative antiarrhythmic effects of mepivacaine and lignocaine. *Br J Anaesth* 1970;42:685–689.

118. Boettner R B, Dunbar R W, Haley J V, Morrow DH. A comparison of the antiarrhythmic effects of bupivacaine and lidocaine. *South Med J* 1972;65:1328–1330.

119. Chapin J C, Kushins L G, Munson E S, Schick L M. Lidocaine, bupivacaine, etidocaine, and epinephrine-induced arrhythmias during halothane anesthesia in dogs. *Anesthesiology* 1980; 52:23–26.

Anesthetic Toxicity, edited by
Susan A. Rice and Kevin J. Fish.
Raven Press, Ltd., New York © 1994.

8

Toxicity of Nitrous Oxide

Donald D. Koblin

*Anesthesiology Service, Veterans Administration Medical Center, San Francisco,
California 94121*

Nitrous oxide and oxygen gas is unquestionably the safest anesthetic in the world; anybody studying the subject clinically and theoretically knows that.
—J.T. Gwathmey, 1906

Although the quotation was written almost a century ago (1), there are many anesthetists who agree with this statement. Nitrous oxide (N_2O) remains a commonly used clinical agent, with its advantages including a lack of odor and lack of airway irritation, a low solubility in blood that permits a rapid induction and emergence from anesthesia, provision of analgesia, and minimal depression of respiration and circulation. However, the safe administration of N_2O requires a knowledge of its unique physicochemical properties, and under certain conditions, the use of N_2O may be harmful.

POTENTIAL FOR PRODUCTION OF HYPOXIA

A key part in the quotation by Gwathmey is the mention of N_2O and oxygen (O_2). N_2O is a weak agent, and a hyperbaric chamber is required to produce the 1.04 atm N_2O (2,3) needed for anesthesia (defined by lack of response to noxious stimuli). Thus, under normal operating room conditions at the ambient pressure of 1 atm, surgical anesthesia cannot be achieved with N_2O alone while coadministering adequate amounts of O_2. Hypoxia may result if N_2O/O_2 mixtures

are administered at concentrations of N_2O > 80% and O_2 concentrations < 20% (or even at higher O_2 concentrations in patients with preexisting pulmonary disease). Although administration of 100% N_2O was still being employed for brief dental procedures as late as the 1960s (4), this technique is unacceptable in modern practice, and current standards require monitoring to ensure adequate oxygenation. Deaths secondary to hypoxia occur in individuals who abuse and breathe 100% N_2O (5).

On recovery from an anesthetic that includes administration of N_2O, the potential for hypoxia exists due to the outpouring of large volumes of N_2O from the blood to alveoli. However, such diffusion hypoxia appears to be of minimal clinical significance, especially if 100% O_2 is provided during the first few minutes of recovery (6).

TOXICITY OF CONTAMINANTS

On rare occasions, patients have died when they received N_2O delivered from commercially prepared tanks that contained impurities, e.g., nitric oxide (NO), nitrogen dioxide (NO_2), nitrogen tetroxide (N_2O_4) (7,8). These impurities can impair oxygenation by direct pulmonary damage as well as through production of methemoglobinemia. Pulmonary toxicity has resulted also from high levels of NO and NO_2 contaminants in those who abuse homemade N_2O prepared from the combustion of ammonium nitrate

(NH_4NO_3) fertilizer (9). Treatment of toxicity produced by these higher oxides of nitrogen includes O_2 therapy to compensate for decreased blood O_2 capacity and reconversion of methemoglobin to oxyhemoglobin using methylene blue (1 to 2 mg/kg).

EXPANSION OF CLOSED GAS SPACES

When N_2O is administered, any closed gas space in the body that contains air will increase in size if the walls surrounding the space are compliant or in pressure if the walls are not compliant (10). This results from N_2O being carried to the closed air space and diffusing from a region of high concentration outside to a region of low concentration inside the space. Nitrogen is transferred from inside to outside the space much slower than N_2O enters because nitrogen is much less soluble in blood and tissues (blood/gas partition coefficients at 37°C of 0.47 for N_2O and 0.015 for nitrogen). The increase in volume or pressure or both of the air space increases with inspired N_2O concentration and duration of exposure.

Expansion of air spaces by N_2O may produce harm. With a pneumothorax, N_2O-induced doubling in size occurs in 10 to 15 minutes and can impair ventilation and circulation (11). Administration of N_2O lowers (by threefold) the volume of i.v. air needed to produce death in animals (12). Although expansion of air emboli in blood vessels by N_2O may produce deleterious effects, especially in coronary arteries (13) where very small air emboli (0.05ml) can limit perfusion and diminish cardiac function, N_2O may be used safely in patients likely to develop air emboli provided that N_2O is discontinued immediately on Doppler detection of an air embolus (14). A unique case of cardiac compromise by N_2O involved the expansion of gas in a pacemaker pocket that led to loss of anodal contact and pacing system malfunction (15).

A closed air space in bowel will expand in the presence of N_2O, with a doubling in volume occurring in about 2 hours (11).

Even in patients without bowel obstruction, N_2O may delay return of normal bowel function if air is present in the bowel at the start of surgery (16). If air in the bowel is not present initially, the use of N_2O during routine intestinal surgery causes a clinically unnoticeable, but statistically significant, increase in circumference of the ileum (17). The expansion of gas spaces in bowel by N_2O may enhance postoperative nausea and vomiting. However, the contribution of N_2O to postoperative emesis will depend on the patient population, the type of surgery performed, and the use of other anesthetics (18).

A potential for injury also exists when N_2O increases pressures in closed air spaces with relatively noncompliant walls. If a patient has blocked eustachian tubes, N_2O will increase middle ear pressure and may result in tympanic membrane rupture (19) or hearing loss (20). Conversely, when N_2O is discontinued at the end of surgery, N_2O rapidly diffuses out of the middle ear and negative pressures may occur and impair hearing (21). However, the development of negative middle ear pressures after N_2O administration is not associated with postoperative vomiting (22).

Intraocular pressure can increase as much as 20 mm Hg when N_2O expands intraocular gases, e.g., air, sulfur hexafluoride (SF_6), that are injected to treat retinal detatchment (23,24). Such a rise in intraocular pressure has the potential to decrease retinal blood flow. Similarly, pressure increases to over 100 mm Hg in endotracheal tube cuffs inflated with air and exposed to N_2O may compromise blood flow to the tracheal mucosa, cause tracheal or laryngeal trauma, and contribute to postoperative sore throat (25).

ADVERSE PHYSIOLOGIC EFFECTS

Acute Administration

In addition to its potential to produce hypoxia and to expand enclosed air-filled spaces, brief exposures to N_2O may disrupt the normal function of major body organs. Like other inhaled anesthetics, N_2O increases respiratory rate, decreases lung tidal volume, and depresses the ventilatory response to hypoxia (10). N_2O increases skeletal muscle activity, and when used as the sole anesthetic under hyperbaric conditions, N_2O produces muscle rigidity, jerky limb movements, and even opisthotonus (2,3). Similar to the volatile anesthetics, N_2O increases intracranial pressure (26). The enhanced sympathetic outflow produced by N_2O (27) may be responsible in part for the tachycardia and hypertension associated with N_2O administration at hyperbaric pressures (3), as well as an increased dysrhythmogenic effect on the myocardium (28) during routine surgical procedures. Although a majority of people enjoy the effects of breathing subanesthetic concentrations of N_2O, about one fourth of individuals dislike breathing N_2O and may have feelings of dysphoria, confusion, fatigue, depression, or anxiety (29).

Chronic Administration

In 1956, Lassen et al. (30) administered a 50% N_2O/50% O_2 mixture for as long as 18 days to patients with tetanus in an attempt to provide pain relief and control spasms. Approximately 6 days after continuous N_2O administration, severe hematologic complications often developed, with pronounced granulocytopenia and thrombocytopenia and with megaloblastic changes on bone marrow biopsy. The authors identified these effects as being similar to those seen with pernicious anemia and treated (without success) these hematologic abnormalities with large doses of vitamin B_{12}. A later investigation demonstrated that megaloblastic bone marrow aspirates could be found in cardiac patients administered 50% N_2O for periods as short as 24 hours (31).

Neurologic disorders associated with prolonged exposure to N_2O, either from its abuse (32,33) or from inadequate scavenging during dental surgeries (33), were reported in the 1970s. Symptoms and signs included numbness and paresthesia in the extremities, loss of balance, unsteady gait, impotence, Lhermitte's sign (an electric shock sensation extending down the spine with head flexion), impairment of touch, vibration or position sense, muscle weakness, and Romberg's sign (when a patient stands more unsteady with the eyes closed). It was recognized that these neurologic abnormalities were similar to those observed with vitamin B_{12} deficiency, but the mechanism of neurotoxicity was unclear. Treatment with vitamin B_{12} injections did not seem to affect the extent of recovery (33).

DISRUPTION OF VITAMIN B_{12}/FOLATE METABOLISM BY N_2O

Oxidation of Vitamin B_{12} (Cobalamin)

Although the first report of a reaction between vitamin B_{12} and N_2O appeared in 1968 (34), the possible clinical significance of this reaction was not recognized until 10 years later, when Amess et al. (31) demonstrated megaloblastic hemopoiesis in cardiac patients receiving N_2O. Banks et al. (34) showed that N_2O oxidized the cobalt atom of vitamin B_{12} at room temperature and in aqueous solution. In the presence of excess cob(I)alamin, the oxidation probably occurs according to the following scheme (35).

$$\text{cob(I)alamin} + N_2O + 2H^+$$
$$\rightarrow \text{cob(III)alamin}$$
$$+ N_2 + H_2O$$
$$\text{cob(III)alamin} + \text{cob(I)alamin}$$
$$\rightarrow 2\,\text{cob(II)alamin}$$

Reaction of N_2O with enzyme-bound cobalamin may differ from that which occurs in aqueous solution, and a scheme has been proposed from model system studies in which a hydroxyl radical is generated (35).

$$\text{cob(I)alamin} + N_2O + H^+$$
$$\rightarrow \text{cob(II)alamin} + N_2 + OH\cdot$$

It was further speculated that the extremely reactive hydroxyl radical may attack amino acids near the active site to produce enzyme inactivation (35). However, it has been pointed out that the above reaction is energetically unfavorable (36), and an alternative explanation is that an unstable hydroxide anion-cobalt ion complex, formed by reaction with N₂O, damages the enzyme (36).

Inactivation of Methionine Synthase

Methionine synthase and methylmalonyl-CoA mutase are the only two enzymes in mammals that require vitamin B_{12} for activity. Methylmalonyl-CoA mutase is a mitochondrial enzyme that uses vitamin B_{12} in its adenosylated form to catalyze the conversion of L-methylmalonyl-CoA to succinyl-CoA. Brief exposures to N₂O do not

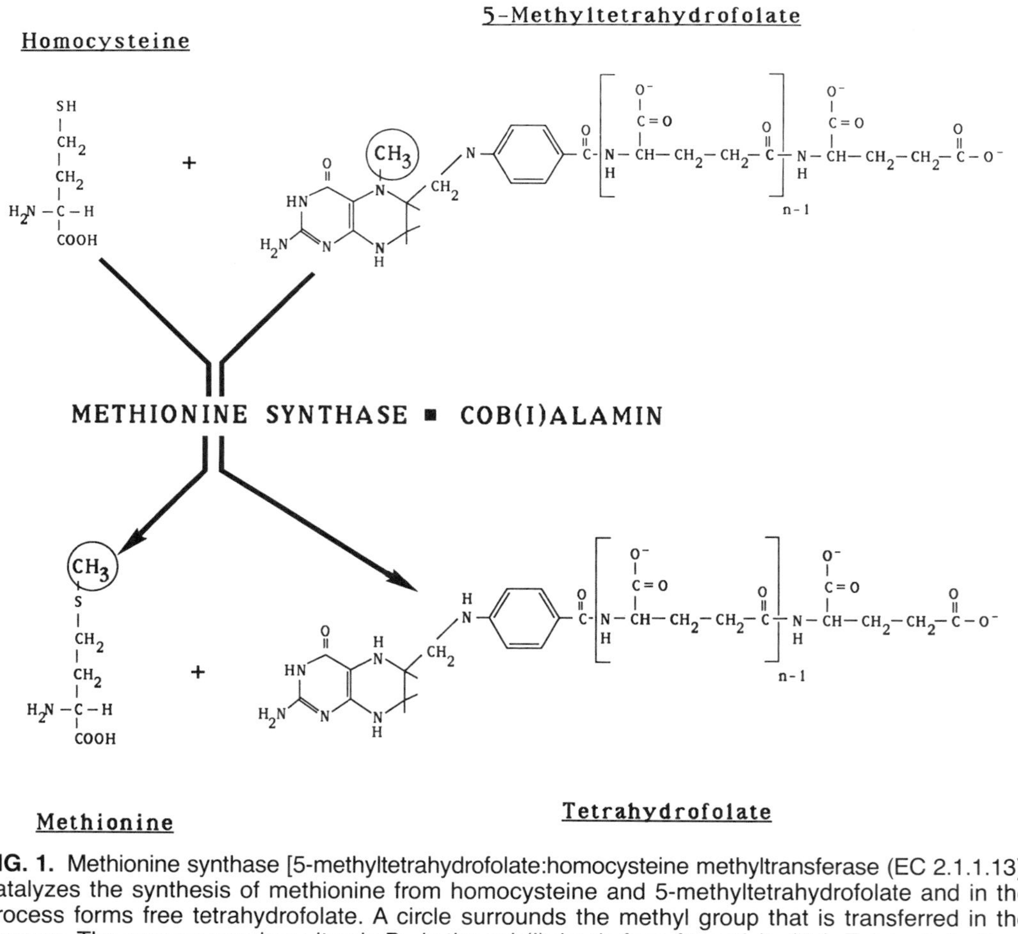

FIG. 1. Methionine synthase [5-methyltetrahydrofolate:homocysteine methyltransferase (EC 2.1.1.13)] catalyzes the synthesis of methionine from homocysteine and 5-methyltetrahydrofolate and in the process forms free tetrahydrofolate. A circle surrounds the methyl group that is transferred in the process. The enzyme requires vitamin B_{12} in the cob(I)alamin form for activity (35). Folate derivatives (i.e., 5-methyltetrahydrofolate and tetrahydrofolate) are shown in a generalized form with a variable glutamate chain length, with the folylpentaglutamate being the major folate in mammalian tissues (74). (Note that references to the literature before the 1980s refer to "methionine synthetase." However, methionine synthase is the correct trivial name for the enzyme and is now more widely accepted.)

inactivate methylmalonyl-CoA mutase (37–40), presumably because the adenosylcobalamin coenzyme is not in the reduced state and is, therefore, not directly susceptible to the oxidative effect of N_2O. Prolonged exposure to 50% N_2O (e.g., >15 days in rats) does decrease methylmalonyl-CoA mutase activity (38), an effect thought to be secondary to the depletion of endogenous vitamin B_{12} and its analogs.

The cytoplasmic enzyme methionine synthase (Fig. 1) adds a methyl group to homocysteine to form methionine and in the process converts methyltetrahydrofolate to tetrahydrofolate. In contrast to methylmalonyl-CoA mutase, methionine synthase is markedly inactivated after brief exposures to N_2O (37,41,42). N_2O-induced inactivation of methionine synthase has been demonstrated in a number of tissues, including liver (35,37–44), kidney (40,45), brain (39–42,45–47), heart (39), ovaries (47), testes (48), placenta (49), intestine (50,51), and bone marrow (45), and in cell cultures (52–54). Inactivation increases with increasing N_2O partial pressure and with duration of N_2O exposure (41–44,55,56). In rodents, exposure to 50% to 80% N_2O inactivates more than 50% of the hepatic enzyme within minutes (Fig. 2). For chronic exposures (several weeks), detectable inactivation of methionine synthase does not occur until N_2O concentrations exceed 500 to 1000 ppm (42,55). The rate of N_2O-induced methionine synthase inactivation depends on the species and tissues examined. For example, the rate of enzyme inactivation is 5 to 10 times slower in human than in rat liver (44) (Fig. 2). For a given species (mice), the rate of enzyme inactivation is about 5 times faster in liver than in brain (56).

Anesthesia *per se* produced by N_2O is not responsible for methionine synthase inactivation. Exposure of rodents to anesthetic concentrations of halothane, enflurane, isoflurane, or xenon for 4 hours does not significantly alter enzyme activity in liver, kidney, or brain (41,42,57). Similarly, a

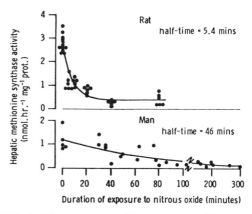

FIG. 2. Time course of inactivation of hepatic methionine synthase in 22 patients undergoing laparotomy and receiving 70% N_2O as a component of their general anesthetic (lower curve) and in rats exposed to 50% N_2O (upper curve). The ordinate represents enzyme activity and is expressed as the nanomoles of methionine produced per hour per milligram protein in the 20,000g supernatant fraction of liver homogenate. (From Royston B D, Nunn J F, Weinbren H K, Royston D, Cormack R S. Rate of inactivation of human and rodent hepatic methionine synthase by nitrous oxide. *Anesthesiology* 1988;68:213–216.

bacterial methionine synthase is unaffected by methoxyflurane, sevoflurane, isoflurane, halothane, enflurane, and trichloroethylene (58). Nor can enzyme inactivation be explained by the coadministration of O_2 with N_2O, since hyperbaric pressures of O_2 have no influence on methionine synthase activity (59).

Recovery of methionine synthase activity is relatively slow and occurs over a period of days (38,40–42,56,57,60–62) (Fig. 3). Four days after a 6-hour exposure to 60% N_2O, methionine synthase activity in rat brain remains significantly decreased (~30%) from control values (60) (Fig. 3). Recovery of enzyme activity presumably requires *de novo* synthesis of the apoenzyme. Recovery of methionine synthase activity following N_2O inactivation has not been studied in humans because of the difficulty in obtaining repetitive samples from vital tissues.

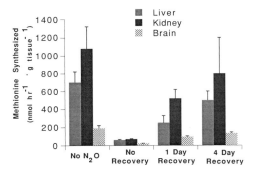

FIG. 3. Methionine synthase activities in livers, kidneys, and brains of rats expressed as nanomoles of methionine produced per hour per gram of tissue. Control rats received "No N₂O" and were only exposed to room air. Other rats were exposed to 60% N₂O for 6 hours and allowed to recover in room air for 1 ("1 Day Recovery") or 4 ("4 Day Recovery") days. Values from the "No Recovery" time point are taken from tissues from rats killed immediately after N₂O exposure. Error bars indicate ± SD. (Adapted from Koblin D D, Everman B W. Vitamin B₁₂ and folate status in rats after chronic administration of ethanol and acute exposure to nitrous oxide. *Alcoholism Clin Exp Res* 1991;15:543–548.

Changes in Vitamin B₁₂ after N₂O

N₂O administration has little or no effect on serum vitamin B₁₂ in patients even after exposures for as long as 24 hours (63–65). Similarly, brief (several hour) exposures of rats to N₂O do not decrease vitamin B₁₂ in serum, liver, kidney, or brain (40,60,66,67). However, prolonged (several weeks) exposures of rats to N₂O result in a marked fall in serum and liver cobalamin and an increase in inactive cobalamin analogs (38,63). It is unclear why brief N₂O exposures, which markedly inactivate methionine synthase (Figs. 2,3), have little influence on tissue levels of vitamin B₁₂. One possible explanation is that the amount of vitamin B₁₂ in a reduced form that is capable of being oxidized by N₂O is a relatively small fraction of the total amount of vitamin B₁₂. Another possibility is that the method used for quantitation (e.g., radioassay binding studies) may not be sensitive enough to distinguish subtle changes in the vitamin B₁₂ molecule induced by N₂O.

Changes in Tissue Folates after N₂O

Inactivation of methionine synthase by N₂O (Fig. 1) prevents the transfer of a methyl group and tends to trap folate in a methylated form (the methyl trap hypothesis) (68,69). Because the activities of the many enzymes involved in one-carbon metabolism depend on a particular type of folate derivative, this trapping in the 5-methyltetrahydrofolate form will influence the production and concentrations of other folate derivatives. After N₂O exposure, folate in plasma (which consists primarily of methylfolate in a monoglutamate form) increases in rats (69) and in patients (Fig. 4) (65,70). The N₂O-induced elevation in plasma folate results from an impaired cellular uptake of methylfolate and is associated with a marked excretion of folate into urine (Fig. 4) and altered amounts of folate coenzymes in tissues (69). In general, N₂O exposure increases the relative amount of 5-methyltetrahydrofolate in tissues and decreases free tetrahydrofolate and formyl(CHO)-tetrahydrofolate (45,62,71–73), although the particular changes produced will depend on the species, the tissue examined, and the N₂O concentration and exposure time. N₂O also may selectively alter the monoglutamate (found principally in plasma and extracellular fluids) and polyglutamate (found in tissues) forms of the coenzyme. Rats exposed to 50% N₂O for 4.5 hours have increased penta- and hexaglutamate forms of hepatic 5-methyltetrahydrofolate and decreased penta- and hexaglutamate forms of free tetrahydrofolate (74). Moreover, the N₂O-induced changes in folate coenzymes are specific at the subcellular level. That is, the increase in the methylated forms of folate and the decrease in the free and formyl forms of folate seen after N₂O exposure are confined to the cytosol of the cell. Mitochondrial folates are not altered by N₂O (75).

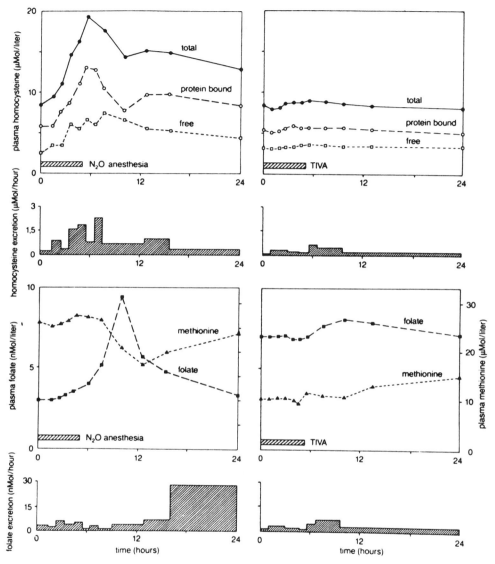

FIG. 4. Time course of changes in plasma homocysteine and folate and excretion of homocysteine and folate in urine in a patient who received 70% N₂O for 5.3 hours as a component of the anesthetic (**left**) and in a patient who was anesthetized for 5.2 hours with total i.v. anesthesia (TIVA) and no exposure to N₂O (**right**). N₂O exposure was associated with increased plasma levels of homocysteine and folate and an enhanced excretion of these compounds in urine. (From Ermens A A M, Refsum H, Rupreht J, et al. Monitoring cobalamin inactivation during nitrous oxide anesthesia by determination of homocysteine and folate in plasma and urine. *Clin Pharmacol Ther* 1991;49:385–393.)

It remains debatable whether the trapping of folate in the methylated form (Fig. 1) can explain all of the metabolic changes seen after N₂O exposure. Although the experiments described are consistent with the methyl trap hypothesis, other studies indicate that methyltetrahydrofolate can be oxidized in N₂O-exposed animals to escape the trap (69,76) and that disruption of metabolic processes by N₂O may occur without the accumulation of methyltetrahydrofolate (77).

Alterations in Amino Acids, Nucleosides, and Their Derivatives

N₂O-induced inactivation of methionine synthase impairs the methylation of homocysteine and thereby leads to a buildup of

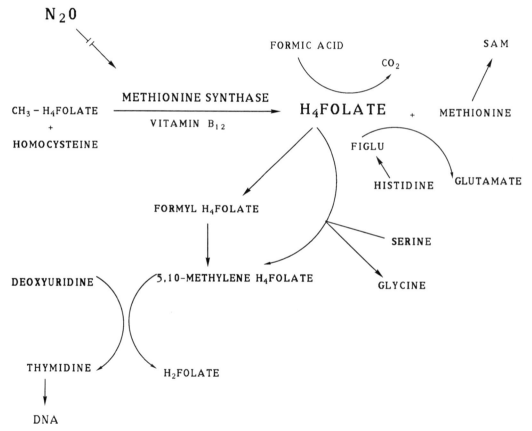

FIG. 5. Inactivation of methionine synthase by N₂O results in decreased formation of free tetrahydrofolate (H₄FOLATE) and methionine. The simplified scheme shown illustrates selected metabolic changes that may occur after N₂O exposure. A decrease in methionine may lead to a decrease in S-adenosylmethionine (SAM). A decrease in H₄FOLATE prevents the oxidation of formate and the breakdown of formiminoglutamic acid (FIGLU), resulting in an accumulation of these metabolites during N₂O exposure. A decrease in H₄FOLATE also may deplete 5,10-methylenetetrahydrofolate (CH₂-H₄FOLATE) and thereby decrease the methylation of deoxyuridylate to deoxythymidylate and impair DNA synthesis. A more complete description of the metabolic processes altered by disruption of the vitamin B₁₂/folate interrelationships can be found in references 68 and 69.

homocysteine and a decrease in methionine (Figs. 1 and 5). The magnitude of the changes in amino acid metabolism seen after N_2O administration will depend on the species and tissue examined, the concentration of N_2O, and the duration of N_2O administration. In humans, N_2O produces about a twofold increase in plasma homocysteine and enhances homocysteine excretion in urine (70) (Fig. 4). Plasma methionine decreases in patients administered N_2O (70,78–80), but most of this decrease can be accounted for by preoperative fasting and a lack of nutritional intake (79,80). S-adenosylmethionine, the derivative used for most biosynthetic methylations in the body, is unchanged in the plasma of patients who receive N_2O for short (~2 hours) time periods (80). Similarly, S-adenosylmethionine is unchanged in the blood, liver, and brain of rats exposed to 50% N_2O for 80 minutes (81). However, prolonged N_2O exposures (several hours to days) decrease S-adenosylmethionine in rat liver (82–84) and in rat (84), mouse (85), and pig (86) brain. Prolonged N_2O exposure is associated also with a reduction in hepatic methionine, as well as a reduction in several other amino acids (84).

Histidine metabolism is markedly affected by N_2O (74), presumably because N_2O decreases the free tetrahydrofolate needed to metabolize formiminoglutamic acid (FIGLU) (a breakdown product of histidine) to glutamate (Fig. 5). The impaired oxidation of histidine is associated with an enhanced excretion of FIGLU in urine (39,87). The elevation in urinary FIGLU excretion after exposure of rats to N_2O may exceed background values by several hundredfold (40,60,87,88) (Fig. 6). Humans also demonstrate an enhanced excretion of FIGLU in urine after N_2O administration (Fig. 7), but the magnitude of this effect is less in humans than in rats (65,89,90). Typically, the enhanced excretion of urinary FIGLU disappears by the first day after N_2O exposure.

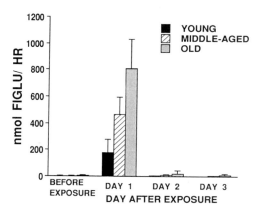

FIG. 6. Urinary formiminoglutamic acid (FIGLU) excretion rates (mean values ± SD) in young (2-month), middle-aged (12-month), and old (24-month) rats on the day immediately before (values are barely visible on the graph) and on days after exposure to 60% N_2O for 6 hours. Values are expressed as the total nanomoles of FIGLU excreted per hour. (From Koblin D D, Tomerson B W, Waldman F M. Disruption of folate and vitamin B_{12} metabolism in aged rats following exposure to nitrous oxide. *Anesthesiology* 1990; 73:506–512.)

Lower free tetrahydrofolate concentrations associated with N_2O treatment may also lead to decreased 5,10-methylene(CH_2)-tetrahydrofolate, a folate derivative needed for the synthesis of deoxythymidine and DNA (Fig. 5). N_2O-induced impairment in DNA synthesis is manifested by an abnormal (elevated) deoxyuridine suppression test (31,78,91–95). That is, a high value for the deoxyuridine suppression test indicates that a relatively high amount (typically more than 5% to 10%) of radioactive thymidine added to the assay medium is incorporated into DNA when precursors are not available for the *de novo* synthesis of thymidine. In healthy patients, abnormal deoxyuridine suppression tests in bone marrow may occur after a 6-hour exposure to N_2O (94). Purine synthesis, which requires the donation of formyl groups from 10-formyltetrahydrofolate, also may be perturbed by N_2O (53,96).

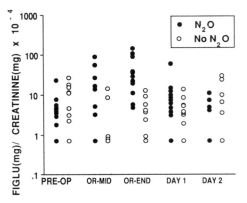

FIG. 7. Ratios of urinary formiminoglutamic acid (FIGLU) to creatinine in patients having resection of acoustic neuromas. The primary anesthetic consisted of isoflurane/oxygen (open circles) or a lesser amount of isoflurane given in a 50% to 70% N_2O/O_2 mixture. The average duration of anesthesia was approximately 10 hours. Patients receiving N_2O had a higher FIGLU/creatinine ratio at the end of the operation (OR-END) compared with those not given N_2O ($p <$ 0.001) and compared with values before anesthesia (PRE-OP) (p = 0.0057). These differences disappeared by the first postoperative day. Note the logarithmic scale of the ordinate. (From Koblin D D, Tomerson B W, Waldman F M, Lampe G H, Wauk L Z, Eger E I II. Effect of nitrous oxide on folate and vitamin B_{12} metabolism in patients. *Anesth Analg* 1990;71:610–617.)

SPECIES DIFFERENCES

Although N_2O inactivates methionine synthase, perturbs folate metabolism, and impairs DNA synthesis in most species, only humans experience megaloblastic anemia after inactivation of cobalamin. The reason for this unique sensitivity of humans is unknown, but possible explanations include a greater dependence in humans on the synthetic pathway for thymidylate, an inability of humans to induce a betaine homocysteine methyltransferase to compensate for the failure of methionine synthase, and a failure of humans to restore polyglutamate forms of folate in cobalamin deficiency (69).

Neuronal toxicity after N_2O administration also differs among species. Humans (32,33,97,98), monkeys (99), swine (46), and fruit bats (100–102) develop disabling neuropathies after prolonged N_2O exposure. In contrast, N_2O does not produce severe neurotoxicity in the rat, even after prolonged and repetitive exposures (e.g., 70% N_2O for 4 hours 5 days a week for 6 months) (103). Nevertheless, N_2O may produce more subtle neurologic changes in rodents, such as the development of a withdrawal syndrome after chronic (104) or acute (105,106) N_2O treatment and reduced cell proliferation in the developing brain (107). The mechanism by which N_2O causes these neurologic changes is unknown. Although it has been hypothesized that a decreased S-adenosylmethionine/S-adenosylhomocysteine ratio and impaired methylation are responsible for the neuropathy produced by N_2O in swine and monkeys (46,99), this does not seem to be the case in the fruit bat (101).

Species differences exist in the biochemical alterations produced by N_2O. As noted previously, N_2O-induced changes in folates, amino acids, and their derivatives depend on the species examined, and inactivation of methionine synthase by N_2O is slower in humans than in rodents (Fig. 2). Differences in the tissue concentrations of folates among species may contribute to the variable responses to N_2O. For example, humans and monkeys given methanol develop a metabolic acidosis and ocular toxicity associated with an accumulation of formic acid (108). In contrast, normal rats are resistant to methanol poisoning (108). However, rats treated with N_2O and administered methanol accumulate formic acid and develop a metabolic acidosis (109). It is thought that the susceptibility of humans and monkeys to methanol poisoning is related to the relatively low levels of hepatic folate in these species (108) because free tetrahydrofolate is required to convert formic acid to carbon dioxide (Fig. 5). Rodents, having relatively high amounts of folate (108), are resistant to methanol poisoning until tissue folate is diminished by N₂O administration (109).

IS THE ROUTINE ADMINISTRATION OF N₂O HARMFUL?

N₂O for Elective Surgical Procedures

From the preceding discussion, it is clear that N₂O produces many physiologic and biochemical changes. In spite of such alterations, no evidence of organ toxicity in mice could be detected after multiple repeated exposures to N₂O (50% N₂O for 4 hours per day 5 days per week for 14 weeks) (110). Overt toxicity in other species requires prolonged N₂O exposures. The question naturally arises whether N₂O-induced biochemical and physiologic perturbations are associated with harm to the patient who routinely receives N₂O during surgery.

This question was addressed in a series of clinical studies by Eger et al. (28,65,111–116), in which approximately 300 patients (undergoing total hip arthroplasty, carotid endarterectomy, transsphenoidal hypophysectomy, or resection of acoustic neuromas) were assigned randomly to receive isoflurane with or without 60% N₂O. Duration of N₂O exposure ranged from approximately 2 hours to 16 hours. No difference in major (e.g., death, myocardial infarction, neuronal injury, hypoxemia, infection) or minor (e.g., nausea, vomiting, headache, earache) untoward clinical outcomes could be detected between anesthetic groups (111–114). Furthermore, N₂O administration did not alter clinical variables measured in practice, including blood pressure, heart rate, rate of recovery from anesthesia, development of postoperative pain, patient satisfaction with anesthesia, and duration of anesthesia or of hospitalization (111,112). Moreover, there was no suggestion of a trend that a larger data cohort would reveal an adverse clinical effect of N₂O (111).

Laboratory evidence of an N₂O-induced

toxicity was looked for in these patients. Using postoperative plasma concentrations of alanine aminotransferase, bilirubin, and alkaline phosphatase as indicators of hepatic injury for individuals having total hip replacements, there was no evidence that N₂O impaired hepatic function (115). Measures of red cell mass (red blood cell count, hemoglobin, mean red cell volume, red cell distribution width, reticulocytes) were not affected by the use of N₂O (116). Similarly, administration of N₂O did not affect the decrease in platelet number observed postoperatively on the rebound thrombocytosis that occurs in the days following anesthesia and surgery (116). There was no evidence of increased numbers of hypersegmented neutrophils after N₂O exposure (116). Patients given N₂O did demonstrate a smaller postoperative rise in leukocytes, but there was no indication that this finding was associated with an adverse clinical outcome (116). The small transient increase in FIGLU/creatinine ratio in patients receiving N₂O (Fig. 7) (65) returned toward control values by the first day after anesthesia.

It is implied from this series of studies that the routine administration of N₂O for elective surgeries is safe and that the use of N₂O does not produce untoward outcomes. Although an occasional patient may prove highly susceptible and develop signs of severe vitamin B₁₂ and folic acid deficiency after N₂O exposure, it seems that this is a rare event.

Chronic Exposure to Trace Levels of N₂O

The question of whether or not the routine administration of N₂O is harmful requires consideration of health care personnel who are chronically exposed to N₂O. In general, operating room and dental personnel chronically exposed to N₂O have normal serum methionine (117) and vitamin B₁₂ and folate concentrations (118,119) and normal excretion of FIGLU (90). However, dentists who use N₂O in a room with inadequate scavenging may develop myeloneuropathy (33) and abnormal bone marrow deoxyuridine suppression tests (119). Anesthetic personnel chronically exposed to high occupational concentrations of N_2O may exhibit decreased peripheral blood leukocyte counts (120). Epidemiologic studies revealed a 1.2-fold to 2.8-fold increase in liver, kidney, and neurologic disease in dentists and dental chairside assistants chronically exposed to N_2O (121). Women employed as dental assistants and exposed to high concentrations of N_2O have a 2.3-fold increase in spontaneous abortion rate (121) and reduced fertility (122,123). However, such findings must be viewed with reference to the limitations of epidemiologic studies (e.g., retrospective study, possibleinaccurate recall of events, possibilities of responder bias). The reproductive toxicity of N_2O is further examined in the chapters by Ebi and Rice and by Rice.

ARE THERE SPECIFIC PATIENT POPULATIONS HIGHLY SUSCEPTIBLE TO N_2O TOXICITY?

Although it is highly unlikely that brief administration of N_2O to patients will produce harm, there are case reports suggesting an association between the routine administration of N_2O and the production of toxicity. Such rare cases are considered here, along with clinical situations in which there are theoretical (but unproven) concerns that the administration of N_2O might produce an unfavorable outcome.

Patients Receiving Multiple Exposures

Because the recovery of methionine synthase activity is relatively slow (Fig. 3), it might be expected that repetitive, brief exposures to N_2O could have a cumulative effect. This appears to have occurred in a patient who developed megaloblastic bone marrow after receiving 50% N_2O for about 15 minutes 3 times each day over a period

of about 3 weeks (124). However, the repetitive administration of N_2O does not always produce untoward effects. Infants have been anesthetized 20 or more times with N_2O (for as long as 2 hours) over 4 to 6 weeks without suffering any apparent harm (125,126).

Patients with a Masked Vitamin B_{12} or Folate Deficiency

Neurologic dysfunction (consistent with subacute combined degeneration of the spinal cord) and megaloblastic anemia developed in 3 patients with masked vitamin B_{12} deficiency weeks to months after a brief exposure (~2 hours) to N_2O (127,128). Two of these patients had previous ileal resections, and 1 had pernicious anemia (127,128). Such associations led to the suggestion that N_2O is a dangerous agent in patients with functional vitamin B_{12} or folate deficiency (127). However, such events seem uncommon, and it is unknown how often patients with these vitamin deficiencies receive N_2O without harmful sequelae. Patients with folate deficiency and low-normal concentrations of serum vitamin B_{12} have received N_2O for several hours during surgical procedures without toxic consequences, as evaluated clinically or from laboratory values (65).

Critically Ill Patients

Patients with sepsis developed abnormal deoxyuridine suppression tests after brief N_2O exposures (129). Moreover, seriously ill patients who received N_2O for as little as 2 hours developed folate deficiency and demonstrated a high incidence of megaloblastic bone marrow changes (130–132) and a high (89%) mortality (130). However, these studies in critically ill patients were not controlled, and it is unclear what role N_2O played in the untoward outcomes of these individuals. Sick patients may develop folate deficiencies and megaloblastic changes even if they do not receive N$_2$O. Perhaps the same morbidity and mortality would have occurred if these patients received another anesthetic in place of N$_2$O.

Patients Receiving Methotrexate

Methotrexate inhibits dihydrofolate reductase, the enzyme that converts dihydrofolate to tetrahydrofolate. Evidence from *in vitro* and animal studies suggests that methotrexate enhances the antifolate and toxic effects of N$_2$O. Bone marrow cells isolated from patients who receive N$_2$O have greater abnormalities in the deoxyuridine suppression test when methotrexate is added to the bone marrow suspension (133). Similarly, N$_2$O increases deoxyuridine suppression test values in fresh leukemic cells isolated from patients and in a human myelomonocytic cell line treated with methotrexate (134). Administration of folate derivatives will rescue lymphoblast cells from methotrexate poisoning alone but not from the combination of N$_2$O and methotrexate (135). In rats, the administration of N$_2$O converts a nonlethal dose of methotrexate into a lethal dose (136,137).

Patients receiving methotrexate for chemotherapy may require surgery and receive N$_2$O as a component of their anesthetic. In a multicenter study that examined treatments for breast cancer, women with operable breast cancer received combination cytotoxic therapy (methotrexate, cyclophosphamide, 5-fluorouracil) at several specific times following mastectomy (138). Mastectomies were performed under general anesthesia, and the anesthetic technique almost always included N$_2$O (138). Untoward outcomes (e.g., death, infection, impaired wound healing, stomatitis, leukopenia) were more common in those patients who received methotrexate within 6 hours of termination of general anesthesia compared to patients who received methotrexate more than 6 hours after anesthesia. It was proposed that these toxic effects arose from the combined antifolate effects of methotrexate and of N$_2$O given during the mastectomy (138). These postoperative complications associated with combined N$_2$O and methotrexate administration were markedly decreased when the treatment protocol was altered to include folinic acid after the first and second doses of chemotherapy (139).

In addition to its use as a chemotherapeutic agent, methotrexate is being employed for treatment of several diseases, including rheumatoid arthritis, asthma, psoriasis, and inflammatory bowel disease. It has been speculated that N$_2$O might help such individuals by promoting the therapeutic effect of methotrexate (140). Conversely, it has been argued that N$_2$O might harm these patients by enhancing the toxic effects of methotrexate (141,142). Solid evidence is not available to support or refute either view.

Patients Undergoing Bone Marrow Transplants

As discussed previously, prolonged exposure (many hours to days) to N$_2$O will cause severe bone marrow depression. Thus, the concern arises that the administration of N$_2$O during anesthesia for bone marrow transplantation might compromise the success of the transplants. However, preliminary studies indicate that brief (<2 hours) exposures to N$_2$O do not impair the growth of bone marrow progenitors in patients receiving autologous transplants (143,144) or delay engraftment of bone marrow (145,146). From these limited data, it appears that N$_2$O can be used safely for the harvesting of bone marrow.

Patients with Impaired Wound Healing

The ability of N$_2$O to interfere with DNA synthesis (Fig. 5) might be expected to be unfavorable for wound healing. However, this supposition is not supported by animal studies. Rats exposed continuously to 20% N_2O for 10 days (147) or to 50% N_2O for 4 hours per day for 7 days (148) did not demonstrate impaired wound healing, as measured by histologic examination or by determination of breaking strengths of wound samples. Furthermore, patients given N_2O for elective surgical procedures do not exhibit a higher incidence of wound infection (111). Nevertheless, it remains possible that specific patient populations having a predilection to poor wound healing (e.g., those with diabetes, uremia, radiation treatment, or receiving chemotherapy) may be susceptible to N_2O. For example, women receiving chemotherapy immediately after mastectomies under general anesthesia with N_2O have a higher incidence of wound healing disorders (138). In contrast, no evidence of impaired wound healing was detected in a mouse model using the combined treatment of radiation exposure and repeated exposures to N_2O (149).

Pregnancy

Pregnancy is associated with a depletion in folate, and the possibility thus arises that administration of N_2O during pregnancy might worsen folate status and compromise the well-being of mother or fetus or both. However, evidence for a harmful effect of N_2O during pregnancy is lacking. Placental methionine synthase is relatively resistant to N_2O, as brief N_2O exposures have no effect on enzyme activity and the half-time for placental methionine synthase inactivation is 5 to 10 hours (49). Although N_2O is a proven teratogen in the rat (see chapter by Rice), analysis of outcomes following general anesthesia during pregnancy failed to reveal a single instance in which N_2O could have been clearly indicated as a cause of fetal abnormality (150). It has been argued that until data are available to suggest otherwise, the continued use of N_2O (for brief operations) during pregnancy is rational (151).

Alcoholism

The chronic intake of alcohol by patients often is associated with abnormalities in folate or vitamin B_{12} metabolism (152). However, the available evidence suggests that brief N_2O administration does not worsen folate/vitamin B_{12} status in alcoholics. In animal studies, acute administration of ethanol to mice has no effect on methionine synthase activity (57). Although chronic administration (6 weeks) of ethanol decreases hepatic (but not kidney or brain) methionine synthase activity in rats by 30% to 40%, exposure of these alcoholic rats to 60% N_2O for 6 hours does not produce severe and lasting disturbances in folate/vitamin B_{12} metabolism (40,60). Clinical studies indicate that N_2O is safe to use in patients with mild alcoholic hepatitis having peripheral surgeries (153). Moreover, the administration of N_2O to alcoholics has been used to treat withdrawal syndromes without the production of adverse side effects (154).

Elderly Patients

Elderly individuals often have deficiencies in vitamin B_{12} or folate or both (155). Although the influence of N_2O on vitamin B_{12} and folate status in the aged has not been examined in detail, it is a general clinical impression that N_2O is safe to use in elderly surgical patients. Patients from 72 to 85 years of age with low folate and low-normal serum vitamin B_{12} concentrations have received N_2O for total hip replacements without the development of untoward outcomes (65). These clinical impressions are supported by animal studies that demonstrate only a slightly greater disruption in folate/vitamin B_{12} metabolism in aged (>24 months old) compared to young rats, and that brief (<6 hour) N_2O administration to aged rats does not result in prolonged and severe metabolic disturbances (Fig. 6) (40,88).

Patients with Acquired Immunodeficiency Syndrome (AIDS)

Patients with AIDS often receive medications that impair folate metabolism and have low concentrations of vitamin B_{12} in their serum (156). These patients not infrequently undergo surgery and receive N_2O. There are no reported cases of exacerbation of vitamin B_{12}/folate deficiency after a patient with AIDS was administered N_2O.

Patients with Genetic Disorders

On extremely rare occasions, patients may need surgery who have hereditary defects in cobalamin metabolism. No information is available concerning the outcome of these patients after N_2O exposure. In a child with methylmalonyl-CoA mutase deficiency undergoing resection of a maxillary tumor, N_2O was purposely avoided to prevent the theoretical (but unproven) risk of methylmalonic acidemia (157).

IS THE TOXICITY OF N_2O USEFUL FOR CHEMOTHERAPY?

Because certain chemotherapeutic agents (e.g., methotrexate) inhibit production of neoplastic cells by perturbing folate-dependent metabolic pathways, N_2O might be expected to have chemotherapeutic properties. N_2O was first tested as a chemotherapeutic agent in 1959, when two patients with chronic myeloid leukemia were treated with 25% N_2O for 5 to 15 days (158). Although N_2O markedly decreased white cell and platelet counts, side effects (anemia, depression, confusion) were associated with N_2O administration, and no long-term beneficial effects could be demonstrated (158). A report several years later (159) described the treatment of patients with acute myelogenous leukemia with 30% to 60% N_2O for 5 weeks. N_2O decreased white cell counts and provided pain relief, but chronic

N_2O administration was associated with bleeding and hyperpyrexia, and the patients died (159). More recently, a patient with chronic myelogenous leukemia treated with 68% N_2O/32% O_2 for 4 days exhibited a marked decrease in leukocyte count and a decrease in spleen size (160). Although the leukocyte count tended to rebound after N_2O was discontinued, satisfactory control of the leukemia was achieved with cytosine arabinoside after N_2O removal (160).

The ability of N_2O to enhance either the chemotherapeutic or toxic effects of a drug probably depends on the concentration of N_2O and its duration of exposure, on the dosage and timing of the chemotherapeutic agent, and on the nutritional status of the patient. As noted previously (138), toxic effects may result if methotrexate is given in its typical dose shortly after patients receive N_2O. Further data are needed before it will be possible to predict whether a patient with cancer will exhibit a favorable therapeutic effect or a toxic side effect when administered N_2O.

REVERSAL OF N_2O TOXICITY

Patients with a masked vitamin B_{12} deficiency who developed neurologic dysfunction and megaloblastic anemia after a single brief exposure to N_2O improved dramatically after cyanocobalamin injections (127, 128). In contrast, individuals who suffer from toxic side effects related to chronic and prolonged administration of N_2O seem less responsive to treatment with vitamin B_{12}. Patients with tetanus who developed megaloblastic anemia after receiving N_2O for many days did not respond to large doses of vitamin B_{12} (30). Similarly, treatment with vitamin B_{12} injections did not promote recovery from myeloneuropathy seen after prolonged N_2O exposure (33). The reason for the ineffectiveness of vitamin B_{12} in these situations is uncertain.

Reversal of N_2O-induced bone marrow abnormalities can be achieved by administration of folates. In general, correction of the N₂O-induced elevations in the deoxyuridine suppression test is most effective with the addition of formylfolates (e.g., folinic acid) and least effective with methyltetrahydrofolate (69,92,94). Intravenous administration of folinic acid (30 mg) reversed the megaloblastic bone marrow changes produced by N₂O in a seriously ill patient (132). Moreover, folinic acid reversed the postoperative complications associated with combined N₂O and methotrexate administration in women undergoing mastectomies (139).

Methionine also may be effective in treating N₂O toxicity. One individual who developed a neuropathy associated with N₂O abuse improved markedly after being started on a methionine-supplemented diet (98). That methionine might be useful in treating N₂O toxicity in the clinical setting is suggested by animal studies that demonstrate a lessening of N₂O-induced biochemical perturbations (76,87) and prevention of neurologic abnormalities in primates chronically exposed to N₂O (99) following methionine administration.

CONCLUSIONS

N₂O continues to be a commonly used agent in anesthetic practice. This popularity persists despite the potential of N₂O to impair oxygenation, to expand closed gas spaces, and to disrupt vitamin B₁₂/folate metabolism through inactivation of the enzyme methionine synthase. The present approach of most anesthesiologists to the clinical use of N₂O is perhaps summarized best by Hornbein (161).

Nitrous oxide may not be as free from toxicity as was once thought, but, despite 140 years of use, little convincing evidence exists that it imposes a risk to the average patient. I shall continue to use nitrous oxide, albeit with a few more concerns and contraindications, until its limitations relative to other alternatives are defined more clearly.

REFERENCES

1. Gwathmey J T. A plea for the scientific administration of anesthetics. *JAMA* 1906;47:1361.
2. Hornbein T F, Eger E I II, Winter P M, Smith G, Wetstone D, Smith K H. The minimum alveolar concentration of nitrous oxide in man. *Anesth Analg* 1982;61:553–556.
3. Russell G B, Snider M T, Richard R B, Loomis J L. Hyperbaric nitrous oxide as a sole anesthetic agent in humans. *Anesth Analg* 1990; 70:289–295.
4. Smith W D A. 410 dental anaesthetics. Part I: Introduction, methods, material and anaesthetic techniques. *Br J Anaesth* 1964;36:620–632.
5. Leadbeatter S. Dental anaesthetic death. An unusual autoerotic episode. *Am J Forensic Med Pathol* 1988;9:60–63.
6. Sugioka K, Cattermole R W, Sebel P S. Arterial oxygen tensions measured continuously in patients breathing 21% oxygen and nitrous oxide or air. *Br J Anaesth* 1987;59:1548–1553.
7. Clutton-Brock J. Two cases of poisoning by contamination of nitrous oxide with higher oxides of nitrogen during anaesthesia. *Br J Anaesth* 1967;39:388–392.
8. Saglam F. Anaesthetic failure due to faulty agents. *Lancet* 1989;i:391.
9. Messina F V, Wynne J W. Homemade nitrous oxide: no laughing matter. *Ann Intern Med* 1982;96:333.
10. Eger E I II, ed. *Nitrous oxide/N₂O.* New York: Elsevier, 1985.
11. Eger E I II, Saidman L J. Hazards of nitrous oxide anesthesia in bowel obstruction and pneumothorax. *Anesthesiology* 1965;26:61–66.
12. Munson E S, Merrick H C. Effect of nitrous oxide on venous air embolism. *Anesthesiology* 1965;27:783–787.
13. Tuman K J, McCarthy R J, Spiess B D, Overfield D M, Ivankovich A D. Effects of nitrous oxide on coronary perfusion after coronary artery air embolism. *Anesthesiology* 1987;67: 952–959.
14. Losasso T J, Muzzi D A, Dietz N M, Cucchiara R F. Fifty percent nitrous oxide does not increase the risk of venous air embolism in neurosurgical patients operated upon in the sitting position. *Anesthesiology* 1992;77:21–30.
15. Lamas G A, Rebecca G S, Braunwald N S, Antman E M. Pacemaker malfunction after nitrous oxide anesthesia. *Am J Cardiol* 1985; 56:995.
16. Scheinin B, Lindgren L, Scheinin T M. Peroperative nitrous oxide delays bowel function after colonic surgery. *Br J Anaesth* 1990;64: 154–158.
17. Boulanger A, Hardy J F. La distension intestinale pendant la chirugie abdominale elective:

doit-on bannir le protoxyde d'azote? *Can J Anaesth* 1987;34:346–350.

18. Watcha M F, White P F. Postoperative nausea and vomiting. Its etiology, treatment, and prevention. *Anesthesiology* 1992;77:162–184.
19. Owens W D, Gustave F, Sclaroff A. Tympanic membrane rupture with nitrous oxide anesthesia. *Anesth Analg* 1978;57:283–286.
20. Hochermann M, Reimer A. Hearing loss after general anaesthesia. *J Laryng Otol* 1987;101: 1079–1082.
21. Blackstock D, Gettes M A. Negative pressure in the middle ear in children after nitrous oxide anaesthesia. *Can Anaesth Soc J* 1986;33:32–35.
22. Montgomery C J, Vaghadia H, Blackstock D. Negative middle ear pressure and postoperative vomiting in pediatric outpatients. *Anesthesiology* 1988;68:288–291.
23. Wolf G L, Capuano C, Hartung J. Nitrous oxide increases intraocular pressure after intravitreal sulfur hexafluoride injection. *Anesthesiology* 1983;59:547–548.
24. Mostafa S M, Wong S H D, Snowdon S L, Ansons A M, Kelly J M, McGalliard J N. Nitrous oxide and internal tamponade during vitrectomy. *Br J Ophthalmol* 1991;75:726–728.
25. Mandoe H, Nikolajsen L, Lintrup U, Jepsen D, Molgaard J. Sore throat after endotracheal intubation. *Anesth Analg* 1992;74:897–900.
26. Algotsson L, Messeter K, Rosen I, Holmin T. Effects of nitrous oxide on cerebral haemodynamics and metabolism during isoflurane anaesthesia in man. *Acta Anaesthesiol Scand* 1992; 36:46–52.
27. Ebert T J. Differential effects of nitrous oxide on baroreflex control of heart rate and peripheral sympathetic nerve activity in humans. *Anesthesiology* 1990;72:16–22.
28. Lampe G L, Donegan J H, Rupp S M, et al. Nitrous oxide and epinephrine-induced arrhythmias. *Anesth Analg* 1990;71:602–605.
29. Dohrn C S, Lichtor J L, Finn R S, et al. Subjective and psychomotor effects of nitrous oxide in healthy volunteers. *Behav Pharmacol* 1992;3:19–30.
30. Lassen H C A, Henriksen E, Neukirch F, Kristensen H S. Treatment of tetanus. Severe bone-marrow depression after prolonged nitrous-oxide anaesthesia. *Lancet* 1956;i:527–530.
31. Amess J A L, Burman J F, Rees G M, Nancekievill D G, Mollin D L. Megaloblastic haemopoiesis in patients receiving nitrous oxide. *Lancet* 1978;ii:339–342.
32. Sahenk Z, Mendell J R, Couri D, Nachtman J. Polyneuropathy from inhalation of N₂O cartridges through a whipped-cream dispenser. *Neurology* 1978;28:485–487.
33. Layzer R B. Myeloneuropathy after prolonged exposure to nitrous oxide. *Lancet* 1978;ii:1227–1230.
34. Banks R G S, Henderson R J, Pratt J M. Reactions of gases in solution. Part III. Some reactions of nitrous oxide with transition metal complexes. *J Chem Soc (A)* 1968;3:2886–2890.
35. Banerjee R V, Matthews R G. Cobalamin-de-

pendent methionine synthase. *FASEB J* 1990;4: 1450–1459.
36. Koppenol W H. Thermodynamic considerations on the generation of hydroxyl radicals from nitrous oxide—no laughing matter. *Free Rad Biol Med* 1991;10:85–87.
37. Deacon R, Lumb M, Perry J, et al. Selective inactivation of vitamin B₁₂ in rats by nitrous oxide. *Lancet* 1978;ii:1023–1024.
38. Kondo H, Osborne M L, Kolhouse J F, et al. Nitrous oxide has multiple deleterious effects on cobalamin metabolism and causes decreases in activities of both mammalian cobalamin-dependent enzymes in rats. *J Clin Invest* 1981;67: 1270–1283.
39. Xue G P, Snoswell A M, Runciman W B. Perturbation of methionine metabolism in sheep with nitrous oxide-induced inactivation of cobalamin. *Biochem Int* 1986;12:61–69.
40. Everman B W, Koblin D D. Aging, chronic administration of ethanol, and acute exposure to nitrous oxide: effects on vitamin B₁₂ and folate status in rats. *Mech Ageing Dev* 1992; 62:229–243.
41. Deacon R, Lumb M, Perry J, et al. Inactivation of methionine synthase by nitrous oxide. *Eur J Biochem* 1980;104:419–422.
42. Koblin D D, Watson J E, Deady J E, Stokstad E L R, Eger E I II. Inactivation of methionine synthetase by nitrous oxide in mice. *Anesthesiology* 1981;54:318–324.
43. Koblin D D, Waskell L, Watson J E, Stokstad E L R, Eger E I II. Nitrous oxide inactivates methionine synthetase in human liver. *Anesth Analg* 1982;61:75–78.
44. Royston B D, Nunn J F, Weinbren H K, Royston D, Cormack R S. Rate of inactivation of human and rodent hepatic methionine synthase by nitrous oxide. *Anesthesiology* 1988;68:213–216.
45. Wilson S D, Horne D W. Effect of nitrous oxide inactivation of vitamin B₁₂ on the levels of folate coenzymes in rat bone marrow, kidney, brain, and liver. *Arch Biochem Biophys* 1986; 244:248–253.
46. Weir D G, Keating S, Molloy A, et al. Methylation deficiency causes vitamin B₁₂-associated neuropathy in the pig. *J Neurochem* 1988;51: 1949–1952.
47. Brennt C E, Smith J R. The inhibitory effects of nitrous oxide and methylmercury *in vivo* on methionine synthase (EC 2.1.1.13) activity in brain, liver, ovary and spinal cord of the rat. *Gen Pharmacol* 1989;20:427–431.
48. Brodsky J B, Baden J M, Serra M, Kundomai Y. Nitrous oxide inactivates methionine synthetase activity in rat testis. *Anesthesiology* 1984;61:66–68.
49. Landon M J, Creagh-Barry P, McArthur S, Charlett A. Influence of vitamin B₁₂ status on the inactivation of methionine synthase by nitrous oxide. *Br J Anaesth* 1992;69:81–86.
50. Keating J N, Weir D G, Scott J M. Demonstration of methionine synthetase in intestinal mucosal cells of the rat. *Clin Sci* 1985;69:287–292.

51. Perry J, Deacon R, Lumb M, Chanarin I. Impaired formylation and uptake of tetrahydrofolate by rat small gut following cobalamin inactivation. *Biochim Biophys Acta* 1987;923:286–290.

52. Rosenblatt D S, Cooper B A, Pottier A, Lue-Shing H, Matiaszuk N, Grauer K. Altered vitamin B_{12} metabolism in fibroblasts from a patient with megaloblastic anemia and homocystinuria due to a new defect in methionine biosynthesis. *J Clin Invest* 1984;74:2149–2156.

53. Boss G R. Cobalamin inactivation decreases purine and methionine synthesis in cultured lymphoblasts. *J Clin Invest* 1985;76:213–218.

54. Christensen B, Refsum H, Garras A, Ueland P M. Homocysteine remethylation during nitrous oxide exposure of cells cultured in media containing various concentrations of folates. *J Pharmacol Exp Ther* 1992;261:1096–1105.

55. Sharer N M, Nunn J F, Royston JP, Chanarin I. Effects of chronic exposure to nitrous oxide on methionine synthase activity. *Br J Anaesth* 1983;55:693–700.

56. Koblin D D, Tomerson B W. Dimethylthiourea, a hydroxyl radical scavenger, impedes the inactivation of methionine synthase by nitrous oxide in mice. *Br J Anaesth* 1990;64:214–223.

57. Koblin D D, Tomerson B W. Methionine synthase activities in mice following acute exposures to ethanol and nitrous oxide. *Biochem Pharmacol* 1989;38:1353–1358.

58. Alston T A. Inhibition of vitamin B_{12}-dependent methionine biosynthesis by chloroform and carbon tetrachloride. *Biochem Pharmacol* 1991;42:R25–R28.

59. Sharer N M, Monk S J, Nunn J F. No effect of hyperbaric oxygen on methionine synthetase activity in rats. *Anesthesiology* 1983;59:440–441.

60. Koblin D D, Everman B W. Vitamin B_{12} and folate status in rats after chronic administration of ethanol and acute exposure to nitrous oxide. *Alcoholism Clin Exp Res* 1991;15:543–548.

61. Baden J M, Serra M, Mazze R I. Inhibition of fetal methionine synthetase activity by nitrous oxide. *Br J Anaesth* 1984;56:523–526.

62. Black K A, Tephly T R. Effects of nitrous oxide and methotrexate administration on hepatic methionine synthetase and dihydrofolate reductase activities, hepatic folates, and formate oxidation in rats. *Mol Pharmacol* 1983;23:724–730.

63. Muir M, Chanarin I. Conversion of endogenous cobalamins into microbiologically inactive cobalamin analogues in rats by exposure to nitrous oxide. *Br J Haematol* 1984;58:517–523.

64. Gokben M, Esener Z. Effect of nitrous oxide on serum vitamin B_{12} levels under surgical anesthesia. *Acta Anaesth Belg* 1985;36:71–77.

65. Koblin D D, Tomerson B W, Waldman F M, Lampe G H, Wauk L Z, Eger E I II. Effect of nitrous oxide on folate and vitamin B_{12} metabolism in patients. *Anesth Analg* 1990;71:610–617.

66. O'Leary P W, Combs M J, Schilling R F. Synergistic deleterious effects of nitrous oxide exposure and vitamin B_{12} deficiency. *J Lab Clin Med* 1985;105:428–431.

67. Van de List, Combs M, Schilling R F. Nitrous oxide and vitamin B_{12} deficiency interact adversely on rat growth. *J Lab Clin Med* 1986;108:346–348.

68. Shane B, Stokstad E L R. Vitamin B_{12}-folate interrelationships. *Annu Rev Nutr* 1985;5:115–141.

69. Chanarin I, Deacon R, Lumb M, Muir M, Perry J. Cobalamin-folate interrelations: a critical review. *Blood* 1985;66:479–489.

70. Ermens A A M, Refsum H, Rupreht J, et al. Monitoring cobalamin inactivation during nitrous oxide anesthesia by determination of homocysteine and folate in plasma and urine. *Clin Pharmacol Ther* 1991;49:385–393.

71. Lumb M, Perry J, Deacon R, Chanarin I. Changes in tissue folates accompanying nitrous oxide-induced inactivation of vitamin B_{12} in the rat. *Am J Clin Nutr* 1981;34:2412–2417.

72. Makar A B, Tephly T R. The role of formate and S-adenosylmethionine in the reversal of nitrous oxide inhibition of formate oxidation in the rat. *Mol Pharmacol* 1987;32:309–314.

73. Ermens A A M, Schoester M, Lindemans J, Abels J. Effect of nitrous oxide on folate coenzyme distribution and *de novo* synthesis of thymidylate in human bone marrow cells. *Tox Vitro* 1992;6:133–137.

74. Brody T, Stokstad E L R. Nitrous oxide provokes changes in folylpenta- and hexagluta-mates. *J Nutr* 1990;120:71–80.

75. Horne D W, Patterson D, Cook R J. Effect of nitrous oxide inactivation of vitamin B_{12}-dependent methionine synthetase on the subcellular distribution of folate coenzymes in rat liver. *Arch Biochem Biophys* 1989;270:729–733.

76. Lumb M, Deacon R, Perry J, Chanarin I. Oxidation of 5-methyltetrahydrofolate in cobalamin-inactivated rats. *Biochem J* 1989;258:907–910.

77. Deacon R, Perry J, Lumb M, Chanarin I. Formate metabolism in the cobalamin-inactivated rat. *Br J Haematol* 1990;74:354–359.

78. Skacel P O, Hewlett A M, Lewis J D, Lumb M, Nunn J F, Chanarin I. Studies on the haemopoietic toxicity of nitrous oxide in man. *Br J Haematol* 1983;53:189–200.

79. Parry T E, Laurence A S, Blackmore J A, Roberts B. Serum valine, methionine and isoleucine levels in patients anaesthetized with and without nitrous oxide. *Clin Lab Haematol* 1985;7:317–326.

80. Nunn J F, Sharer N M, Bottiglieri T, Rossiter J. Effect of short-term administration of nitrous oxide on plasma concentrations of methionine, tryptophan, phenylalanine and S-adenosyl methionine in man. *Br J Anaesth* 1986;58:1–10.

81. Royston B D, Bottiglieri T, Nunn J F. Short-term effect of nitrous oxide on methionine and S-adenosyl methionine concentrations. *Br J Anaesth* 1989;62:419–424.

82. Makar A B, Tephly T R. Effect of nitrous oxide

and methionine treatments on hepatic S-adenosylmethionine and methylation reactions in the rat. *Mol Pharmacol* 1983;24:124–128.

83. Lumb M, Sharer N, Deacon R, et al. Effects of nitrous oxide-induced inactivation of cobalamin on methionine and S-adenosylmethionine metabolism in the rat. *Biochim Biophys Acta* 1983;756:354–359.

84. Vina J R, Davis D W, Hawkins R A. The influence of nitrous oxide on methionine, S-adenosylmethionine, and other amino acids. *Anesthesiology* 1986;64:490–494.

85. Dorris R L. The effect of nitrous oxide on S-adenosylmethionine levels in mouse brain. *J Pharm Pharmacol* 1991;43:369–370.

86. Molloy A M, Weir D G, Kennedy G, Kennedy S, Scott J M. A new high performance liquid chromatographic method for the simultaneous measurement of S-adenosylmethionine and S-adenosylhomocysteine. Concentrations in pig tissues after inactivation of methionine synthase by nitrous oxide. *Biomed Chromatog* 1990;4:257–260.

87. Deacon R, Perry J, Lumb M, Chanarin I. Increased urinary excretion of formiminoglutamic acid in nitrous oxide-treated rats and its reduction by methionine. *Eur J Biochem* 1983; 129:627–628.

88. Koblin D D, Tomerson B W, Waldman F M. Disruption of folate and vitamin B$_{12}$ metabolism in aged rats following exposure to nitrous oxide. *Anesthesiology* 1990;73:506–512.

89. Hawkins R A, Snider M T, Russell G B, Davis D W, Biebuyck J F. Does nitrous oxide inactivation of methionine synthase decrease folic acid activity in man? *Anesthesiology* 1987;67: A292.

90. Armstrong P, Rae P W H, Gray W M, Spence A A. Nitrous oxide and formiminoglutamic acid: excretion in surgical patients and anaesthetists. *Br J Anaesth* 1991;66:163–169.

91. McKenna B, Weir D G, Scott J M. The induction of functional vitamin B$_{12}$ deficiency in rats by exposure to nitrous oxide. *Biochim Biophys Acta* 1980;628:314–321.

92. Deacon R, Chanarin I, Perry J, Lumb M. The effect of folate analogues on thymidine utilization by human and rat marrow cells and the effect on the deoxyuridine suppression test. *Postgrad Med J* 1981;57:611–616.

93. O'Sullivan H, Jannings F, Ward K, McCann S, Scott J M, Weir D G. Human bone marrow biochemical function and megaloblastic hematopoiesis after nitrous oxide anesthesia. *Anesthesiology* 1981;55:645–649.

94. Kano Y, Sakamoto S, Sakuraya K, et al. Effects of leukovorin and methylcobalamin with N$_2$O anesthesia. *J Lab Clin Med* 1984;104:711–717.

95. Healy C E, Drown D B, Sharma R P. Short-term toxicity of nitrous oxide on the immune, hemopoietic, and endocrine systems in CD-1 mice. *Toxic Indust Health* 1990;6:57–70.

96. Deacon R, Perry J, Lumb M, Chanarin I. Effect of cobalamin inactivation on folate-dependent transformylases involved in purine synthesis in rats. *Biochem J* 1985;227:67–71.

97. Heyer E J, Simpson D M, Bodis-Wollner I, Diamond S P. Nitrous oxide: clinical and electrophysiological investigation of neurologic complications. *Neurology* 1986;36:1618–1622.

98. Stacy C B, Di Rocco A, Gould R J. Methionine in the treatment of nitrous oxide-induced neuropathy and myeloneuropathy. *J Neurol* 1992; 239:401–403.

99. Scott J M, Dinn J J, Wilson P, Weir D G. Pathogenesis of subacute combined degeneration: a result of methyl group deficiency. *Lancet* 1981;ii:334–337.

100. Metz J, van der Westhuyzen J. The fruit bat as an experimental model of the neuropathy of cobalamin deficiency. *Comp Biochem Physiol* 1987;88A:171–177.

101. Viera-Makings E, Metz J, van der Westhuyzen J, Bottiglieri T, Chanarin I. Cobalamin neuropathy. Is S-adenosylhomocysteine toxicity a factor? *Biochem J* 1990;266:707–711.

102. Viera-Makings E, Chetty N, Reavis S C, Metz J. Methylmalonic acid metabolism and nervous system fatty acids in cobalamin-deficient fruit bats receiving supplements of methionine, valine, and isoleucine. *Biochem J* 1991;275:585–590.

103. Dyck P J, Grina L A, Lambert E H, et al. Nitrous oxide neurotoxicity studies in man and rat. *Anesthesiology* 1980;53:205–209.

104. Koblin D D, Dong D E, Eger E I II. Tolerance of mice to nitrous oxide. *J Pharmacol Exp Ther* 1979;211:317–325.

105. Harper M H, Winter P M, Johnson B H, Koblin D D, Eger E I II. Withdrawal convulsions in mice after nitrous oxide. *Anesth Analg* 1980; 59:19–21.

106. Dolin S J, Little H J. Effects of "nitrendipine" on nitrous oxide anesthesia, tolerance, and physical dependence. *Anesthesiology* 1989;70: 91–97.

107. Rodier P M, Aschner M, Lewis L S, Koeter H B W M. Cell proliferation in developing brain after brief exposure to nitrous oxide or halothane. *Anesthesiology* 1986;64:680–687.

108. Black K A, Eells J T, Noker P E, Hawtrey C A, Tephly T R. Role of hepatic tetrahydrofolate in the species difference in methanol toxicity. *Proc Natl Acad Sci USA* 1985;82:3854–3858.

109. Eells J T, Makar A B, Noker P E, Tephly T R. Methanol poisoning and formate oxidation in nitrous oxide-treated rats. *J Pharmacol Exp Ther* 1981;217:57–61.

110. Rice S A, Mazze R I, Baden J M. Effects of subchronic intermittent exposure to nitrous oxide in Swiss Webster mice. *JEPTO* 1985;6:271–282.

111. Eger E I II, Lampe G H, Wauk L Z, Whitendale P, Cahalan M K, Donegan J H. Clinical pharmacology of nitrous oxide: an argument for its continued use. *Anesth Analg* 1990; 71:575–585.

112. Lampe G H, Wauk L Z, Donegan J H, et al.

Effect on outcome of prolonged exposure of patients to nitrous oxide. *Anesth Analg* 1990; 71:586–590.

113. Kozmary S V, Lampe G H, Benefiel D, et al. No finding of increased myocardial ischemia during or after carotid endarterectomy under anesthesia with nitrous oxide. *Anesth Analg* 1990;71:591–596.

114. Lampe G H, Wauk L Z, Whitendale P, et al. Postoperative hypoxemia after nonabdominal surgery: a frequent event not caused by nitrous oxide. *Anesth Analg* 1990;71:597–601.

115. Lampe G H, Wauk L Z, Whitendale P, Way W L, Murray W, Eger E I II. Nitrous oxide does not impair hepatic function in young or old surgical patients. *Anesth Analg* 1990;71: 606–609.

116. Waldman F M, Koblin D D, Lampe G H, Wauk L Z, Eger E I II. Hematologic effects of nitrous oxide in surgical patients. *Anesth Analg* 1990; 71:618–624.

117. Nunn J F, Sharer N, Royston D, Watts R W E, Purkiss P, Worth H G. Serum methionine and hepatic enzyme activity in anaesthetists exposed to nitrous oxide. *Br J Anaesth* 1982; 54:593–597.

118. Salo M, Rajamaki A, Nikoskelainen J. Absence of signs of vitamin B$_{12}$–nitrous oxide interaction in operating theatre personnel. *Acta Anaesth Scand* 1984;28:106–108.

119. Sweeney B, Bingham R M, Amos R J, Petty A C, Cole P V. Toxicity of bone marrow in dentists exposed to nitrous oxide. *Br Med J* 1985; 291:567–569.

120. Peric M, Vranes Z, Marusic M. Immunological disturbances in anaesthetic personnel chronically exposed to high occupational concentrations of nitrous oxide and halothane. *Anaesthesia* 1991;46:531–537.

121. Cohen E N, Brown B W, Wu M L, et al. Occupational disease in dentistry and chronic exposure to trace anesthetic gases. *J Am Dent Assoc* 1980;101:21–31.

122. Rowland A S, Baird D D, Weinberg C R, Shore D L, Shy C M, Wilcox A J. Reduced fertility among women employed as dental assistants exposed to high levels of nitrous oxide. *N Engl J Med* 1992;327:993–997.

123. Baird P A. Occupational exposure to nitrous oxide—not a laughing matter. *N Engl J Med* 1992;327:1026–1027.

124. Nunn J F, Sharer N M, Gorchein A, Jones J A, Wickramasinghe S N. Megaloblastic haemopoiesis after multiple short-term exposure to nitrous oxide. *Lancet* 1982;i:1379–1381.

125. Brett C M, Wara W M, Hamilton W K. Anesthesia for infants during radiotherapy. *Anesthesiology* 1986;64:402–405.

126. Griswold J D, Vacanti F X, Goudsouzian N G. Twenty-tree sequential out-of-hospital halothane anesthetics in an infant. *Anesth Analg* 1988;67:779–781.

127. Schilling R F. Is nitrous oxide a dangerous anesthetic for vitamin B$_{12}$-deficient subjects? *JAMA* 1986;255:1605–1606.

128. Berger J J, Modell J H, Sypert G W. Megaloblastic anemia and brief exposure to nitrous oxide—a causal relationship? *Anesth Analg* 1988; 67:197–198.

129. Van Achterbergh S M, Vorster B J, Heyns A D P. The effect of sepsis and short-term exposure to nitrous oxide on the bone marrow and the metabolism of vitamin B$_{12}$ and folate. *SAMJ* 1990;78:260–262.

130. Amos R J, Amess J A L, Hinds C J, Mollin D L. Incidence and pathogenesis of acute megaloblastic bone marrow change in patients receiving intensive care. *Lancet* 1982;ii:835–839.

131. Amos R J, Amess J A L, Hinds C J, Mollin D L. Investigations into the effect of nitrous oxide anaesthesia on folate metabolism in patients receiving intensive care. *Chemioterapia* 1985;4:393–399.

132. Nunn J F, Chanarin I, Tanner A G, Owen E R T C. Megaloblastic bone marrow changes after repeated nitrous oxide anaesthesia. *Br J Anaesth* 1986;58:1469–1470.

133. Kano Y, Sakamoto S, Sakuraya K, et al. Effect of nitrous oxide on human bone marrow cells and its synergistic effect with methionine and methotrexate on functional folate deficiency. *Cancer Res* 1981;41:4698–4701.

134. Ermens A A M, Kroes A C M, Schoester M, van Lom K, Lindemans J, Abels J. Effect of cobalamin inactivation on folate metabolism of leukemic cells. *Leukemia Res* 1988;12:905–910.

135. Dudman N P B, Slowiaczek P, Tattersall H N. Methotrexate rescue by 5-methyltetrahydrofolate in lymphoblast cell lines. *Cancer Res* 1982;42:502–507.

136. Kroes A C M, Ermens A A M, Lindemans J, Abels J. Enhanced therapeutic effect of methotrexate in experimental rat leukemia after inactivation of cobalamin (vitamin B$_{12}$) by nitrous oxide. *Cancer Chemother Pharmacol* 1986;17: 114–120.

137. Ermens A A M, Schoester M, Spijkers L J M, Lindemans J, Abels J. Toxicity of methotrexate in rats preexposed to nitrous oxide. *Cancer Res* 1989;49:6337–6341.

138. Ludwig Breast Cancer Study Group. Toxic effect of early adjuvant chemotherapy for breast cancer. *Lancet* 1983;ii:542–544.

139. Goldhirsch A, Gelber R D, Tattersall M N H, Rudenstam C M, Cavalli F. Methotrexate/nitrous oxide toxic interaction in perioperative chemotherapy for early breast cancer. *Lancet* 1987;ii:151.

140. Ueland P M, Refsum H, Wesenberg F, Kvinnsland S. Methotrexate therapy and nitrous oxide anesthesia. *N Engl J Med* 1986;314:1514.

141. Kroes A C M, Ermens A A M, Lindemans J, Abels J. More on methotrexate–nitrous oxide interaction. *N Engl J Med* 1986;315:895.

142. Gillman M A. Anti-neoplastic synergism of nitrous oxide and methotrexate in patients. *Br J Anaesth* 1988;60:349–350.

143. Truffa-Bachi J, Bonnet D, Guigon M, Benhamou E, Cosset M F, Auquier A. Effect of short nitrous oxide exposure on human bone

marrow progenitors. *Anesthesiology* 1992;77: A405.

144. Lederhaas G, Negrin R, Brodsky J B, Brock-Utne J G. Safety of nitrous oxide for bone marrow harvests. *Anesthesiology* 1992;77:A1074.

145. McCloskey G F, Rinder H M, Rappeport J M. Nitrous oxide and bone marrow donation. *Anesthesiology* 1992;77:A1049.

146. Fausel D, Ryckman J V, Schubert A, Bolwell B, Green R. The influence of nitrous oxide on time of bone marrow engraftment. *Anesthesiology* 1992;77:A1073.

147. Shah N K, Kripke B J, Sanzone C F, Cosman E B. Histological evaluation of cutaneous wound healing in presence of nitrous oxide in rats. *Anesth Analg* 1978;57:527–533.

148. Algie T A, Seth A, Barbenel J C, Galloway D J, Gray W M, Spence A A. Nitrous oxide and wound healing. *Br J Anaesth* 1985;57:621–623.

149. Irish C L, Weisleider L, Mazer C D, Bell R S. Effect of nitrous oxide on impaired wound healing in mice. *Can J Anaesth* 1991;38:S135.

150. Crawford J S, Lewis M. Nitrous oxide in early human pregnancy. *Anaesthesia* 1986;41:900–905.

151. Mazze R I. Nitrous oxide during pregnancy. *Anaesthesia* 1986;41:897–899.

152. Gimsing P, Melgaard B, Andersen K, Vilstrup H, Hippe E. Vitamin B₁₂ and folate function in chronic alcoholic men with peripheral neuropathy and encephalopathy. *J Nutr* 1989;119:416–424.

153. Zinn S E, Fairley H B, Glenn J D. Liver function in patients with mild alcoholic hepatitis, after enflurane, nitrous oxide-narcotic, and spinal anesthesia. *Anesth Analg* 1985;64:487–490.

154. Daynes G. The initial management of alcoholism using oxygen and nitrous oxide: a transcultural study. *Int J Neurosci* 1989;49:83–86.

155. Pennypacker L C, Allen R H, Kelly J P, et al. High prevalence of cobalamin deficiency in elderly outpatients. *J Am Geriatr Soc* 1992;40: 1197–1204.

156. Burkes R L, Cohen H, Krailo M, Sinow R M, Carmel R. Low serum cobalamin levels occur frequently in the acquired immune deficiency syndrome and related disorders. *Eur J Haematol* 1987;38:141–147.

157. Sharar S R, Haberkern C M, Jack R, Scott C R. Anesthetic management of a child with methylmalonyl-coenzyme A mutase deficiency. *Anesth Analg* 1991;73:499–501.

158. Lassen H C A, Kristensen H S. Remission in chronic myeloid leukemia following prolonged nitrous oxide inhalation. *Dan Med Bull* 1959;6: 252–255.

159. Eastwood D W, Green C D, Lambdin M A, Gardner R. Effect of nitrous oxide on the white cell count in leukemia. *N Engl J Med* 1963; 268:297–299.

160. Ikeda K, Aosaki T, Furukawa Y, et al. Antileukemic effect of nitrous oxide in a patient with chronic myelogenous leukemia. *Am J Hematol* 1989;30:114.

161. Hornbein T F. Epilogue. In: Eger E I II, ed. *Nitrous oxide/N₂O*. New York: Elsevier, 1985: 355–357.

Anesthetic Toxicity, edited by
Susan A. Rice and Kevin J. Fish.
Raven Press, Ltd., New York © 1994.

9

Reproductive and Developmental Toxicity of Anesthetics in Animals

Susan A. Rice

*Susan A. Rice and Associates, Inc., Sunnyvale, California 94087, and Department of
Anesthesia, Stanford University School of Medicine, Stanford, California 94305*

Interest in the reproductive and developmental effects of the anesthetics stems from concern for the pregnant surgical patient and the anesthetic-exposed health care worker. Although most human operatories in the United States, Canada, the U.K., Europe, and Japan scavenge waste anesthetic gases, there are still techniques that offer the potential for relatively high exposure, such as administration by mask.

Epidemiologic studies of reproductive and developmental outcome are summarized in the chapter by Ebi and Rice. Some studies show an association between adverse reproductive or developmental outcomes and anesthetic administration, but none establish a causal relationship. This chapter summarizes selected laboratory studies designed to assess the role of anesthetics in reproductive and developmental toxicity.

REPRODUCTIVE AND DEVELOPMENTAL TOXICITY

Reproductive toxicity is the manifestation of abnormalities in the ability to conceive and produce liveborn offspring that is induced by drugs, chemicals, and physical forces (e.g., heat). Developmental toxicity is the manifestation of abnormalities in the development of the conceptus that is induced by these same agents.

Reproductive toxicity may result in failure of ovulation, prevention of fertilization, interference with ovum or early embryo transfer, or failure of or abnormality in implantation. The outcome of developmental toxicity is death, morphologic malformation, growth retardation, or functional disorder of a biochemical, physiologic, or behavioral nature. Teratogenicity is one form of developmental toxicity. Teratogenic changes are alterations in cell, tissue, organ, and system formation, whereas other toxicologic changes are degenerative and are not directly related to the formation of cells, tissues, and organs.

One can think of toxic (including teratogenic) effects as being either reversible or irreversible. Reversible effects result in only transient changes in the organism because of inherent repair mechanisms or redundant functions. Irreversible effects either cause death or produce long-lasting changes in the organism. Resorption in rodents and spontaneous abortion in humans are the result of irreversible lethal effects. Irreversible effects may also be compatible with life. Structural, behavioral, and functional abnormalities are the result of specific teratogenic effects. Embryonic, fetal, and organ system growth retardation generally are the result of general toxic effects. An agent that is a selective developmental toxicant (i.e., teratogen) produces adverse effects in offspring without causing severe toxic effects in the mother. The distinction between teratogenic and general toxicologic changes is unclear at times. For example, runting or increased body size may result from either teratogenic or toxicologic mechanisms.

The traditional teaching of teratology is that teratogenesis occurs only during organogenesis and histogenesis. It was thought that exposure during preimplantation, the period of blastocyst formation, results either in early death or in repair and complete recovery. This tenet has been challenged with recent evidence that certain agents can cause an increased incidence of malformations following exposure of the early postfertilization conceptus (1). The mechanism is unclear, and malformations following anesthetic exposure during this early developmental period have not been reported.

With the possible exception of the preceding information, susceptibility to teratogenic insult and the type of developmental abnormality and its severity are dependent on the developmental stage, the intensity and duration of exposure, and the specificity of the teratogen for its target cell or tissue. Different combinations of stage, exposure, and specificity result in different patterns of effects. Both the severity of abnormalities and the number of affected individuals are increased in a dose-dependent manner when teratogens are administered during a susceptible period.

Susceptibility of a specific tissue, organ, or biochemical or physiologic system depends on the period during which it undergoes organogenesis and histogenesis. The organism is especially sensitive to morphologic abnormalities during organogenesis and to growth retardation, functional disorders, and transplacental carcinogenesis during histogenesis. Once the formation of a particular cell or tissue type or physiologic or biochemical system is complete, a teratogen cannot exert a teratogenic effect. Therefore, the end of histogenesis for a system precludes any teratogenic action on that system by a drug or chemical. The rel-

ative timing of organogenesis and histogenesis is different for each system, and because histogenesis continues into the neonatal period, the neonate as well as the fetus is susceptible to teratogenic action. For example, in both humans and other species, including rat, the brain continues developing into the postnatal period; thus the vulnerable period is extended well past birth. Animal studies unequivocally demonstrate behavioral abnormalities in the absence of gross morphologic abnormalities. The CNS is particularly vulnerable to the toxic effects of drugs administered during development because the specialized CNS cell population is produced over an extended period of time. What is even more important is that the CNS has little or no ability to replace injured or missing neurons. The brain regions actively forming at the time of exposure will be most affected.

A precise molecular mechanism has not been accepted unequivocally for any teratogenic agent. In spite of this lack of agreement on a mechanism for any specific compound, there is agreement that the following molecular mechanisms may be involved in teratogenesis. The teratogen may cause a mutation, interfere in mitosis, alter nucleic acid integrity or function, alter essential biosynthesis by limiting or removing precursors and substrates, alter energy sources, inhibit essential enzymes, alter cellular osmolality, interact with cellular receptors, interfere with intercellular communication, or alter membrane characteristics (2–5). There are many mechanisms that produce abnormal development. Some, such as mutations that result in specific biochemical abnormalities and chromosomal nondisjunction, are well established. Others, such as interferences with cell membranes, are less certain mechanisms of teratogenicity. The pathogenesis of malformations at the molecular level is transferred to higher levels of organization, that is, to cells and tissues. The pathogenic mechanisms at these levels may then be categorized into general mechanisms: cell death, excessive or reduced cell proliferation, reduced biosynthesis of compounds essential for growth, impeded morphogenic movement, altered cell interactions, and mechanical disruption or rearrangement of cells and tissues.

Part of the difficulty in determining mechanisms of action for teratogens and other developmental toxicants is identifying the initiating adverse event. Identifying causes and investigating mechanisms in humans are inherently difficult because of ethical issues, apart from the practical considerations. *In vivo* and *in vitro* mammalian and nonmammalian test systems have been developed to study under controlled conditions the potential of agents to produce developmental toxicity. These tests help to identify the mutagenic, carcinogenic, reproductive, teratogenic, and functional effects of many agents.

As discussed in the chapter by Lukas, it is impossible to determine which species will be the most appropriate in terms of predicting which adverse effects may be caused in humans with a particular agent. This emphasizes the necessity to evaluate effects in multiple species. The differences in species reactions could be due to differences in timing of exposure, species differences in critical periods, metabolism, developmental patterns, placentation, or mechanisms of action. Table 1 summarizes some reproductive and developmental characteristics of humans and four species used for reproductive and developmental studies. The role of the genotype and its in-

teractions with environmental factors in teratogenic susceptibility also must be considered because it has long been recognized that equivalent exposure to a specific teratogen produces morphologic abnormalities in some, but not all, exposed individuals.

The following sections of this chapter summarize the results of selected studies of experimental mammalian and nonmammalian models to evaluate the potential reproductive and developmental toxicity of anesthetics.

Inhaled Anesthetics

The inhaled anesthetics have been studied in many mammalian and nonmammalian test systems. Because of the large literature base on this topic, only selected studies are included in the summaries and discussions. There are many review articles for the interested reader (6–9).

Mutagenicity

Mutagenicity has received much attention in recent years in the scientific community and the lay press. The mutagenic potential of drugs and chemicals relates not only to the potential for carcinogenicity but also to teratogenesis and the possible threat of producing genetic abnormalities that are passed to future generations. Mutations are changes in the genetic information in cells. Changes in germ cells can be passed from

TABLE 1. *Reproductive and developmental characteristics of selected species*[a]

Species	Placenta	Implantation (days)	Gestation (days)	Early differentiation ends (day)	Organogenesis (days)	Primitive streak (day)
Mouse	Hemotrichorial	4.5–5	19–20	9	7–16	7–8
Rat	Hemotrichorial	5.5–6	21–22	10	9–17	8.5–9
Rabbit	Hemodichorial	7–7.5	30–32	9	7–20	7–8
Hamster	Hemotrichorial	4.5–5	16	8	7–14	6–7
Human	Hemomonochorial	6–10	267–270	21	20–55	14–20

[a]Data gathered from various sources including references 95 and 96.

one generation to the next; changes in somatic cells cannot.

Only the inhaled anesthetics have been tested extensively for mutagenic activity. These agents have been examined in a variety of test systems, including bacteria, yeast, *Drosophila, Tradescantia,* mammalian cells in culture, and intact mammals (8–11). The only mutagenic anesthetics are those that contain a vinyl moiety (a double-bonded carbon structure) or acquire a vinyl group via metabolism. Only divinyl ether and fluroxene produce unequivocal positive mutagenic responses, and only trichloro-ethylene produces a weak mutagenic response in test systems. These findings appear consistent with the high reactivity and mutagenicity of vinyl compounds as a class (12). The anesthetics currently in use are not mutagenic from all the existing data.

In Vitro *Developmental Test Systems*

Many *in vitro* test systems have been developed to assess developmental toxicity. Several of these test systems appear especially relevant because of the use of technology to overcome problems in female and male fertility (e.g., oocyte retrieval, embryo transfer).

To test the effects of anesthetics on fertilization and subsequent development, sea urchin (*Lytechinus variegatus*) eggs were incubated with halothane, enflurane, or methoxyflurane (13). Anesthetic concentrations ranged from 0.3 to 2.5 mM, which corresponded to concentrations in the gas phase of 0.58% to 4.8% for halothane, 0.63% to 5.22% for enflurane, and 0.1% to 0.85% for methoxyflurane. After 15 minutes of incubation, sperm were introduced, and fertilization proceeded. The eggs were removed from the anesthetic solution and allowed to develop through the first cell division, at which time they were evaluated. At the highest concentration (2.5 mM), all the anesthetics significantly increased the percent of eggs exhibiting an abnormal (asymmetric) cleavage pattern, which fore-

tells of embryonic death before gastrulation. Embryo cleavage was least affected by enflurane, with only a 2% increase in abnormal cleavage. Methoxyflurane increased abnormal cleavage by 32%, and halothane-exposed embryos exhibited a 96% increase in abnormal cleavage. Halothane, but not the other agents, also produced significant toxic effects at concentrations as low as 0.3 mM. The mechanism for producing an abnormal cleavage pattern is unclear because it is not directly related to the anesthetic potency of these agents in humans.

Drosophila melanogaster flies derived from larvae exposed during development (metamorphosis) to 20% or 40% nitrous oxide (N_2O) exhibited no morphologic abnormalities (14). Enflurane, isoflurane, or halothane at 0.1% or 0.2% likewise produced no abnormalities. However, both enflurane and isoflurane decreased the number of flies and increased the duration of metamorphosis. These end points correspond to the mammalian equivalent of increased postimplantation loss and delayed maturation.

Chetkowski and Nass (15) examined the effects of N_2O and isoflurane on mouse embryo development. B6C3F$_1$ mice, a mouse strain used in many *in vitro* fertilization (IVF) programs for quality control, were superovulated and then mated. Two-cell embryos were collected, randomly assigned to treatment groups, and incubated in phosphate-buffered saline exposed for 30 minutes to 60% N_2O, 1.5% isoflurane, or 60% N_2O in combination with 0.75% isoflurane. The embryos were allowed to develop for 72 hours, at which time 79% of controls had developed to the blastocyst stage. Blastocyst development was unaffected by N_2O but was significantly reduced to 82% of that of controls by concomitant N_2O and isoflurane exposure. When cells were incubated with 1.5% isoflurane, a further decrease, to approximately 55% of control values, was observed. The authors reported anecdotally that the cleavage rate of 187 mature nonatretic oocytes collected during 22 laparoscopies showed no adverse effects of N_2O-narcotic anesthesia administered at the time of oocyte retrieval for IVF procedures.

Embryo culture is a technique that has gained more acceptance in recent years. At present, there are no standardized, validated testing methods for screening teratogenic agents, but the technique is well established in the research arena. The most significant results related to this technique and the anesthetics are for N_2O. These results are similar to those observed with *in vivo* testing, and, therefore, they are discussed in the following section on *in vivo* systems.

Mammalian **In Vivo** *Test Systems*

A problem always encountered with epidemiologic studies and often encountered with clinical studies is that the timing of mating and conception is known only within weeks. With animal studies, the timing can be easily pinpointed within hours. Thus, *in vivo* animal models can offer a significant advantage in determining causation of an exposure and an adverse outcome.

There are several differences between humans and rodents that require clarification. For the purpose of this discussion, the day that a copulatory plug is found in mated female rats or mice or sperm are observed in a vaginal smear is defined as day 0 of gestation (GD 0). The rat and mouse have a bipartite uterus and multiple pregnancies and, unlike humans, do not abort but rather resorb embryonic and early fetal wastage. Thus, resorptions are the rodent equivalent of human spontaneous abortions. Fetuses found dead at birth or dead at the time of cesarean section are the equivalent of human stillbirths. Delayed ossification is an indication of delayed fetal maturation and not necessarily a teratogenic effect. Decreased fetal weight or length may be the result of either teratogenesis or delayed maturation.

Potent Volatile Anesthetics

The potent volatile anesthetics have been studied sufficiently in the postimplantation period to suggest that there are no adverse morphologic effects at subanesthetic concentrations. Adverse behavioral effects have been documented at subanesthetic concentrations in rats but not humans. At anesthetic concentrations, however, both teratogenic and behavioral effects are observed in animal models. It is unclear if these adverse outcomes are the result of direct anesthetic effects on the conceptus or indirect anesthetic effects via physiologic changes in the mother or conceptus. Table 2 briefly summarizes selected reproductive and developmental effects observed in some studies of the potent volatile agents.

The majority of studies on the potent volatile anesthetic agents have been performed with halothane. An exhaustive review was published by Baeder and Albrecht (9). The summary presented in this chapter includes a number of studies that exemplify the range of concentrations studied and the observations made.

Several studies have been performed at trace and subanesthetic concentrations. Male Sprague-Dawley (SD) rats were exposed to 10 ppm halothane 5 days/week over 36 or 64 days and then were mated to unexposed females (16). Fetal weights were slightly decreased in the presence of larger litters in the 36-day but not the 64-day exposure group. No adverse effects were seen when females were exposed for 8 hours/day to 10 ppm for 5 days/week throughout pregnancy and over a 31-day period before mating with unexposed males. SD rats were exposed to halothane at concentrations ranging from 0.005% to 0.32% for 8 hours/day on GD 8–12 or to 0.16% throughout gestation (17). Only the group exposed to 0.16% throughout gestation exhibited decreased fetal weights. Exposure of SD rats to 0.16% or 0.32% halothane for 8 hours/day throughout gestation likewise resulted in decreased fetal weights and some slight

TABLE 2. Reproductive and developmental toxicity of the potent volatile anesthetics: Adverse effects on selected end points[a]

Anesthetic	Concentration[b] (%)	(ppm)	Species	Exposure period (days)[c]	Exposure duration	Reproductive toxicity	Maternal toxicity Death	Maternal toxicity Weight	Developmental toxicity (embryo or fetus) Death	Weight	Maturation	Major malformations Skeletal	External or Visceral	Reference
Enflurane	0.002	20	Rat	Premating and 0–20	8 h/d[d] 5 d/week	N[e]	N	N	N	Y	N	N	—	16
	0.02	200	Rat	Premating and 0–20	8 h/d 5 d/week	N	N	N	N	N	N	N	—	34
	0.05	500	Mouse	7–12	1 h/d	N	N	N	N	N	—	N	N	36
	0.32	3,200	Rat	9–14	1 h/d	N	N	N	N	Y	—	N	N	35
	0.75	7,500	Mouse	0–20	8 h/d	N	N	Y	N	Y	—	N	Y	36
	1.00	10,000	Mouse	7–12	1 h/d	N	N	N	N	Y	—	N	N	37
	1.25	12,500	Rat	6–15	4 h/d	N	N	N	N	N	N	N	N	36
	1.65	16,500	Rat	9–14	1 h/d	N	N	Y	N	Y	N	N	N	36
			Rat	8–10	6 h/d		N	Y	N	Y	N	N	N	38
				11–13	6 h/d									
				14–16	6 h/d									
Halothane	0.001	10	Rat	Premating and 0–20	5 d/week 8 h/d	N	N	N	N	N	N	N	—	16
	0.01	100	Rat	8–12	8 h/d	—	N	N	N	N	—	N	—	17
	0.16	1,600	Rat	8–12	8 h/d	—	N	N	N	N	—	N	—	
				0–20	8 h/d	—	N	N	N	Y	N	N	—	
	0.16	1,600	Rat	0–20	8 h/d	—	—	—	—	—	Z	N	Z	18
	0.30	3,000	Mouse	6–15	4 h/d	—	—	—	—	—	Y	N	Z	20
				Premating and 1–17	4 h/d	Y	Y	Y	N	Y	Y	—	—	19
	0.32	3,200	Rat	8–12	8 h/d	—	N	N	N	N	Y	N	—	17
				0–20	8 h/d	—	—	—	—	Y	?/	N	—	
	0.80	8,000	Rat	6	12 h	—	N	N	N	N	?	N	—	22
				6.5	12 h	—	N	N	N	N	?	N	—	
				7.0	12 h	—	N	N	N	N	?	N	—	
				7.5	12 h	—	N	N	N	N	?	N	—	
				8.0	12 h	—	N	N	N	N	?	N	—	
				8.5	12 h	—	N	N	N	N	?	N	—	
				9.0	12 h	—	N	N	N	N	?	N	—	
				9.5	12 h	—	Y	N	Y	N	?	Y[g]	—	
				10.0	12 h	—	Y	Y	Y	Y	Y	Y[g]	Y	
	1.00	10,000	Mouse	6–15	4 h/d	Y	—	—	—	Y	Y	Y	Y	20
				Premating and 1–17	4 h/d	Y	Y	Y	Y	Y	Y	N	N	19

Agent	Conc. (%)	Conc. (ppm)	Species	Days[c]	Duration[d]									Ref.[a]
Halothane and N₂O	1.35	13,500	Rat	1–5	1 h/d	N	N	N	N	N	N	N	N	21
	1.43	14,300	Rat	6–10	1 h/d	N	N	N	N	N	N	N	N	
	2.16	21,600	Rabbit	11–15	1 h/d	N	N	Y	N	N	N	N	N	
	2.30	23,000	Rabbit	6–9	1 h/d	N	N	N	N	N	N	N	N	23
	0.0001	1	Rabbit	10–14	1 h/d	N	N	N	N	N	N	N	N	
	0.005	50	Rat	15–18	1 h/d	Y	N	N	N	N	N	—	—	
				Premating and 1–15	7 h/d	N	N	N	N	N	N	N	N	
	0.001	10	Rat	Premating and 6–15	7 h/d	Y	N	Y	N	—	—	N	N	
	0.05	500	Rat	Premating and 1–15	7 h/d	N	N	N	Y	Y	Y	N	N	
	0.60	6,000	Hamster	6–15	3 h	N	N	N	N	—	—	—	—	24
	60.0	600,000	Hamster	8	3 h	N	N	N	N	N	N	N	N	
				9	3 h	N	N	N	Y	—	—	N	—	
				10	3 h	N	N	Y	Y	Y	—	Y	N	
Isoflurane	0.06	600	Mouse	6–15	4 h/d	N	N	N	Y	Y	N	Z	Z	40
	0.60	6,000	Mouse	6–15	4 h/d	N	N	N	Y	Y	Y	N	N	
	1.05	10,500	Rat	8–10	6 h/d	N	N	N	Z	Z	Z	N	N	37
				11–13	6 h/d	N	N	N	Y	Y	Y	N	N	
				14–16	6 h/d	N	N	N	N	N	N	N	N	
	1.63	16,300	Rat	1–5	1 h/d	N	N	N	N	N	N	N	N	41
	1.66	16,600	Rat	6–10	1 h/d	N	N	N	N	N	N	N	N	
	1.73	17,300	Rat	11–15	1 h/d	N	N	N	N	N	N	N	N	
	2.28	22,800	Rabbit	6–9	1 h/d	N	N	N	N	N	N	N	N	
	2.31	23,100	Rabbit	10–14	1 h/d	N	N	N	N	N	N	N	N	
	2.34	23,400	Rabbit	15–19	1 h/d	N	N	N	Y	Y	Y	N	N	
Methoxyflurane	0.0002	2	Mouse	6–15	4 h/d	N	N	N	Y	Y	Y	N	N	43
	0.006	60	Mouse	6–15	4 h/d	N	N	N	Y	Y	Y	N	N	
	0.01	100	Rat	0–20	8 h/d	—	—	—	—	Y	Y	—	—	18
	0.04	400	Rat	0–20	8 h/d	—	—	—	—	—	Y	—	—	35
	0.08	800	Rat	0–20	8 h/d	—	—	—	Y	—	Y	—	—	
	0.20	2,000	Mouse	6–15	4 h/d	N	N	N	Y	Y	Y	N	N	43

[a]Selected studies of reproductive and developmental toxicity.
[b]Not all concentrations are presented for each study listed.
[c]Days refer to days of pregnancy or gestation.
[d]h, hour; d, day.
[e]N, no significant effect; Y, significant effect or trend (e.g., when an adverse effect is present but numbers are low due to death or reproductive failure);—, the end point was not evaluated or information was not provided.
[f]?, decreased ossification cited but not quantified or related to a single day.
[g]Skeletal anomalies cited; unknown if major or minor.

developmental retardation indicated by delayed ossification at the highest concentration (18). No morphologic abnormalities were observed from external examination; viscera were not examined.

In two studies from the same laboratory, Swiss Webster (SW) mice were exposed to 0.1%, 0.3%, or 1% halothane for 4 hours/day over varied periods. In the study of reproductive effects, male and female rats were exposed for 5 days/week for 9 weeks before mating (19). The copulatory rate was decreased for females exposed to 1% halothane. The pregnancy rate for those that did copulate was decreased following exposure to 0.3% or 1% halothane. Males were not affected at exposures of 0.3% but did not sire any litters at exposure concentrations of 1%. Subsequent matings with untreated females showed no reduced reproductive indices for males. In the study of developmental toxicity, mice exposed on GD 6–15 to the subanesthetic concentrations of 0.1% or 0.3% produced no significant increases in major malformations or minor anomalies (20). Exposure at these subanesthetic concentrations for 9 weeks before mating and on GD 1–17 resulted in an increased incidence of delayed ossification and developmental variants at the 0.3% exposure level. Premating exposure to 1% halothane prevented conception and implantation in all but one dam. That dam had 4 fetuses, all with severe growth retardation. Exposure to 1% halothane only on GD 6–15 was lethal to 14 of 23 pregnant rats. Embryo lethality was 100% for 8 of the 9 remaining dams. In the one surviving litter, 5 of 5 fetuses suffered major malformations.

No adverse reproductive or teratogenic effects were observed, however, following exposure to halothane at anesthetizing concentrations in a study of two species (21). SD rats were exposed to approximately 1.4% halothane for 1 hour on 5 consecutive days starting on GD 1, 6, or 11, and New Zealand rabbits were exposed to approximately 2.2% to 2.3% halothane for 1 hour on GD 6–9, 10–14, or 15–18. No adverse effects were observed. Adverse reproductive effects likewise did not occur following exposure and subsequent mating to unexposed animals. Adverse effects have been reported, however, for SD rats exposed to 0.8% halothane for a single 12-hour period beginning in either the AM or PM on GD 6–10 (22). Both halothane-exposed and control dams lost weight up to 24 hours postexposure. Resorptions were significantly increased following daytime exposure on GD 7 (7.0) or GD 9 (9.0). Vertebral anomalies and lumbar ribs or rudiments were increased following daytime exposure on GD 8 (8.0) or nocturnal exposure on GD 9 (9.5). Lumbar ribs or rudiments also were increased following exposure on GD 10.0. Visceral examinations were not performed.

A few studies examined the combination of halothane and N_2O. In a study of trace concentrations, female and male SD rats were exposed to 1 ppm halothane with 50 ppm N_2O or to 10 ppm halothane with 500 ppm N_2O for 7 hours/day for 5 days/week for 12 weeks before mating. Pregnant rats were then again exposed on GD 1–15 or 6–15 (23). In rats exposed on GD 6–15, there were no significant increases in visceral or skeletal abnormalities in offspring, but both concentrations were associated with delayed skeletal ossification. Fetal weights and lengths were decreased at the higher concentrations. In rats exposed on GD 1–15 and allowed to deliver naturally, both concentrations significantly decreased the number of corpora lutea and the implantation efficiency and significantly increased the postimplantation loss. In study of near-anesthetizing concentrations, hamsters were exposed to 0.6% halothane with 60% N_2O for 3 hours on GD 8, 9, or 10 (24). Resorptions were increased following exposure only on GD 10, whereas fetal length and weight were decreased following exposure on either GD 9 or 10.

Several studies using trace concentrations of halothane have demonstrated significant behavioral effects. SD rats exposed chronically to 10 ppm halothane from conception to 60 days of age had enduring learning deficits when tested on a shock-motivated light–dark discrimination task and a food-motivated symmetric maze (25–27). Cerebral tissue showed electron microscopic evidence of neuronal degeneration, synaptic malformation, disruption of the nuclear envelope, and cell death (28). Albino, Norwegian rats were exposed for 8 hours/day for 5 days/week to 100 ppm halothane or continuously to 25 or 100 ppm halothane from GD 2 to postnatal day 60 (29). At 150 days of age, there was no effect in rats exposed to 25 ppm, but exposure at 100 ppm significantly decreased cognitive performance in a radial-arm maze. DUB/ICR mice exposed to subanesthetic 0.5% concentrations of halothane on GD 13 for 6 hours exhibited hypoactivity as young adults (30,31).

Significant behavioral effects have been observed following halothane exposure at anesthetic concentrations during gestation. On days 3, 10, or 17 of pregnancy, SD rats were anesthetized with 1.2% to 1.25% halothane for 2 hours. At 75 days of age or older, male offspring exposed on GD 3 or 10 were hyperalgesic and committed significantly more errors than expected in learning a shock-motivated, visual discrimination task. They also committed more errors than animals exposed on GD 17 (27,32). Mice exposed to 1% halothane for 30 minutes/day on GD 6 and 11 or on GD 14 and 17 took longer to learn a maze than did controls (33). Mice exposed to 2% halothane on GD 6 and 11 failed to learn the maze; those exposed on GD 14 and 17 exhibited slower learning.

Developmental and reproductive studies of enflurane have been conducted for concentrations ranging from trace to anesthetizing. Exposure of female SD rats to 20 or 200 ppm enflurane 5 days/week throughout gestation and over 28 days before mating with untreated males produced no in-

creased incidences of resorptions or major skeletal malformations in offspring. Visceral examinations were not performed (16,34). Fetuses exposed to 200 ppm enflurane exhibited an increased incidence of supernumerary ribs. Additional male rats were exposed to 20 or 200 ppm enflurane 5 days/week over 29 or 63 days, respectively, before mating with unexposed females. Both females and males exposed to 20 ppm, but not to 200 ppm, enflurane produced fetuses with slightly decreased weights. The decrease could be attributed to corresponding increased litter sizes.

SD rats exposed to 0.32% enflurane for 8 hours/day throughout gestation exhibited decreased fetal weights, but no other adverse effects were observed (35). Wistar rats exposed for 1 hour/day to 0.05% or 1.25% enflurane on GD 9–14 and ddY mice exposed for 1 hour to 0.05% to 0.75% enflurane on GD 7–12 exhibited no adverse reproductive or developmental effects (36). Similarly, no major skeletal or visceral malformations were observed following exposure of SW mice to concentrations as high as 1.0% enflurane for 4 hours/day on GD 6–15 (37). Six hours of exposure to 1.65% enflurane daily on GD 8–10, 11–13, or 14–16 had no significant teratogenic effects on SD rats (38). However, a significantly decreased weight gain in dams was observed for exposures on GD 14–16, and decreased fetal weights were observed for exposures on GD 8–10 and GD 14–16. Implantations were unaffected, and resorptions were not increased.

Two studies have examined the behavioral effects of prenatal enflurane exposure. Anesthetizing concentrations of enflurane (2% or 4%) administered to mice for 30 minutes on GD 6 and 11 or on GD 14 and 17 resulted in offspring exhibiting delayed learning in a maze (33). Subanesthetic exposure of Fischer 344 rats to enflurane (0.15%) for a greater period and duration, 6 hours/day from conception for 21 days, showed no adverse treatment effects on behavioral measures, activity, or shock-avoidance learning in offspring tested from 2 days to 90 weeks of age (39).

Few studies have been conducted with either isoflurane or methoxyflurane. Exposure of SW mice to 0.06% isoflurane for 4 hours/day on GD 6–15 produced no adverse effects, whereas decreased fetal weight, decreased ossification, and minor renal changes were seen following exposure to 0.6% isoflurane (40). Cleft palate was observed in 12% of these offspring. Data presented from other studies by these authors showed that exposure of mice to halothane or enflurane at concentrations equipotent to that of 0.6% isoflurane resulted in only 1.2% and 1.9% cleft palates, respectively, suggesting that the depth of anesthesia alone was not responsible for the increased rate of cleft palate in mice. Because mice can be prone to development of cleft palate, the rat was investigated to confirm teratogenic effects in a second species. To target specific periods of organ and system development for sensitivity to isoflurane, SD rats were exposed to 1.05% isoflurane for 6 hours/day on GD 8–10, 11–13, or 14–16 (38). No teratogenic effects were observed, although there were significant decreases in the weights of dams and fetuses exposed on GD 8–10 or 14–16. A similar lack of teratogenic and reproductive effects was observed for SD rats exposed to approximately 1.6% to 1.7% isoflurane for 1 hour on 5 consecutive days starting on GD 1, 6, or 11 and for New Zealand white rabbits exposed for 1 hour on 4 consecutive days beginning on GD 6, 10, or 15 to approximately 2.3% isoflurane (41). Delayed preweaning development of swimming ability and negative geotaxis and surface righting reflexes observed in SW mice exposed to 0.4%, but not 0.1%, isoflurane 4 hours/day on GD 6–15 are the only behavioral effects thus far reported (42).

SW/ICR mice exposed for 4 hours/day to 2, 60, or 2000 ppm (0.2%) methoxyflurane on GD 6–15 exhibited decreased fetal weight, decreased ossification, and delayed renal maturation at the highest concentration. Malformations were not increased (43). Exposure of SD rats to 0.01%, 0.04%, or 0.08% methoxyflurane for 8 hours/day throughout gestation resulted in decreased fetal weights and slight developmental retardation, indicated by delayed ossification at the highest concentration (18). There were no morphologic abnormalities observed by external examination.

Nitrous Oxide (N$_2$O)

Unlike the potent volatile anesthetics, N$_2$O is teratogenic to experimental animals without achieving anesthetizing concentrations. Relatively prolonged exposure, however, is required. Increased incidences of fetal resorptions and fetal visceral and skeletal abnormalities are observed when concentrations of 50% to 75% N$_2$O are delivered for 24-hour periods on selected days during organogenesis or when concentrations of 0.1% to 0.5% are delivered throughout pregnancy. Behavioral effects have been observed in some studies at concentrations and for durations of exposure below those that produce morphologic abnormalities. Studies of the reproductive, teratogenic, and behavioral effects of N$_2$O are discussed, followed by a summary of the biochemical effects related to and measured in the pregnant animal and her offspring.

Current interest in the teratogenic effects of N$_2$O started with two studies in the late 1960s that examined the effects of relatively high concentrations of N$_2$O administered for a prolonged period (44,45). Fink et al. (44) reported increased rates of resorptions, rib and vertebral abnormalities, and visceral malformations for SD rats exposed to 45% to 50% N$_2$O continuously on GD 8–9, 8–11, or 8–13. A 24-hour exposure to 70% N$_2$O on a single day of GD 5–10 resulted in a significantly increased incidence of skeletal abnormalities, including shortened and missing ribs and incomplete vertebral ossification (45). Exposure on GD 11 had no effect. No visceral abnormalities were observed, but too few litters were examined to draw valid conclusions.

Using a unique approach, Lane et al. (46) compared N_2O with xenon in an attempt to separate the physiologic effects of N_2O from its teratogenic effects. Xenon was used as an anesthetic control because it is an inert gas and has anesthetic potency similar to that of N_2O. Another group of rats served as exposure controls and received nitrogen. SD rats inhaled 70% to 75% N_2O, 70% to 75% xenon, or 70% to 75% nitrogen for 24 hours on GD 8. The two control groups had less than a 4% incidence of visceral malformations. The N_2O-exposed group, however, had a 15% incidence of visceral malformations and significantly increased incidences of resorptions, skeletal abnormalities, delayed skeletal maturation, and fused ribs. A comparable study by Mazze et al. (47), without a xenon control, resulted in a similar incidence of abnormalities in SD rats exposed for 24 hours on GD 8 to 75% N_2O. N_2O concentrations of 25% and lower had no adverse effects.

Using this model of exposure to a high concentration for a 24-hour period, several additional studies were conducted to define the day of greatest susceptibility to N_2O-induced teratogenesis. SD rats were exposed on 1 day of GD 6–12 for a single 24-hour period to 60% N_2O (48). Major visceral malformations, including hydrocephalus, and major and minor skeletal malformations, including fusion of ribs and severe deformity of vertebrae, were significantly increased following exposure on GD 9. Evidence of altered laterality (i.e., increased incidence of right-sided aortic arch and left-sided umbilical artery) was observed following exposure on GD 8, and subsequent studies confirmed this finding (49,50). Exposure on either GD 8 or 11 resulted in a 10-fold increased resorption rate (48). The increased fetal wastage observed following exposure on GD 8 or 11 was suggested by the authors to result from failure of the embryo to change dependence from the yolk sac to the chorioallantoic placenta rather than to result from the teratogenic effects of N_2O.

Inhalation of N_2O concentrations even as low as 0.1% produced significant effects in Wistar rats continuously exposed on GD 1–19 (51,52). The pattern of increased rates of resorptions, decreased fetal size, and skeletal abnormalities (primarily of the vertebrae and ribs) was similar to that observed following exposure to higher concentrations. No adverse effects were evident following continuous exposure to 0.05% N_2O (52).

Increased spontaneous motor activity at both 1 and 5 months of age was observed in SD rats exposed to 75% N_2O for 8 hours on GD 14 and 15 (53). This exposure regimen resulted in only transient growth effects without associated teratogenic effects (54). No alterations in reproductive or developmental indices or in growth were observed in SW mice exposed to 5%, 15%, or 35% N_2O for 4 hours/day on GD 6–15. In the period before weaning, righting and orienting reflexes and locomotion were unaffected, and swimming ability was accelerated. The overall activity across 25, 50, and 75 days of age was increased and tends to support the observations made by Mullenix et al. (53) in rats. Offspring of N_2O-exposed mice were hyporeactive in the startle reflex compared to controls following auditory and tactile stimuli on postnatal days 60 and 95 (55). In order to evaluate the behavioral effects in a second species, SD rats were exposed at the same concentrations, durations, and GD as were the mice. Rats, however, exhibited an overall hyperreactive startle response compared to controls in response to auditory stimuli at various ages up to 150 days (55,56). As discussed previously in this chapter and in the chapter by Lukas, the difference in responses between mice and rats could be the result of species-specific susceptibilities or the relatively longer gestational exposure of mice compared to rats.

The pathogenesis of N_2O-induced teratogenesis in animals is not known. N_2O has both physiologic and biochemical effects, which are discussed in the chapter by Koblin. Methionine synthase (MS) is inhibited by N_2O. This inhibition, in turn, results in the disruption of several pathways involved in one-carbon metabolism. N_2O oxidizes vitamin B_{12}, which is an essential cofactor of MS. In its oxidized form, the vitamin irreversibly inactivates MS because it cannot be displaced from the MS-B_{12} enzyme complex (57). The leading theory for the pathogenesis of N_2O-induced teratogenesis is that MS inhibition causes substantial deficiencies of intracellular components necessary for embryonic and fetal development and growth.

MS in essence controls the production of methionine, nonmethylated folates, and DNA (see chapter by Koblin). MS regulates the formation of methionine and tetrahydrofolate (H_4-folate), which are key components of two essential metabolic pathways. MS facilitates transfer of a methyl group (—CH_3) from 5-methyltetrahydrofolate (5-CH_3-H_4-folate) to homocysteine, thus producing methionine and H_4-folate. S-adenosylmethionine is produced, which is essential for many methylation reactions, including the production of active formate and the synthesis of polyamines with ornithine decarboxylase. Active formate and H_4-folate are needed for the synthesis of folinic acid (10-formyl-H_4-folate). DNA synthesis is dependent on deoxyuridine 5'-monophosphate (5'-MP) methylation to deoxythymidine 5'MP (dTMP), which in turn requires 5,10-methylene-H_4-folate derived from folinic acid (58–60).

The extent of N_2O-induced inhibition of MS depends on the N_2O concentration, the exposure duration, and the species (61). At a concentration of 50%, the half-time of MS inactivation by N_2O is approximately 5 minutes in rats (62). Because oxidized vitamin B_{12} is irreversibly bound to MS, recovery of activity requires resynthesis of the enzyme, which takes 3 to 4 days in rats. In humans,

the half-time of inactivation is approximately 45 minutes (62). This does not seem to offer any significant protective effect, however, because MS activity is very low even after several hours of routine anesthesia using N_2O. The decrease in dTMP synthesis likewise takes somewhat longer to develop in humans than in rodents but also lasts several days. These high N_2O concentrations are relevant for the surgical patient and the N_2O abuser but not the occupationally exposed health care professional. Experimental data from animals suggest that N_2O has no biochemical effect below a threshold concentration between 0.01% (1000 ppm) and 0.05% (52,63).

The majority of studies of MS inhibition have been performed in adult rodents (58, 64–66), but N_2O-induced inhibition of MS in tissues of the pregnant rat, embryo, or fetus also has been documented. MS activity in livers of SD dams was significantly depressed following 30 minutes of exposure to 10% N_2O on GD 19 (67). MS activity in fetal liver was significantly decreased only after 60 minutes. MS was significantly depressed after 15 minutes in dams and 30 minutes in fetuses when 50% N_2O was administered to mimic concentrations that might be used for cesarean section. Following 60-minutes exposure to 50% N_2O, activity in fetal liver recovered within 72 hours, while activity in maternal liver remained significantly depressed.

The extent and duration of N_2O effects on embryonic and fetal growth and tissue contents of protein, DNA, and folates were examined in SD rats exposed to 35% N_2O for hours on GD 13 (68). Embryos or fetuses were examined immediately following exposure or 24 or 48 hours after exposure. No effects were observed in weight, protein, DNA, or total folates. Nonmethylated reduced folates (e.g., tetrahydrofolate) as a percent of total folates decreased about 30% immediately following exposure, whereas methylated folates (e.g., 5-methyltetra-hydrofolate) were significantly increased. Groups of SD rats were exposed for 4 hours on 1, 2, or 3 successive days starting on GD 13 (69). Folates were examined each day at the termination of exposure and 24 hours after the last exposure on GD 15. Methylated folates increased on GD 13 and 15, and total folates increased on GD 15. Twenty-four hours after the last exposure, methylated and nonmethylated folates were not different from controls; only total folates were significantly elevated. Thus, single 4-hour exposures and multiple 4-hour exposures alter folate metabolism, which is recovered within 24 hours (68,69; S.A. Rice and A. Carughi, unpublished observations).

MS activity was significantly depressed in embryonic and maternal liver of SD rats following continuous exposure to 50% N_2O for 4, 24, or 48 hours culminating on GD 14 (70). Methylated folates in N_2O-exposed embryos increased to 83% to 87% of total folates compared to 76% in controls. Twenty-four hours of exposure to 50% N_2O on GD 10 did not alter maternal S-adenosylmethionine or S-adenosylhomocysteine concentrations or ornithine decarboxylase activity (71). Ornithine decarboxylase activity, however, was increased in embryos, thus suggesting the possible involvement of polyamine synthesis in N_2O teratogenesis.

The duration of N_2O exposure also is directly related to the duration of depressed dTMP synthesis (72). Bone marrow, the only actively growing tissue in the adult rat, exhibited significantly depressed rates of dTMP synthesis in pregnant rats exposed to N_2O for 24 hours at 75% and 7.5%, but not at the lowest concentration of 0.75% (73). Embryonic dTMP synthesis significantly declined following exposure to 25% N_2O for 24 hours on GD 8 (47). Concomitant teratogenic effects were not evident. The synthesis of embryonic DNA and RNA likewise was significantly depressed, and the embryonic contents of DNA and RNA were significantly decreased following 24-hour exposure to 50% N_2O (74,75).

These experimental results suggest that impaired DNA synthesis resulting from MS inhibition is not solely responsible for N_2O-induced teratogenic effects because significant effects on cellular components are measured when N_2O is administered at concentrations and for periods that are not associated with teratogenesis. In addition, folinic acid, which should bypass any disruption in folate metabolism caused by inhibition of MS, does not prevent most of the adverse reproductive and teratogenic effects of N_2O, but surprisingly isoflurane and halothane can (76,77). In addition to the previously discussed lack of effect of folinic acid and the mitigating effects of the anesthetics, an α_1-adrenergic antagonist, phenoxybenzamine, has been shown to reduce the incidence of resorptions, but not abnormalities, following exposure to 60% N_2O (78).

The mechanism by which N_2O produces behavioral deficits in prenatally exposed offspring is also unknown. Behavioral abnormalities have not been observed in the absence of MS inhibition. The CNS may be more susceptible to the adverse effects of N_2O because MS is the only enzyme in the brain that synthesizes methionine (61), and dihydrofolate reductase (the only other enzyme that can produce H_4-folate) is present in very low concentrations.

The mechanisms of N_2O-induced effects are being investigated actively because an understanding of these mechanisms will help to assure patient and health care worker safety. Additionally, an understanding of these mechanisms will help to clarify the role of vitamin B_{12}, folates, and one-carbon chemistry in development.

Other General Anesthetics

The teratogenicity of the barbiturates used as anesthetics is not well studied. It is not known if neonatal depression following maternal exposure is related to the few reported developmental effects of the barbiturates. Most studies have examined phenobarbital in its context as an anticonvulsant. Phenobarbital is discussed here only briefly because the duration of administration for these studies is very different from that which would be used for anesthesia. The few published studies of the other barbiturates are discussed.

The teratogenic potential of phenobarbital was identified in the 1960s in studies by McColl et al. (79,80). Dietary administration of phenobarbital (0.16% w/w) for 3 days before mating and throughout pregnancy produced 78% mortality in SD offspring. Eighty percent of examined dead offspring had centrum of the vertebra that were duplicated (79). In a later study, skeletal and aortic arch defects were observed in the offspring of rabbits treated with 50 mg/kg phenobarbital orally on GD 8–16 (80). Intravenous administration of New Zealand white rabbits with 40 mg/kg of sodium pentobarbital on GD 6, 7, 8, or 9 did not significantly increase the malformation incidence (81). Resorption rates, however, were slightly increased in does treated on either GD 8 or 9. When laparotomy and exposure of the uterine horns were performed under this phenobarbital-induced anesthesia, significant increases in resorptions were observed. The greatest effects occurred following anesthesia and surgery on the earlier days. The literature related to adverse outcome associated with prenatal phenobarbital administration has been reviewed extensively (82–84).

Shepard (85) has cited two studies by Tanimura et al. (86,87). The offspring of mice treated i.p. with 60 to 140 mg/kg of thiamylal sodium on GD 10 exhibited increased malformations of the foot joint (86). Polydactyly and malformation of the tail also were observed. Injection on a single day of GD 7–9 or 11–14 or at doses below 60 mg/kg did not produce increased malformations. Thiopental administration to pregnant mice at doses up to 100 mg/kg on GD 11 produced some reduction in fetal weight above 50 mg/kg (87). Rats injected i.p. with 50 or 100 mg thiopental on GD 4 showed no

increased rates of resorptions or malformations (88). A slightly increased incidence of limb defects was observed in rats following i.p. injection of 50 mg/kg hexobarbital on GD 5 (88).

There is relatively little information on the other general anesthetic agents. One study showed no adverse effects in rats treated daily with i.m. ketamine at 120 mg/kg on GD 9–13 (89). Another study showed no effect in pregnant rats treated with a single dose of 12 mg/kg of etomidate (90).

Local Anesthetics

Little is known about the potential reproductive and developmental toxicity of the local anesthetics because few experimental studies have been performed. The animal studies performed have not revealed any teratogenic effects, but there are some behavioral effects at high concentrations of the local anesthetics.

In Vitro *Developmental Test Systems*

The effect of local anesthetics on IVF was investigated with SW mouse oocytes exposed *in vitro* to lidocaine, chloroprocaine, or bupivacaine for 30 minutes at concentrations ranging from 0.01 to 100 μg/ml (91). The oocytes were then washed and inseminated. Effects were examined at 24, 48, and 72 hours. Chloroprocaine adversely affected fertilization and embryo development at concentrations as low as 0.1 μg/ml. Lidocaine produced effects at 1.0 μg/ml, and bupivacaine required a concentration of 100 μg/ml.

In Vivo *Developmental Test Systems*

Lidocaine injected i.p. daily at 56 mg/kg on GD 5–7, 9–11, 12–14, or 15–17 in SD rats produced no adverse fetal effects (92). No significant effects were observed in offspring of SD rats administered lidocaine at 100 or 250 mg/kg/day by constant infusion for 2 weeks before mating and throughout pregnancy (93). Administration at a rate of 500 mg/kg/day on GD 3–17 produced a reduction in fetal weight but no teratogenic effects.

Some behavioral effects have been documented for offspring of rats exposed during pregnancy to lidocaine and mepivacaine at doses near the recommended maximum for humans. Offspring of Long-Evans hooded rats injected in the masseter muscle with 6 mg/kg lidocaine containing epinephrine (1 : 100,000) on day 11 of pregnancy resulted in offspring exhibiting poor performance on a visual discrimination task and impaired learning of a water maze. Rats similarly treated with 6 mg/kg of mepivacaine produced offspring that were hypoactive in the open field (94).

SUMMARY

Adverse reproductive and developmental effects in experimental animals associated with the anesthetic agents generally are observed only after long periods of continuous exposure to subanesthetic concentrations or multiple exposures to anesthetizing concentrations. A reasonable explanation for many observed adverse effects is the alteration of maternal fetal physiology. Because few studies have made an attempt to monitor physiologic responses to any significant degree, the question of cause and effect remains unanswered.

Statistically significant behavioral effects are observed in offspring of mice and rats exposed to nonteratogenic concentrations of several of the anesthetics. In general, the effects are evident when animals are exposed to high concentrations for moderate times or to lower concentrations for extended periods. Gestational exposure to halothane results in significant behavioral effects under a number of different expo-

sure conditions. However, the mechanism is unclear because anatomic observations have not correlated with the severity of impairment in behavioral testing (28,29), thus implying a complex relationship between brain development and behavioral manifestations (29).

The extent to which the results of animal studies of anesthetic reproductive and developmental toxicity can be extrapolated to humans is not apparent. In addition to the difficulties inherent in extrapolating animal data to humans, there is a general lack of documentation in humans of adverse reproductive and development effects, even at anesthetizing concentrations.

REFERENCES

1. Kimmel C A, Generoso W M, Thomas R D, Bakshi K S. A new frontier in understanding the mechanisms of developmental abnormalities. *Toxicol Appl Pharmacol* 1993;119:159–165.
2. Wilson J G. Current status of teratology. In: Wilson J G, Fraser K C, eds. *Handbook of teratology. Vol. 1 General principles and etiology.* New York: Plenum Press, 1977:47–74.
3. Kimmel G L. Developmental aspects of chemical interaction with cellular receptors. In: Kimmel C A, Buelke-Sam J, eds. *Developmental toxicology.* New York: Raven Press, 1981:115–130.
4. Trosko J E, Cjhang C-C, Netzloff M. The role of inhibited cell-cell communication in teratogenesis. *Teratogen Carcinogen Mutagen* 1982;2:31–45.
5. Welsch F, Stedman D B. Inhibition of metabolic cooperation between Chinese hamster V79 cells by structurally diverse teratogens. *Teratogen Carcinogen Mutagen* 1984;4:285–301.
6. Ferstandig L L. Trace concentrations of anesthetic gases: a critical review of their disease potential. *Anesth Analg* 1978;57:328–345.
7. Eger E I, II. *Nitrous oxide/N_2O.* New York: Elsevier Science Publishing Company, Inc., 1985.
8. Baden J M, Rice S A. Metabolism and toxicity of inhaled anesthetics. In: Miller R D, ed. *Anesthesia,* 3rd ed. New York: Churchill Livingstone, 1990;1:135–170.
9. Baeder C, Albrecht M. Embryotoxic/teratogenic potential of halothane. *Int Arch Occup Environ Health* 1990;62:263–271.
10. Baden J M. Chronic toxicity of inhalation anaesthetics. *Clin Anaesth* 1983;1:441–454.
11. Baden J M, Simmon V F. Mutagenic effects of inhalation anesthetics. *Mutat Res* 1980;75:169–189.

12. Simmon V F, Baden J M. Mutagenic activity of vinyl compounds and derived epoxides. *Mutat Res* 1980;78:227–231.

13. Hinkley R E, Wright B D. Comparative effects of halothane, enflurane, and methoxyflurane on the incidence of abnormal development using sea urchin gamates as an *in vitro* model system. *Anesth Analg* 1985;64:1005–1009.

14. Kundomal Y R, Baden J M. Toxicity and teratogenicity of inhaled anesthetics in *Drosophila melanogaster*. *Toxicol Lett* 1985;25:287–291.

15. Chetkowski R J, Nass T E. Isofluorane inhibits early mouse embryo development *in vitro*. *Fertil Steril* 1988;49:171–173.

16. Halsey M J, Green C J, Monk S J, et al. Maternal and paternal chronic exposure to enflurane and halothane: fetal and histological changes in the rat. *Br J Anaesth* 1981;53:203–215.

17. Pope W D B, Halsey M J, Lansdown A B G, Bateman P E. Lack of teratogenic dangers with halothane. *Acta Anaesthesiol Belg* 1975;26(suppl): 169–173.

18. Pope W D B, Halsey M J, Lansdown A B G, et al. Fetotoxicity in rats following chronic exposure to halothane, nitrous oxide, or methoxyflurane. *Anesthesiology* 1978;48:11–16.

19. Wharton R S, Mazze R I, Baden J M. Hitt B A, Dooley J R. Fertility, reproduction and postnatal survival in mice chronically exposed to halothane. *Anesthesiology* 1978;48:167–174.

20. Wharton R S, Wilson A I, Mazze R I, Baden J M, Rice S A. Fetal morphology in mice exposed to halothane. *Anesthesiology* 1979;51: 532–537.

21. Kennedy G L, Smith S H, Keplinger M L, Calandra J C. Reproductive and teratologic studies with halothane. *Toxicol Appl Pharmacol* 1976; 35:467–474.

22. Basford A B, Fink B R. The teratogenecity of halothane in the rat. *Anesthesiology* 1968;29: 1167–1173.

23. Coate W B, Kapp R W, Ulland B M, Lewis T R. Toxicity of low-concentration long-term exposure to an airborne mixture of nitrous oxide and halothane. *J Environ Pathol Toxicol* 1979;2:209–231.

24. Bussard D A, Stoelting R K, Peterson C, Ishaq M. Fetal changes in hamsters anesthetized with nitrous oxide and halothane. *Anesthesiology* 1974;41:275–278.

25. Quimby K L, Ashkenase L J, Bowman R E, et al. Enduring learning deficits and cerebral synaptic malformation from exposure to 10 parts of halothane per million. *Science* 1974;185:625–627.

26. Quimbly K L, Katz J, Bowman R E. Behavioral consequences in rats from chronic exposure to 10 ppm halothane during early development. *Anesth Analg* 1975;54:628–633.

27. Bowman R E, Smith R F. Behavioral and neurochemical effects of prenatal halothane. *Environ Health Perspect* 1977;2:189–193.

28. Chang L W, Dudley A W J, Katz J. Pathological changes in the nervous system following *in utero*

exposure to halothane. *Environ Res* 1976;11: 40–51.

29. Levin E D, DeLuna R, Uemura E, Bowman R E. Long-term effects of developmental halothane exposure on radial arm maze performance in rats. *Behav Brain Res* 1990;36:147–154.

30. Koeter H W M, Rodier P M. Behavioral effects in mice exposed to nitrous oxide or halothane: prenatal vs. postnatal exposure. *Neurobehav Toxicol Teratol* 1986;8:189–194.

31. Rodier P M, Koeter H B W M. General activity from weaning to maturity in mice exposed to halothane or nitrous oxide. *Neurobehav Toxicol Teratol* 1986;8:195–199.

32. Smith R F, Bowman R E, Katz J. Behavioral effects of exposure to halothane during early development in the rat: sensitive period during pregnancy. *Anesthesiology* 1978;49:319–323.

33. Chalon J, Tang C K, Ramanathan S, et al. Exposure to halothane and enflurane affects learning function of murine progeny. *Anesth Analg* 1981;60:794–797.

34. Green C J, Monk S J, Knight J F, et al. Chronic exposure of rats to enflurane 200 p.p.m.: no evidence of toxicity or teratogenicity. *Br J Anaesth* 1982;54:1097–1104.

35. Pope W D B, Persaud T V N. Foetal growth retardation in the rat following chronic exposure to the inhalation anaesthetic enflurane. *Experientia* 1978;34:1332.

36. Saito N, Urakawa M, Ito R. Influence of enflurane on fetus and growth after birth in mice and rats (Japanese). *Oyo Yakuri* 1974;8:1269–1276.

37. Wharton R S, Mazze R I, Wilson A I. Reproductive and fetal development in mice chronically exposed to enflurane. *Anesthesiology* 1981; 54:505–510.

38. Mazze R I, Fujinaga M, Rice S A, et al. Reproductive and teratogenic effects of nitrous oxide, halothane, isoflurane, and enflurane in Sprague-Dawley rats. *Anesthesiology* 1986;64: 339–344.

39. Peters M A, Hudson P M. Postnatal development and behavior in offspring of enflurane-exposed pregnant rats. *Arch Int Pharm Ther* 1982;256:134–144.

40. Mazze R I, Wilson A I, Rice S A, Baden J M. Fetal development in mice exposed to isoflurane. *Teratology* 1985;32:339–345.

41. Kennedy G L, Smith S H, Keplinger M L, Calandra J C. Reproductive and teratologic studies with isoflurane. *Drug Chem Toxicol* 1977;1:75–88.

42. Rice S A. Behavioral effects of *in utero* isoflurane exposure in young SW mice. *Teratology* 1986;33:100C.

43. Wharton R S, Sievenpiper T S, Mazze R I. Developmental toxicity of methoxyflurane in mice. *Anesth Analg* 1980;59:421–425.

44. Fink B R, Shepard T H, Blandau R J. Teratogenic activity of nitrous oxide. *Nature* 1967; 214:146–148.

45. Shepard T H, Fink B R. Teratogenic activity of nitrous oxide in rats. In: Fink B R, ed. *Toxicity*

of anesthetics. Baltimore: Williams & Wilkins, 1968:308–323.

46. Lane G A, Nahrwold M L, Tait A R, et al. Anesthetics as teratogens: nitrous oxide is fetoxic, xenon is not. *Science* 1980;210:899–901.

47. Mazze R I, Wilson A I, Rice S A, Baden J M. Reproduction and fetal development in rats exposed to nitrous oxide. *Teratology* 1984;30:259–266.

48. Fujinaga M, Baden J M, Mazze R I. Susceptible period of nitrous oxide teratogenicity in Sprague-Dawley rats. *Teratology* 1989;40:439–444.

49. Fujinaga M, Baden J M, Shepard T H, Mazze R I. Nitrous oxide alters body laterality in rats. *Teratology* 1990;41:131–135.

50. Baden J M, Fujinaga M. Effects of nitrous oxide on day 9 rat embryos grown in culture. *Br J Anaesth* 1991;66:500–503.

51. Vieira E. Effect of the chronic administration of nitrous oxide 0.5% to gravid rats. *Br J Anaesth* 1979;51:283–287.

52. Vieira E, Cleaton-Jones P, Austin J C, et al. Effects of low concentration of nitrous oxide on rat fetuses. *Anesth Analg* 1980;59:175–177.

53. Mullenix P J, Moore P A, Tassinari M S. Behavioral toxicity of nitrous oxide in rats following prenatal exposure. *Toxicol Ind Health* 1986;2: 273–287.

54. Tassinari M, Mullenix P, Moore P. The effects of nitrous oxide after exposure during middle and late gestation. *Toxicol Ind Health* 1986;2:261–271.

55. Rice S A. Effects of prenatal N_2O exposure on startle reflex reactivity. *Teratology* 1990;42:373–381.

56. Rice S A. Startle reflex reactivity of rats perinatally treated with methimazole or prenatally exposed to N_2O. *Teratology* 1989;39:508.

57. Deacon R, Lumb M, Perry J, et al. Inactivation of methionine synthase by nitrous oxide. *Eur J Biochem* 1980;104:419–422.

58. Eells J T, Black K A, Makar A B, et al. The regulation of one-carbon oxidation in the rat by nitrous oxide and methionine. *Arch Biochem Biophys* 1982;219:316–326.

59. Lumb M, Sharer N, Deacon R, et al. Effects of nitrous oxide-induced inactivation of cobalamin on methionine and S-adenosylmethionine metabolism in the rat. *Biochim Biophys Acta* 1983; 756:354–359.

60. Vina J R, Davis D W, Hawkins R A. The influence of nitrous oxide on methionine, S-adenosylmethionine, and other amino acids. *Anesthesiology* 1986;64:490–495.

61. Nunn J F, Chanarin I. Nitrous oxide inactivates methionine synthetase. In: Eger EI II, ed. *Nitrous oxide/N_2O*. New York: Elsevier Science Publishing Company, Inc., 1985:211–233.

62. Royston B D, Nunn J F, Weingren H K, Royston D, Cormack R S. Rate of inactivation of human and rodent hepatic methionine synthase by nitrous oxide. *Anesthesiology* 1988;68:213–216.

63. Sharer N M, Nunn J F, Royston J P, Chanarin I. Effects of chronic exposure to nitrous oxide on methionine synthase activity. *Br J Anaesth* 1983; 55:693–701.

64. Lumb M, Perry J, Deacon R, et al. Recovery of tissue folates after inactivation of cobalamin by nitrous oxide. The significance of dietary folate. *Am J Clin Nutr* 1981;34:2418–2422.

65. Brody T, Watson J E, Stokstad E L R. Folate pentaglutamate and folate hexaglutamate mediated one-carbon metabolism. *Biochemistry* 1982;21:276–282.

66. Black K A, Tephly T R. Effects of nitrous oxide and methotrexate administration on hepatic methionine synthetase and dihydrofolate reductase activities, hepatic folates, and formate oxidation in rats. *Mol Pharmacol* 1983;23:724–730.

67. Baden J M, Serra M, Mazze R I. Inhibition of fetal methionine synthase by nitrous oxide. *Br J Anaesth* 1984;56:523–530.

68. Carughi A, Rice S A. Embryonic and fetal folates in N_2O-exposed rats. *FASEB J* 1990;4: A873.

69. Rice S A, Carughi A. Embryonic and fetal folates following N_2O exposure. *Toxicologist* 1990; 10:40.

70. Hansen D K, Billings R E. Effects of nitrous oxide on maternal and embryonic folate metabolism in rats. *Dev Pharmacol Ther* 1985;8:43–54.

71. Hansen D K, Knowles B J, Fullerton F R, Poirier L A. Effect of nitrous oxide exposure on maternal and embryonic S-adenosylmethionine levels and ornithine decarboxylase activity. *Life Sci* 1993;52:1669–1675.

72. Deacon R, Perry J, Lumb M, Chanarin I. The effect of nitrous oxide-induced inactivation of vitamin B_{12} on thymidylate synthetase activity of rat bone marrow cells. *Biochem Biophys Res Commun* 1981;102:215–218.

73. Baden J M, Rice S A, Serra M, Kelley M, Mazze R. Thymidine and methionine synthesis in pregnant rats exposed to nitrous oxide. *Anesth Analg* 1983;62:738–741.

74. Hansen D K, Billings R E. Effects of nitrous oxide on macromolecular content and DNA synthesis in rat embryos. *J Pharmacol Exp Ther* 1986;238:985–989.

75. Hansen D K, Grafton T F. Effect of nitrous oxide on embryonic macromolecular synthesis and purine levels. *Teratogen Carcinogen Mutagen* 1988;8:107–115.

76. Fujinaga M, Baden J M, Yhap E O, Mazze R I. Reproductive and teratogenic effects of nitrous oxide, isoflurane, and their combination in Sprague-Dawley rats. *Anesthesiology* 1987;67: 960–964.

77. Mazze R I, Fujinaga M, Baden J M. Halothane prevents nitrous oxide teratogenicity in Sprague-Dawley rats; folinic acid does not. *Teratology* 1988;38:121–127.

78. Fujinaga M, Baden J M, Suto A, Myatt J K, Mazze R I. Preventive effects of phenoxybenzamine on nitrous oxide-induced reproductive toxicity in Sprague-Dawley rat. *Teratology* 1991; 43:151–157.

79. McColl J D, Globus M, Robinson S. Drug-induced skeletal malformations in the rat. *Experientia* 1963;19:183–184.
80. McColl J D, Robinson S, Globus M. Effect of some therapeutic agents on the rabbit fetus. *Toxicol Appl Pharmacol* 1967;10:244–252.
81. Johnson W E. Fetal loss from anesthesia and surgical trauma in the rabbit. *Toxicol Appl Pharmacol* 1971;18:773–779.
82. Middaugh L D. Prenatal phenobarbital: effects on pregnancy and offspring. In: Riley EP, Vorhees CV, eds. *Handbook of behavioral teratology.* New York: Plenum Press, 1986:243–266.
83. Finnell R H, Shields H E, Chernoff G F. Variable patterns in anticonvulsant drug-induced malformations in mice: comparisons of phenytoin and phenobarbital. *Teratogen Carcinogen Mutagen* 1987;7:541–549.
84. Yanai J, Fares F, Gavish M, et al. Neural and behavioral alterations after early exposure to phenobarbital. *Neurotoxicology* 1989;10:543–554.
85. Shepard T. *Catalog of teratogenic agents.* Baltimore: Johns Hopkins University Press, 1989.
86. Tanimura T. Effect of administration of thiamylal sodium to pregnant mice upon the development of their offspring. *Kaibogaku Zasshi Acta Anat Nippon* 1965;40:323–328.
87. Tanimura T, Owaki Y, Nishimura H. Effects of administration of thiopental sodium to pregnant mice upon the development of their offspring. *Okajimas Folia Anat Jpn* 1967;43:219–226.
88. Persaud T V N. Tierexperimentelle Untersuchungen zur Frage de teratogenen Wirkung von Barbituraten. *Acta Biol Med Ger* 1965;14:89–90.
89. El-Karim A H B, Benny R. Embryotoxic and teratogenic action of ketamine hydrochloride in rats. *Ains Shams Med J* 1976;27:459–463.
90. Doenicke V A, Heinrigh G, Boll H, et al. Teratogene Shaden durch Narkotika. In: Henschel W F, Lehmann C, eds. *Schadigungen des Anaesthesie-Personals durch Nakose-Gase und -Dampfe.* Berlin: Springer-Verlag, 1975:90–106.
91. Schnell V L, Sacco A V, Savoy-Moore R T, Ataya K M, Moghissi K S. Effects of oocyte exposure to local anesthetics on *in vitro* fertilization and embryo development in the mouse. *Reprod Toxicol* 1992;6:323–327.
92. Ramazzotto L J, Curro F A, Paterson J A, et al. Toxicological assessment of lidocaine in the pregnant rat. *J Dent Res* 1985;64:1214–1218.
93. Fujinaga M, Mazze R I. Reproductive and teratogenic effects of lidocaine in Sprague-Dawley rats. *Anesthesiology* 1986;65:626–632.
94. Smith R F, Wharton G G, Kurtz S L, Mattran K M, Hollenbeck A R. Behavioral effects of mid-pregnancy administration of lidocaine and mepivacaine in the rat. *Neurobehav Toxicol Teratol* 1986;8:61–68.
95. Hoar R M, Monie I W. Comparative development of specific organ systems. In: Kimmel C A, Buelke-Sam J, eds. *Developmental toxicology. Target organ toxicology series.* New York: Raven Press, 1981:13–33.
96. Schardein J L. *Chemically induced birth defects.* New York: Marcel Dekker, Inc., 1985.

Anesthetic Toxicity, edited by
Susan A. Rice and Kevin J. Fish.
Raven Press, Ltd., New York © 1994.

10

Reproductive and Developmental Toxicity of Anesthetics in Humans

Kristie L. Ebi and *Susan A. Rice

*EMF Health Studies Program, Environment Division, Electric Power Research Institute,
Palo Alto, California 94304 and *Susan A. Rice and Associates, Inc.,
Sunnyvale, California 94087 and Department of Anesthesia, Stanford University School of
Medicine, Stanford, California 94305*

Reports of adverse reproductive and developmental effects of the anesthetic agents are of potential concern for surgical patients and health care workers alike. By various estimates, between 0.5% and 2.0% of pregnant women undergo anesthesia and surgery for reasons unrelated to their pregnancy. In the United States alone, this translates to approximately 50,000 women a year. The number of health care workers exposed to anesthetics is much larger, especially when one considers that this group encompasses physicians, veterinarians, dentists, nurses, technicians, and assistants. Differences in anesthetic exposure between patients and health care workers are apparent. Surgical patients are exposed to high anesthetic concentrations for brief time periods, whereas occupationally exposed workers are exposed to low anesthetic concentrations for prolonged time periods.

This chapter summarizes the results of epidemiologic studies that assessed the adverse reproductive and developmental effects of anesthetic exposure on the pregnant surgical patient and the occupationally exposed female and male health care worker.

PATIENT EXPOSURE TO ANESTHETICS

Collaborative Perinatal Project

The main objective of the Collaborative Perinatal Project (1) was to determine whether there were factors during pregnancy or delivery that were related to the risk of cerebral palsy or other neurologic outcomes. For 7 years starting in 1959, data were collected on 55,908 pregnancies of women admitted to 12 collaborating medical centers. The selection procedures were not uniform in all clinics. Common disqualifications were a woman's intention to leave the locality soon, residence in certain areas, and delivery on the first day of registration. A woman could be a participant more than once. The sample was reduced to 50,282 mother–infant pairs after excluding refusals, losses to follow-up, pregnancy terminations before the twentieth week, twin and triplet pregnancies, pregnancies with clinical evidence of maternal rubella, participants missing certain information, and ethnic groups other than white, black, or Puerto Rican. Data were collected by interview and from physicians throughout pregnancy and at specific intervals during childhood. There were 3248 children with malformations of more than minor importance. The study identified 9 malformed infants in 218 mother–infant pairs exposed to general anesthetics, nitrous oxide (N_2O), or oxygen (O_2). The rate of congenital malformations adjusted for mother's ethnic group and survival of the child was not increased when anesthetics were analyzed as a group [rate ratio (RR) = 0.66] or as individual anesthetics and O_2 (range of RRs = 0.47 to 1.33). Additionally, there was no suggestion that any of the local anesthetics, with the possible exception of mepivacaine (RR = 2.66; $p<0.01$), were teratogens. Because only 82 mother–infant pairs were exposed to mepivacaine, no other local anesthetic increased the incidence of abnormalities, and because of the large number of statistical comparisons, the teratogenic potential of mepivacaine requires further investigation.

Anesthetic Exposure During Nonobstetric Surgery

Seven retrospective studies published over the past 30 years evaluated reproductive and developmental outcomes in pregnant women undergoing anesthesia and nonobstetric surgery. These studies were designed to investigate whether exposure to anesthesia and surgery during pregnancy affected the rates of pregnancy loss and congenital malformations. Selected characteristics of the studies are summarized in Table 1. This chapter does not address studies that evaluated only pregnancy outcome following nonobstetric surgery without consideration of the role of anesthesia exposure.

The first study appeared in 1963. Smith (2) reviewed every record from a U.S. Naval Hospital and identified 67 pregnant women who underwent regional or general anesthesia for any reason except delivery of an infant. Total mortality after anesthesia for the fetuses of these women was 15%—

10% fetal mortality in the first, 15% in the second, and 25% in the third trimester. There were 10 fetal fatalities, 4 among 16 appendectomies, all associated with appendiceal abscesses. In addition, there were 4 fetal fatalities among 10 cases of Shirodkar procedures, and 2 fetal fatalities following other surgical procedures. Nine fetal fatalities followed surgical procedures with spinal anesthesia, and 1 followed a surgical procedure with general anesthesia. No fetal anomalies were observed.

In 1965, Shnider and Webster (3) evaluated the clinical experience and pregnancy outcome of 147 pregnant women undergoing surgical procedures. These women were 1.6% of 9063 patients delivered of infants during a 49-month period at a medical center. Hospital records of 8926 nonsurgical patients were reviewed for pregnancy outcome. Most of the surgical procedures were the result of medical and obstetric abnormalities. Eighteen patients underwent a Shirodkar procedure, 13 had an appendectomy, 18 had intraperitoneal operations excluding appendectomies, 29 had extraperitoneal major operations, and 69 underwent minor operations. The operations were divided fairly evenly among the pregnancy trimesters. General anesthesia was administered to 60 patients, spinal or epidural anesthesia to 18, local anesthesia to 50, and no anesthesia to 19. Agents included N_2O, thiopental, meperidine, halothane, and cyclopropane.

Premature delivery within 14 days after surgery was reported for 6.4% of first trimester, 8.6% of second trimester, and 11.9% of third trimester patients. Congenital abnormalities were reported for 8.5% of first trimester, 3.4% of second trimester, and 4.8% of third trimester patients. The overall rate was 5.4% and was not statistically different from the 6.0% rate reported for the nonsurgical patients. Overall, perinatal mortality was significantly higher for the surgical than for the nonsurgical patients (7.5% vs 2.1%). However, 6 of the 11 perinatal deaths followed Shirodkar procedures. When these fatalities were excluded, the rate of perinatal mortality for the offspring of surgical patients was 3.8%, not significantly different from the rate for the nonsurgical group. Similarly, a statistically significantly higher percentage of infants with birthweights under 2500 g was reported for the surgical group (15.6% vs 10.0%). Eight of the 23 low birthweight infants were born to mothers who underwent Shirodkar procedures. When these infants were excluded, the rate of low birthweight among offspring of surgical patients was 11.6%, not statistically different from the nonsurgical group. The authors concluded that the reason for surgery was probably a far more important factor in producing adverse pregnancy outcomes than either the surgical procedure or the anesthetic.

Shnider and Webster (3) also reported data from the 1961 Obstetrical Statistical Cooperative Study of 60,912 obstetric patients. Overall, 2.4% of the patients had an operation during pregnancy. Among 50 pregnant women who underwent appendectomies, rates of congenital abnormalities and perinatal mortality were similar to rates for women without surgical complications during pregnancy, and the rate of low birthweight infants was lower (8.0% vs 17.5%). Among the 81 women who underwent Shirodkar procedures, the rate of congenital abnormalities was slightly increased, and the rates of perinatal mortality and low birthweight were elevated over the rates observed for nonsurgical women (19.7% vs 3.3% and 45.7% vs 17.5%, respectively).

Brodsky et al. (4) mailed questionnaires to 29,514 male dentists and 30,272 female dental assistants concerning anesthetic practice and exposure, pregnancy history of the respondent or spouse for the years 1968 to 1978, and exposure to anesthetics during surgical procedures that occurred in each trimester of each pregnancy. Questionnaire response rates were 73.3% for the dentists and 70.0% for the dental assistants. There were 12,929 pregnancies with complete data. Pregnancies were considered to have occupational exposure if either parent worked with anesthetics for the year before conception. Anesthetics were administered to 187 women during the first trimester and 100 women during the second trimester of gestation. After adjusting for maternal age and smoking history, the rates of spontaneous abortion in the first trimester were $8.0 \pm 3.4\%$ in the surgical group and $5.1 \pm 0.2\%$ in the comparison group ($p = 0.01$). The rates in the second trimester were $6.9 \pm 3.9\%$ in the surgical group and $1.4 \pm 0.1\%$ in the comparison group ($p < 0.01$). The rate of spontaneous abortion in the first trimester for the surgical group was about the same as that observed for pregnancies occupationally exposed to anesthetics. The rate for the 65 pregnancies with both surgical and occupational exposure was $14.8 \pm 3.2\%$ ($p < 0.01$). The rate of spontaneous abortion in the second trimester for occupationally exposed pregnancies ($2.6 \pm 0.3\%$) was statistically significant and less than the rate in the surgical group. There were no pregnancies in the second trimester with both surgical and occupational exposure. There were no significant increases in the rates of congenital abnormalities reported for infants born to women who had surgery during pregnancy ($3.1 \pm 1.6\%$ first trimester, $5.8 \pm 4.2\%$ second trimester, and $4.5 \pm 0.2\%$ comparison group). The rates of congenital abnormalities reported for offspring of women with both surgical and occupational exposure were elevated over the comparison rate but were not significant.

Aldridge and Tunstall (5) reviewed the clinical records of all patients in Aberdeen who had insertion of Shirodkar sutures. All third trimester procedures were excluded. From 1978 through 1984 there were 175 pregnancies in 130 women. All women were parous, and 110 had a history of 226 previous abortion(s). N_2O was administered to

TABLE 1. *Summary of epidemiologic studies of reproductive and developmental outcomes following exposure to anesthetics for nonobstetric surgery*

Agent or procedure	Definition of exposure	Data collection instrument	Study type	Study population	Comparison population	Outcome(s) investigated	Results[a]	Potential covariates considered	Ref
Anesthesia	General or regional anesthesia for nonobstetric surgery during pregnancy	Hospital chart review	Retrospective, U.S.A. 1957–1961	24 pregnant women who underwent general anesthesia and 43 pregnant women who underwent regional anesthesia	18,248 live births and 255 stillbirths	*Fetal mortality* Appendectomy Shirodkar Intraperitoneal Miscellaneous *Congenital abnormalities*	Increased Increased? Increased? Negative? Negative? Negative	None	2
Anesthesia	Nonobstetric surgery during pregnancy	1. Hospital chart review for information on obstetric history, surgery, and pregnancy outcome 2. Data provided by the Obstetrical Statistical Cooperative from 17 hospitals	Retrospective, U.S.A. 1959–1964 ‌1961	1. 147 pregnant women who underwent surgery 2. Data on 50 pregnant women who underwent appendectomies and 81 pregnant women who underwent Shirodkar procedures	1. 8,926 women who did not undergo surgery 2. 59,456 pregnancies without surgical procedures	*Premature delivery* *Congenital abnormalities* *Perinatal mortality* *Low birthweight* Appendectomies *Congenital abnormalities* *Perinatal mortality* *Low birthweight* Shirodkar procedure *Congenital abnormalities* *Perinatal mortality* *Low birthweight*	Increased Negative Negative Negative ‌ Negative? Negative? Decreased ‌ Increased Increased Increased	Types of surgery: results exclude women who underwent Shirodkar procedures None None	3
Anesthesia	Nonobstetric surgery during 1st or 2nd trimester of pregnancy	Postal questionnaire concerning occupational anesthetic exposure, reproductive history, exposure to anesthetics for surgery, and pregnancy outcome	Retrospective survey, U.S.A. 1968–1978	287 pregnant women who underwent surgery	12,642 pregnancies in women who did not undergo surgery	*Spontaneous abortion* 1st trimester 2nd trimester With occupational exposure 1st trimester 2nd trimester *Congenital abnormalities* With occupational exposure	Positive Positive Positive Negative Negative Negative	Maternal age and smoking history	4
Anesthesia and N_2O	Insertion of Shirodkar suture during 1st or 2nd trimester of pregnancy	Record review for information on obstetric history, type of anesthetic, and pregnancy outcome	Retrospective, Scotland 1978–1984	175 pregnancies (176 fetuses) in 130 women who underwent surgery	Background rate in population	*Spontaneous abortion* *Neonatal mortality/stillbirth* *Congenital abnormalities* *Preterm delivery*	Negative Negative Negative Increased	Maternal smoking	5

178

Exposure	Description	Methods	Study	Exposed group	Comparison group	Outcome	Result[a]	Controls	#
Anesthesia and N_2O	General anesthesia for surgery during 1st or 2nd trimester of pregnancy	Hospital chart review for information on obstetric history, type of anesthetic, and pregnancy outcome	Retrospective, England 1968+	1. 375 patients (383 fetuses) who received general anesthesia for cervical cerclage 2. 58 patients (59 fetuses) who received general anesthesia for operations other than cervical cerclage	114 patients (115 fetuses) who received regional anesthesia for cervical cerclage 114 patients (115 fetuses) who received regional anesthesia for cervical cerclage	*Spontaneous abortion* *Low birthweight* *Congenital abnormalities* *Spontaneous abortion* *Low birthweight* *Congenital abnormalities*	Negative? Negative? Negative? Negative Negative? Negative?	None None	6
Anesthesia	Nonobstetric surgery during pregnancy	Review of health insurance records for information on surgery, type of anesthesia, and pregnancy outcome; data from congenital abnormalities surveillance program	Case-control, Canada 1971–1978	2,565 pregnant women who underwent surgery	2,565 pregnant women with a pregnancy-related condition who did not undergo surgery	*Congenital abnormalities* *Spontaneous abortion* Spinal block Local anesthesia General anesthesia Ob/gyn procedures Abnormal procedures Other surgical procedures	Negative Negative Negative Negative Positive Positive Negative Positive	Controls matched on maternal age and geographic area of residence	7

Anesthesia	Nonobstetric surgery during pregnancy	Record linkage of 3 Swedish health care registries for information on surgery, type of anesthesia, and pregnancy outcome	Retrospective, Sweden 1973–1981	5,405 pregnant women who underwent surgery	Expected national rates for 1973–1981	*Congenital abnormalities*
						  1st–2nd trimesters
						  3rd trimester
						  All trimesters
						Stillbirth
						Birthweight
						  < 1500 g
						  < 2500 g
						Prematurity rate
						Dead at 168 hours
						  1st trimester
						  2nd–3rd trimester
						  All trimesters
						All adverse outcomes
						  General anesthesia
						  Type of operation
							Negative
							Positive
							Negative
							Negative
							
							Positive
							Positive
							Positive
							
							Positive
							Positive
							Negative
							Positive
							Positive
							
							Negative
							Negative
								Infant's year of birth, maternal age and parity, delivery unit (except for birthweight), and infant gender (for birthweight only)	8

[a]Positive, statistically significant association; Negative, no association; Increased, rate increased over comparison rate; Decreased, rate decreased below comparison rate; ?, appears likely but inconclusive because necessary data not provided.

all women for 20 to 30 minutes as one component of the general anesthetic technique. There were 30 spontaneous preterm deliveries, 11 (14.8%) in women with parity 1 to 2, and 19 (18.6%) in women with parity 3 or more. These rates were elevated over the population background rates of 3.6% and 6.5%, respectively. There were 6 infants with minor and 4 infants with major congenital abnormalities, many with known genetic and embryologic origins. The authors concluded that there was no evidence to suggest that administration of N_2O was associated with an increased incidence of congenital abnormalities. The overall incidence of congenital abnormalities was the same as the Scottish norm. The rates of spontaneous abortion and neonatal mortality/stillbirth did not appear to be elevated above the background rates.

Crawford and Lewis (6) evaluated the administration of N_2O to 375 women (383 fetuses) undergoing cervical cerclage and 58 women (59 fetuses) undergoing other surgical procedures in the first two trimesters of pregnancy. In addition, 364 of the women also received halothane, trichloroethylene, methoxyflurane, or enflurane. Among women undergoing cervical cerclage, the mean duration of anesthesia was 22.3 minutes (range 10 to 65 minutes). There were 10 (3.4%) infants with congenital abnormalities among the 298 fetuses exposed before completion of the sixteenth week of gestation, and there were 4 (4.7%) infants with congenital abnormalities among the 85 fetuses exposed after the sixteenth week of gestation. The rate of spontaneous abortion was 9.7% ($n=37$), with most ($n=28$) spontaneous abortions occurring during the first trimester. The rate of low birthweight was 3.2% ($n=11$) among the remaining infants. These rates were similar to the rates among 114 cases where cervical cerclage was inserted under regional analgesia (congenital abnormalities 6.1%, spontaneous abortion 9.6%, and low birthweight 3.8%). Among women undergoing other surgical procedures, the mean duration of anesthesia was 37.6 min-

utes (range 15 to 80 minutes). There was 1 (2.9%) infant with a congenital abnormality among the 35 fetuses exposed before completion of the sixteenth week of gestation, and there were 3 (12.5%) infants with congenital abnormalities among the 24 fetuses exposed after the sixteenth week of gestation. None of the 59 fetuses aborted or were stillborn, and only 1 infant was low birthweight. The authors concluded that none of the fetal abnormalities among the 442 infants could be clearly linked to N_2O exposure. Exposure to the other anesthetics was not evaluated.

Duncan et al. (7) conducted a case-control study using data from a Canadian congenital abnormalities monitoring surveillance system and health insurance data from the province of Manitoba. The population of Manitoba was estimated at 1 million. All hospitalizations for pregnancy-related conditions were determined for the period 1971 through 1978. Cases were 2565 pregnant women undergoing a surgical procedure, including procedures performed under local anesthesia and traumatic injuries. Controls were 2565 pregnant women with a pregnancy-related condition (not defined) but without any surgical procedure. Controls were matched to cases on geographic area and age (± 2 years). There were 82 infants with congenital abnormalities, 43 (1.7%) born to cases and 39 (1.5%) born to controls. This difference was not statistically significant, even after stratification by timing of exposure, type of anesthetic, and surgical procedure. There were 181 (7.1%) spontaneous abortions among cases and 166 (6.5%) among controls, not statistically significant. There was a significant increase in the rate of spontaneous abortion among cases who received a general anesthetic [estimated RR = 1.58, 95% confidence interval (CI) = 1.19–2.09]. The increased risk was associated with obstetric or gynecologic procedures and with other nonabdominal surgical procedures. The findings for the obstetric/gynecologic surgery were not explained by Shirodkar procedures.

Mazze and Kallen (8) published a study based on the computer linkage of three Swedish health care registries for the years 1973 to 1981. There were 5405 women who underwent nonobstetric operations (0.75%) in the population of approximately 720,000 pregnant women; 2252 women (41.6%) underwent surgery during the first trimester, 1881 (34.8%) during the second trimester, and 1272 (23.5%) during the third trimester (up to the day before delivery). Women who underwent cervical cerclage operations were excluded from analysis, as were multiple births for the analysis of birthweight. General anesthesia was reported for 2929 women (54.2%), and N_2O was administered in more than 98% of these cases, two thirds of the time with an i.v. anesthetic agent and one third of the time with a potent inhaled agent. Rates of pregnancy outcomes were standardized for several potential covariates (Table 1) and compared with Swedish national data.

The overall incidence of all congenital abnormalities was approximately 5%, and the incidence, excluding minor and inconsistently classified abnormalities, was 1.9%. These rates were similar to the Swedish national rates. The observed number of congenital abnormalities in offspring of women who underwent surgery during the first trimester was almost identical to the expected number (44 vs 42.6). Although the incidence of all abnormalities was significantly increased among offspring of women who underwent surgery during the third trimester (32 observed vs 20.9 expected), the authors concluded that this finding could not be of biologic significance because the operations took place several months after in utero development of the malformed organs.

The rate of stillborn infants was not increased in any of the trimester subgroups or in the total surgical population. However, the number of infants with birthweights of less than 1500 g was increased over the expected number for the total surgical population and for women who underwent surgery during the first two trimesters (ratios

of observed/expected ranged from 1.7 to 3.2). The number of infants with birthweights of less than 2500 g was increased for the total surgical population and for women who underwent surgery in all three trimesters (ratios of observed to expected ranged from 1.4 to 2.2). Reduced birthweight was due to both prematurity and intrauterine growth retardation. The overall prematurity rate was 7.5% for infants of mothers who underwent surgery vs a control rate of 5.1% ($p<0.001$). For each gestational age, the mean birthweight of infants of surgical mothers was less than the mean birthweight of infants of the control group. The number of liveborn infants who died within 168 hours after birth was significantly increased when surgery occurred during the second and third trimester, and 70% (40/57) of the deaths occurred in infants weighing less than 1500 g.

The overall incidence of adverse outcomes associated with general anesthesia was significantly less than predicted (odds ratio = 0.62, 95% CI = 0.38–0.99). There was no association between adverse outcomes and specific type of anesthesia or type of operation.

REPRODUCTIVE AND DEVELOPMENTAL OUTCOMES FOLLOWING OCCUPATIONAL EXPOSURE TO ANESTHETICS

Several reviews have been published of epidemiologic studies of reproductive and developmental outcomes following occupational exposure to the inhaled anesthetics, including an excellent review by Tannenbaum and Goldberg (9) and meta-analysis by Buring et al. (10). Selected characteristics of 19 epidemiologic studies of reproductive and developmental outcomes are summarized in Table 2.

The first published study of health effects associated with occupational exposure to anesthetics appeared in the Russian literature in 1967 (11). According to Tannenbaum and Goldberg (9), Vaisman surveyed 345

TABLE 2. Summary of epidemiologic studies of reproductive and developmental outcomes following occupational exposure to anesthetics

Agent	Definition of exposure	Data collection instrument	Study type	Study population	Comparison population	Outcome(s) investigated	Results[a]	Potential covariates considered	Ref
Waste anesthetics	Employment	Postal questionnaire	Retrospective survey, Denmark	Pregnancies conceived during employment: 229 in nurse anesthetists, 26 in female anesthesiologists, and 137 in wives of male anesthesiologists	Pregnancies conceived before employment: 85 in nurse anesthetists, 8 in female anesthesiologists, and 119 in wives of male anesthesiologists	*Spontaneous abortion* Nurse anesthetists Female anesthesiologists Wives of male anesthesiologists *Premature deliver* Nurse anesthetists Female anesthesiologists Wives of male anesthesiologists *Sex ratio*	Negative Negative Positive Negative Negative Positive Increased females	Unknown	12
Waste anesthetics	1. Any exposure in the OR within preceding 5 years 2. Any exposure in the OR within preceding 6 years	1. Personal interview concerning obstetric history and pregnancy outcome 2. Postal questionnaire	Retrospective survey, U.S.A. 1. 1966–1970 2. 1965–1970	1. 67 OR nurses 2. 50 female anesthesiologists	1. 92 general duty nurses 2. 81 female physicians	*Spontaneous abortion* Nurses Anesthesiologists *Average week of gestation at abortion* Nurses Anesthesiologists *Congenital abnormalities*	Positive Positive Decreased Decreased Negative	None	13
Waste anesthetics	Employment in anesthesia during 1st or 2nd trimester of pregnancy	Postal questionnaire concerning obstetric history and pregnancy outcome	Retrospective survey, U.K.	893 pregnancies in 563 married female anesthesiologists	1,835 pregnancies in 828 married female physicians	*Stillbirth* *Congenital abnormalities* Anesthesiologists employed vs not employed *Ratio of spontaneous abortions to total pregnancies* Employed anesthesiologists *Sex ratio* *Infertility due to unknown cause*	Negative Negative Positive Negative Positive Negative Positive	None	14
Waste anesthetics	Employment as an anesthesia or scrub nurse	Postal questionnaire concerning obstetric history, exposure to x-rays and halothane, and pregnancy outcome	Retrospective survey, Finland 1965–1972	257 pregnancies in 58 anesthesia and 124 scrub nurses	150 pregnancies in 75 casualty department and 43 intensive care unit nurses	*Spontaneous abortion* *Average week of gestation at abortion* *Low birthweight* *Congenital abnormalities*	Positive Negative Negative Negative	None	15
Waste anesthetics	For females, exposure during 1st trimester of pregnancy and work in OR during previous calendar year; for males, work in OR during year prior to pregnancy	Postal questionnaire concerning occupational experience, reproductive history, and pregnancy outcome	Retrospective survey, U.S.A. 1972–1974	18,568 pregnancies in 29,810 exposed OR personnel from 4 societies	5,620 pregnancies in 10,420 unexposed physicians, nurses, and their wives from 2 societies plus unexposed individuals and their wives from study population	*Spontaneous abortion* Female respondents *Average week of gestation at abortion* *Sex ratio at abortion* Wives of male respondents *Congenital abnormalities* Female respondents Wives of male respondents	Positive Negative Negative Negative Postive Positive	Maternal age and smoking history at conception	16

Agent	Exposure	Method	Study design, country	Exposed group	Comparison group	Outcome	Association	Confounders / matching	Ref.
Waste anesthetics	OR employment during pregnancy	Postal questionnaire and telephone interview concerning exposure, obstetric history, and pregnancy outcome	Retrospective survey, U.S.A.	434 births to 268 nurses who practiced anesthesia during pregnancy	1. 261 births to nurses who did not practice anesthesia during pregnancy 2. Published incidence rates	*Congenital abnormalities*		Age	17
						Total cutaneous abnormalities	Positive		
						Total noncutaneous abnormalities	Positive		
						Hemangiomas	Positive		
						Musculoskeletal	Positive		
						Inguinal hernia	Positive		
						All others	Negative		
Waste anesthetics	Exposure to anesthetics at least 3 hours weekly during calendar year preceding wife's pregnancy	Postal questionnaire concerning weekly exposure to anesthetic gases and pregnancy history of wife	Retrospective survey, U.S.A.	1,668 male dentists and oral surgeons exposed to anesthetics	1,560 male dentists and oral surgeons not exposed to anesthetics	*Spontaneous abortion*	Positive	Age and smoking habit of wife at time of pregnancy; also pregnancy history of wife and reluctance to answer survey	18
						Congenital abnormalities	Negative		
Waste anesthetics	OR employment during 1st trimester of pregnancy	Postal questionnaire concerning occupation of respondents and their wives, obstetric history of wives, and pregnancy outcome	Retrospective survey, U.K.	Married male anesthesiologists reporting at least one pregnancy for their wives; 5,891 pregnancies with only paternal exposure and 166 pregnancies with only maternal exposure	Male doctors registered in 1972; 7,296 pregnancies without paternal or maternal exposure	*Spontaneous abortion* — Paternal exposure	Negative	None	19
						Spontaneous abortion — Maternal exposure	Positive		
						During 1st pregnancy — Paternal exposure	Negative		
						During 1st pregnancy — Maternal exposure	Positive		
						During 2nd pregnancy — Paternal exposure	Negative		
						During 2nd pregnancy — Maternal exposure	Negative		
						Average week of gestation at abortion — Paternal exposure	Negative		
						Average week of gestation at abortion — Maternal exposure	Negative		
						Major congenital abnormalities — Paternal exposure	Negative		
						Major congenital abnormalities — Maternal exposure	Negative		
						Minor congenital abnormalities — Paternal exposure	Positive		
						Minor congenital abnormalities — Maternal exposure	Negative		
						Total congenital abnormalities — Paternal exposure	Positive		
						Total congenital abnormalities — Maternal exposure	Negative		
						Involuntary infertility — Paternal exposure	Positive		
						Stillbirth — Paternal exposure	Negative		
Waste anesthetics	OR employment during 1st trimester of pregnancy	Postal questionnaire concerning occupation of respondents and their wives, obstetric history of wives, and pregnancy outcome	Case-control, U.K.	1. 4,074 pregnancies with paternal exposure 2. Pregnancies with maternal exposure a. 435 b. 368	1. 4,074 pregnancies without paternal or maternal exposure 2. Pregnancies without paternal or maternal exposure a. 435 b. 772	*Spontaneous abortion*	Negative	Matched on maternal smoking habits, birth order, maternal age at birth, and year of father's birth (father's age at time of response for study population 2b)	19
						Congenital abnormalities	Positive		
						Major abnormalities	Negative		
						Minor abnormalities	Positive		
						Stillbirth	Negative		
						Spontaneous abortion 2a and 2b study populations	Positive		
						Congenital abnormalities 2a and 2b study population	Positive		
						2b study population	Negative		
						Stillbirth 2a and 2b study population	Negative		

TABLE 2. *Continued.*

Agent	Definition of exposure	Data collection instrument	Study type	Study population	Comparison population	Outcome(s) investigated	Results[a]	Potential covariates considered	Ref
Waste anesthetics	Appointment as an anesthesiologist at time of conception	Postal questionnaire concerning exposure, obstetric history, and pregnancy outcome	Retrospective survey, U.K.	670 pregnancies conceived while women employed as anesthesiologists	1,977 pregnancies conceived while women employed had no medical appointments	*Spontaneous abortion* / *Stillbirth* / *Low birthweight* / *Congenital abnormalities* / Cardiovascular system / Other malformations	Positive / Increased / Positive / / Positive / Negative	Maternal age and smoking habits at conception and parity	20
Waste anesthetics	Member of the Finnish Society of Anesthesiologists	Postal questionnaire concerning exposure, obstetric history, and pregnancy outcome	Retrospective survey, Finland 1961–1976	248 pregnancies in anesthesiologists' families	266 pregnancies in pediatricians' families (no OR exposure)	*Spontaneous abortion* / *Average week of gestation at abortion* / *Mean birthweight* / *Congenital abnormalities* / Musculoskeletal / Other	Negative / Decreased / Decreased / Negative / Increased / Negative	Selected results analyzed separately by smoking habits	21
Waste anesthetics	Women working in OR during pregnancy who gave birth in 1973 or 1975	Information on occupational exposure and infant diagnoses obtained from registry data; employment in OR obtained from hospitals; computerized delivery records for 1973, 1975	Cohort Sweden, 1973 and 1975	494 women who worked throughout pregnancy, 37 women who worked more than half of their pregnancies, and 10 women who worked less than half of their pregnancies	19,127 women employed in medical work who were delivered in 1973 or 1975	*Birthweight* / *Perinatal death rate* / *Congenital abnormalities* / *Pregnancy duration in weeks*	Negative / Negative / Negative / Decreased	Maternal age and parity	22
Waste anesthetics	Physicians who spent half or more time working in anesthesia practice	Postal questionnaire concerning obstetric and relevant occupational histories	Retrospective survey, England	277 children born to 186 anesthesiologists and their wives	92 children born to anesthesiologists and their wives not occupationally exposed to anesthesia	*Spontaneous abortion* / Maternal exposure / Paternal exposure / *Decreased birthweight* / *Congenital abnormalities* / Major disorders (girls) / Central nervous system / Bony disorders / Harelip/cleft palate / Locomotor system / Circulatory system	Positive / Positive / Increased / Positive / Increased / Positive / Increased / Increased / Increased / Increased / Negative	None	23
N₂O	Exposure in year preceding pregnancy; light exposure was 1–8 hours weekly and heavy exposure was more than 8 hours weekly	Postal questionnaire concerning occupational exposure, obstetric history, and pregnancy outcome	Retrospective survey, U.S.A.	Wives of 21,634 male dentists, and 21,202 female chairside assistants	Those not exposed in any years before conception, including year of conception	*Spontaneous abortion* / Wives of male dentists / Female chairside assistants / N₂O only / *Congenital abnormalities* / Wives of male dentists / Female chairside assistants / Light exposure / Heavy exposure / N₂O only / Musculoskeletal abnormalities / All other abnormalities	Positive / Positive / Positive / Negative / Positive / Increased / Positive / Positive / Negative	Maternal age and smoking history and history of previous spontaneous abortion or congenital abnormalities	24

184

Agent	Exposure	Study design	Population	Outcome	Result	Comments	Ref.
Waste anesthetics	Exposure to anesthetic gases by one or both parents either during or in the year before pregnancy	Postal questionnaire concerning respondent's professional career, and obstetric history and pregnancy outcome of respondent or their wives	Retrospective survey, Belgium	Pregnancies in 149 anesthesiologists and their wives and 240 OR nurses and their wives	*Sum of all abnormal pregnancies* *Congenital abnormalities* *Premature birth* *Stillbirth* *Spontaneous abortion* *Sex ratio*	Negative Negative Negative Negative Negative Increased males	Maternal smoking habits	25
Waste anesthetics	Employment for at least 3 continuous months in hospital departments where exposure to anesthetic gases was possible	Postal questionnaire concerning employment history and pregnancies and their outcome; more detailed questionnaire sent to women reporting a birth or spontaneous abortion	Retrospective cohort, Sweden 1970–1979	185 pregnancies in 152 women employed in hospital departments with possible exposure	*Spontaneous abortion* Period up to 16 weeks Nonresponse considered *Congenital abnormalities*	Negative Positive Negative Negative?	Maternal age and smoking habits; also stress, heavy work, x-ray exposure, and medication	26
Waste anesthetics	Employment during 1st trimester of pregnancy in anesthesia, surgery, intensive care, OR or internal medicine department of a general hospital	Head nurses sent a questionnaire to ascertain exposure during 1st trimester; registry data for outcomes	Case-control Finland, 1973–1979	1. 469 employed nurses who had a spontaneous abortion 2. 38 employed nurses who gave birth to an infant with congenital abnormalities	*Spontaneous abortion* *Congenital abnormalities*	Negative Negative	Matched on maternal age and hospital; also other potential exposures Matched on maternal age and hospital; also other potential exposures	27
Waste anesthetics and N₂O	Exposure index was product of hours in surgery and a subjective factor for presence of anesthetic odor	Postal questionnaire concerning reproductive history and occupational experience of respondents and their wives; additional questionnaire sent for senior female veterinary assistants	Case-control, U.S.A.	278 spontaneous abortions and stillbirths, and 98 live births with congenital abnormalities that occurred to female veterinarians and veterinarian assistants and wives of male veterinarians 642 normal pregnancies chosen on a stratified random basis	*Spontaneous abortion* Female veterinarians Female assistants Wives of male veterinarians N₂O Female veterinarians Female assistants Wives of male veterinarians *Congenital abnormalities* Female veterinarians	Increased Increased Negative Negative Increased Positive Negative	Pregnancy order, maternal age at pregnancy, and use of diagnostic x-rays	28

TABLE 2. *Continued.*

Agent	Definition of exposure	Data collection instrument	Study type	Study population	Comparison population	Outcome(s) investigated	Results[a]	Potential covariates considered	Ref
Waste anesthetics	Exposure at least 2 hours weekly in hospital OR or recovery room	Self-administered questionnaire or interview of reproductive history and pregnancy outcome	Retrospective survey, Ontario, Canada 1981–1985	10,232 pregnancies in 6,336 exposed staff and 2,225 pregnancies in 1,443 randomly sampled staff	3,656 pregnancies in 2,202 unexposed staff	*Spontaneous abortion* Maternal exposure Paternal exposure *Congenital abnormalities* Maternal exposure Paternal exposure	 Positive Positive Positive Positive	Birth order, maternal age, maternal smoking and alcohol consumption during pregnancy, and previous spontaneous abortion (except for congenital abnormalities)	29
N₂O	Exposure at least 5 hours weekly to scavenged or unscavenged N₂O	Telephone interviews of reproductive history and occupational exposures	Retrospective survey, U.S.A. 1987–1988	Female dental assistants pregnant within previous 4 years; 127 exposed to scavenged N₂O and 63 exposed to unscavenged N₂O	215 unexpected female dental assistants who were pregnant within previous 4 years	*Ratio of conception rate for exposed relative to unexposed in each menstrual cycle of unprotected intercourse* Scavenged Unscavenged *Mean time to conception* Scavenged Unscavenged *Spontaneous abortion* Unscavenged	 Negative Positive Negative Increased Increased	Age, race, family income, exercise, body mass, alcohol, smoking, recreational drugs, douching, history of IUDs, age at menarche, history of PID, frequency of intercourse, lifetime number of sexual partners, and recent use of oral contraceptives; also, other occupational exposures	30

[a]Positive, statistically significant association; Negative, no association; Increased, rate increased over comparison rate; Decreased, rate decreased below comparison rate; ?, appears likely but inconclusive because necessary data not provided.

anesthesiologists. Among the 110 female respondents, there were 31 pregnancies, 18 (58%) of which ended in spontaneous abortion. A subsequent study by Askrog and Harvald (12) is in Danish. Based on the abstract and tables, the authors sent questionnaires to 174 male and female anesthesiologists and 578 nurse anesthetists regarding their or their wives reproductive history. Among satisfactory responses there were 212 pregnancies that started before (unexposed pregnancies) and 392 that started during employment in an anesthetic department. The rate of spontaneous abortion for the exposed group was 18.6 per 100 pregnancies compared with a rate of 9.0 for the unexposed pregnancies ($p<0.001$). Wives of male anesthesiologists had a rate of 20.4 for pregnancies that started during paternal employment compared with 7.6 for pregnancies that started before paternal employment ($p<0.001$). The rate of spontaneous abortion, however, was not significantly increased for female anesthesiologists or nurse anesthetists. The rate of premature delivery for the exposed group was 6.4 per 100 pregnancies compared with a rate of 1.4 for the unexposed pregnancies ($p<0.01$). This rate also was increased for the wives of male anesthesiologists but not for female anesthesiologists and nurse anesthetists. The frequency of congenital malformations was similar between the exposed and unexposed groups. The authors noted that the exposed group had a decreased number of male children.

Cohen et al. (13) reported the results of an epidemiologic survey of spontaneous abortion among 67 operating room (OR) nurses and 50 female anesthesiologists. The control group consisted of 92 general duty nurses and 81 female physicians practicing in specialties other than anesthesia. All women were married and aged 25 to 50 years. The rate of spontaneous abortion among the OR nurses was 29.7% compared with 8.8% among the controls ($p<0.05$). Similar results were reported for the physicians. The rate of spontaneous abortion

among the anesthesiologists was 37.8% compared with 10.3% among the controls ($p<0.005$). For both nurses and physicians, the average week of spontaneous abortion was 8 weeks for the exposed groups and 10 weeks for the control groups. No differences were noted in the rate of congenital malformations.

Knill-Jones et al. (14) mailed questionnaires to 1241 female anesthesiologists and 1678 female practicing physicians whose names were taken from the 1970 U.K. Medical Register. Obstetric information was usable for 563 married female anesthesiologists and 828 practicing female physicians. The groups were similar in the rates of stillbirths, neonatal deaths, and congenital abnormalities, and in the sex ratio of their offspring. The data were analyzed further by whether the anesthesiologists were or were not employed during the first and second trimesters of gestation. The incidence of congenital abnormalities among live births was significantly greater when the mother had been employed than when she had not (6.5% vs 2.5%, $p<0.02$) but did not differ significantly from the incidence in the control group (4.9%). The groups were similar in the type of abnormality reported. The ratio of spontaneous abortions to total pregnancies did not differ for all anesthesiologists (i.e., employed and unemployed) compared with controls, but the ratio differed significantly between employed anesthesiologists and controls (18.2% vs 14.7%, $p<0.025$). The ratio did not differ significantly between anesthesiologists employed and not employed during the first two trimesters (18.2% vs 13.7%). Overall, 12% of anesthesiologists and 6% of controls had infertility for which there was no known cause ($p<0.001$).

Rosenberg and Kirves (15) mailed questionnaires to 300 married Finnish female nurses between the ages of 24 and 40 years. There were 506 pregnancies among the women, 99 prior to employment. Both OR scrub nurses and nurse anesthetists were considered exposed to anesthetics. Nurses employed in intensive care units or casualty departments were considered unexposed; nurses previously employed in ORs were excluded from analysis. The rates of spontaneous abortion among pregnancies conceived during employment were 21.5% among scrub nurses, 15.0% among nurse anesthetists, 16.7% among intensive care nurses, and 8.3% among casualty department nurses. The overall difference in rates between exposed (19.5%) and unexposed (11.4%) nurses was statistically significant ($p<0.05$). The rates of spontaneous abortion among pregnancies conceived before employment ranged from 10.3% among scrub nurses to 21.5% among nurse anesthetists. The average week of gestation at abortion did not differ significantly between the exposed and unexposed nurses. The mean birthweight of delivered infants was lowest in nurse anesthetists, although the difference was not statistically significant. No infants were reported to have gross abnormalities.

Because of the concerns raised by these studies, the American Society of Anesthesiologists (ASA) appointed an ad hoc committee to prepare a study protocol to investigate the health of OR personnel (16). The National Institute for Occupational Safety and Health (NIOSH) approved and funded the study. Questionnaires were mailed to 49,585 OR personnel in the United States, including all members of the ASA, the American Association of Nurse Anesthetists (AANA), and the Associations of OR Nurses and OR Technicians (AORN/T). These individuals represented essentially all male and female OR personnel exposed to waste anesthetics in the United States. Questionnaires also were mailed to 23,911 members of the American Academy of Pediatrics and to a 10% sample of the American Nursing Association (ANA). The questionnaire covered exposure and pregnancy outcomes for the previous 10 years. The response rates ranged from 41.8% among female members of the ANA to 75.7% among female members of the ASA. The overall response rate was 54.7%. Cases without any controls with OR exposure for the relevant pregnancy were excluded from their respective groups. The comparison group consisted of 10,420 unexposed individuals from the control societies as well as unexposed cases. Rates were directly standardized for maternal age and smoking habits at the time of pregnancy. There were 18,568 pregnancies among the 29,810 responding members of the ASA, AANA, and AORN/T, and 5620 pregnancies among the 10,420 responding members of the other societies. Rates of spontaneous abortion per 100 pregnancies among female respondents of the ASA and AORN/T (17.1 ± 2.0 and 19.5 ± 0.9, respectively) were statistically significantly higher ($p<0.01$) than among female respondents of the comparison societies (8.9 ± 1.8 and 15.1 ± 0.9). The rate was elevated among female respondents of the AANA (17.0 ± 0.9) but was not significant ($p = 0.07$). Spontaneous abortion rates also were compared between exposed and unexposed female members of each society, and the rates were elevated for exposed women who were members of the AANA ($p = 0.06$) and AORN/T ($p<0.01$). The rate was increased for exposed women who were members of the ASA (17.1 ± 2.0 vs 15.7 ± 3.3) but was not significant ($p = 0.35$). No significant differences were found in the average week of gestation at the time of abortion, nor was there any evidence of a change in the sex ratio between the exposed and comparison groups.

Similar analyses for the various societies were performed to compare the rate of congenital abnormalities in offspring of female respondents in the exposed and unexposed groups. Skin abnormalities were excluded. The rates per 100 liveborn babies were increased only among female members of the ASA (5.9 ± 1.4 vs 3.0 ± 1.1, $p<0.07$) and AANA (9.6 ± 0.8 vs 7.6 ± 0.7, $p<0.03$) vs the female members of their comparison societies. The rate was significantly increased for exposed vs unexposed respondents within the AANA (9.6 ± 0.8 vs 5.9 ± 1.0,

$p<0.01$) but not for respondents from the other societies.

The rates of spontaneous abortion and congenital malformations also were compared for wives of male respondents. Wives of respondents who were members of the AORN/T had a significantly elevated rate of spontaneous abortion (18.4 ± 4.1 vs 10.0 ± 3.3, $p = 0.04$). No significant differences were found in the rates of spontaneous abortion between the other exposed and unexposed groups (rates ranged from 10.0 ± 3.3 to 12.6 ± 0.8). The authors concluded that there was little evidence that male exposure resulted in spontaneous abortion in their wives. The rates of congenital abnormalities for infants born to wives of males employed in the OR were consistently higher than the rates for infants born to wives of unexposed males from the comparison societies. Only the difference for male physicians was statistically significant (5.4 ± 0.4 vs 4.2 ± 0.5, $p = 0.04$).

For both male and female respondents, a category of congenital abnormality was defined that included atrial septal defect, patent ductus, congenital hip, cleft palate or lip, clubfoot, pyloric stenosis, anencephaly, spina bifida, and hydrocephalus. The rates of this group of abnormalities per 100 live births were increased in both female respondents ($p = 0.06$) and wives of male respondents ($p = 0.03$) who were members of the ASA (1.24 ± 0.47 and 1.56 ± 0.21, respectively) when compared with members of the AAP (0.21 ± 0.21 and 0.90 ± 0.24). The authors concluded that the increased risk of congenital abnormalities among OR personnel may be due to environmental hazards as well as to genetic differences between the exposed and unexposed groups.

Corbett et al. (17) mailed questionnaires to 621 female nurse anesthetists to determine the incidence of congenital abnormalities. The response rate was 84.5%. There were 695 births among the 268 respondents who were mothers; the mother practiced anesthesia during 434 pregnancies and the mother did not practice anesthesia during 261 pregnancies. Congenital abnormality rates were compared between the exposed and unexposed pregnancies and with published incidence rates. The rates of one or more congenital abnormalities were 16.4% among exposed vs 5.7% among unexposed pregnancies ($p<0.005$). Excluding anomalies of the skin, the rates were 8.8% vs 3.8% ($p<0.025$). Rates also were compared for various organ systems and differed significantly for the following organ systems: skin, cavernous hemangiomas, musculoskeletal, and inguinal hernia. Rates were not significantly different for cardiovascular, urogenital, gastrointestinal, central nervous system, and miscellaneous systems.

Cohen et al. (18) mailed questionnaires to all 2642 male members of the American Society of Oral Surgeons and to a 4% sample of the membership of the American Dental Association ($n = 4797$). The questionnaire was based on the ASA questionnaire. The response rates were 65.4% for the oral surgeons and 38.9% for the general dentists. There were 1291 oral surgeons and 377 general dentists in the exposed group and 209 oral surgeons and 1351 general dentists in the unexposed group. Rates of spontaneous abortion and congenital malformations during the previous 10 years were standardized for maternal age and smoking habit at the time of pregnancy. The rates of spontaneous abortion were significantly increased in the wives of exposed dentists (16.0 ± 1.8 vs 9.0 ± 1.0 per 100 pregnancies, $p<0.01$). The rates of congenital abnormalities were similar among the wives of exposed and unexposed dentists (4.7 ± 1.1 vs 4.1 ± 0.4 per 100 live births, $p = 0.26$).

Knill-Jones et al. (19) conducted a questionnaire survey of 7949 male doctors residing in the United Kingdom, including all anesthesiologists and every tenth male doctor in the 1972 Medical Register. Doctors who qualified before 1932 were excluded. The overall response rate was 70.1%. The questionnaire was based on the ASA questionnaire and included questions on the exposure of either parent in an OR during each trimester of pregnancy. There were 4602 married doctors who reported one or more pregnancies for their wives; 26% were anesthesiologists. Results on several reproductive and developmental outcomes were reported by the presence of paternal and maternal exposure. No association was reported between paternal exposure and the following reproductive outcomes: spontaneous abortion, abortion during the first, second, or third and subsequent pregnancy, average week of gestation at abortion, and major congenital abnormalities. There was an increase in the frequency of minor congenital abnormality among pregnancies with paternal exposure (3.1%) compared with unexposed pregnancies (2.4%, $p<0.02$). The rate of all congenital abnormalities in pregnancies with paternal exposure was 4.5% compared with 3.6% in pregnancies without maternal or paternal exposure ($p<0.05$). There were no significant differences in the types of congenital abnormalities reported between pregnancies without exposure and those in which one or both parents were exposed. The rate of involuntary infertility did not differ among male anesthesiologists, other hospital doctors, and doctors not working in hospitals.

Positive associations were reported between maternal exposure and spontaneous abortion (15.5% vs 10.9%, $p<0.01$) and abortion during the first trimester (16.1% vs 7.7%, $p<0.001$). No association was reported between maternal exposure and the following reproductive outcomes: abortion during the second or third and subsequent pregnancy, average week of gestation at abortion, and minor and major congenital abnormalities. The rate of all congenital abnormalities in pregnancies with maternal exposure was 5.5% compared with 3.6% in unexposed pregnancies ($p>0.05$). When either parent was exposed during pregnancy, the rate of stillbirth was similar in exposed and unexposed pregnancies.

Knill-Jones et al. (19) also conducted a case-control study that matched 4074 pregnancies with paternal exposure to an equal number of pregnancies without maternal or paternal exposure. Cases and controls were matched on birth order, maternal smoking habits, maternal age at the time of birth, and year of father's birth. The rates of spontaneous abortion and stillbirth were similar between cases and controls. The rate of all congenital abnormalities was significantly increased in cases (4.5% vs 3.2%, $p<0.01$) primarily due to an increased rate of minor congenital abnormalities among the cases (3.1% vs 2.1%, $p<0.02$). Pregnancies with maternal exposure were matched using the same criteria; there were 435 case-control pairs. In addition, 386 (73.8%) of these cases were matched with two controls each using two different orderings of the file to give two different control groups. For all three sets of matched data, the rate of spontaneous abortion was significantly increased among cases compared with controls (14.5% to 14.9% vs 5.5% to 9.2%, $p<0.01$). The rate of all congenital abnormalities was significantly increased only in the 435 case-control pairs and not in the case-control pairs with two controls per case. The increase was due to increased reporting of both major and minor abnormalities. The stillbirth rate was similar between cases and controls.

Pharoah et al. (20) analyzed pregnancy outcome among women in anesthetic practice as part of a survey of all 7992 women on the 1975 Medical Register who were first registered in England and Wales in 1950 or later. Among the 5700 respondents who completed the questionnaire (72.0%), 2313 had never been pregnant or were pregnant for the first time. The remaining 3387 women reported 9301 pregnancies; 670 pregnancies were conceived while the women were engaged in anesthesia practice, and 1997 pregnancies were conceived while the women had no medical appointments. After standardizing for age, the rate of spontaneous abortion was 13.8% in practicing anesthesiologists and 12.0% in women without a medical appointment at the time of conception ($p<0.05$). When examined by parity, the stillbirth rate was increased, but not significantly, among anesthesiologists compared with women without a medical appointment (17.3 vs 10.3 per 1000 total births). After adjusting for parity, infants born to anesthesiologists had a lower mean birthweight (3347 ± 524 vs 3430 ± 491, $p<0.01$). The difference persisted when stillbirths and infants with congenital abnormalities were excluded from the analysis and when smokers and nonsmokers were examined separately. The rates of various types of congenital abnormalities were compared. Abnormalities of the heart and great vessels were significantly higher (13.8% vs 3.6%, $p<0.05$) among children of anesthesiologists than among the rest of the infants. No significant differences were found for other malformations: Down syndrome, neural tube defect, cleft lip/palate, talipes, congenital dislocation of the hip, hydrocele, hypospadias, epispadias, and genitourinary.

Rosenberg and Vanttinen (21) mailed questionnaires to all 212 members of the Finnish Society of Anesthesiologists and to 356 members of the Finnish Society of Pediatricians. The response rates were 85% and 64%, respectively. During the period 1961 to 1976, there were 248 pregnancies in anesthesiologists' families and 266 pregnancies in pediatricians' families while the parents were not working in an OR. The rate of diagnosed spontaneous abortion was 10.1% when either parent worked in an OR and 13.2% in the comparison group. The rate was similar for male anesthesiologists and pediatricians with OR employment, but the rate was 9.3% for female anesthesiologists and 18.8% ($n=3$) for female pediatricians with OR employment (not significant). Diagnosed spontaneous abortion occurred about 2 weeks earlier in anesthesiologists' than in pediatricians' families (8.2 ± 0.65 vs 10.9 ± 0.6 weeks, not significant). Exposure to halothane among anesthesiologists was subjectively evaluated to be slightly lower in cases of spontaneous abortion compared with exposure in the pe-

riod immediately before and during full-term pregnancies. The mean birthweight of infants born to anesthesiologists and their wives was slightly smaller than the mean birthweight of infants born to pediatricians and their wives. There were 29 reported congenital abnormalities among infants born to anesthesiologists and their wives and 28 among infants born to pediatricians and their wives. There were 6 congenital luxations of the hip joint and 3 congenital inguinal hernias in infants of anesthesiologists compared with no such abnormalities among infants of pediatricians.

Ericson and Kallen (22) linked records on all women employed in health care in Sweden with computerized delivery records for all women who bore a child during 1973 and 1975. For women with potential exposure to waste anesthetics, the location of work for each woman was requested from the employing hospitals. There were 541 offspring of women who worked in ORs for at least part of their pregnancy. The number of threatened abortions, the observed distribution of birthweights, the number of perinatal deaths, and the number of infants with congenital abnormalities were similar to the expected numbers. There were 36 pregnancies with duration of less than 37 weeks where 26 were expected. For pregnancy duration less than 32 weeks, the observed number was 2 and the expected number was 5.

Tomlin (23) mailed questionnaires to all 340 anesthesiologists in the West Midlands region of England to determine their obstetric and relevant occupational histories. Each anesthesia department was visited to collect and verify the completed questionnaires. Response rates were 92.6% for male and 91.6% for female anesthesiologists. Within the previous 20 years, 186 anesthetists had tried to establish a family. The rate of spontaneous abortion when either parent was occupationally exposed was 18.2% compared with 9.8% among the controls ($p<0.05$). The rate when there was maternal exposure was 29.3% ($p<0.05$), and the rate when there was paternal exposure was 15.8% ($p = 0.10$). Infants born to exposed women weighed 10% less than the expected mean birthweight; girls were particularly underweight. Anesthesiologists bore 26 offspring (9.3%) with a congenital abnormality or developmental problem (increased over the rates in various comparison populations). A significantly greater proportion of girls had major congenital or developmental disorders ($p < 0.05$). The rates of various congenital abnormalities were compared with the rates in several populations. The rates for abnormalities of the central nervous system, hip dysplasias, foot or ankle, and cleft lip/palate were increased, whereas rates for circulatory abnormalities were not.

Cohen et al. (24) surveyed 138,278 U.S. dentists to determine the use of inhaled anesthetics, and the response rate was 77.9%. A questionnaire based on the ASA questionnaire was sent to a stratified systematic sample of 30,650 respondents, including all 1136 female respondents. The questionnaire asked each dentist to supply, in the returned questionnaire, the names of assisting personnel so they could be surveyed. Questionnaires were sent to 30,547 chairside assistants. The response rate for dentists was 73.6% and for chairside assistants was 70.0%. Study results relating to anesthetic exposure during surgical procedures were reported by Brodsky et al. (4). Respondents who were older than 65 years or who worked only in a hospital setting were excluded from the analysis. Users of anesthetics tended to be younger and have greater exposure to amalgam restorations than nonusers. After adjusting for maternal age, smoking and pregnancy history, the rates of spontaneous abortion in wives of dentists were 6.7 ± 0.3 for nonusers, 7.7 ± 0.6 for light users, and 10.2 ± 1.0 for heavy users of inhaled anesthetic. The rates for female chairside assistants were 8.1 ± 0.5 for nonusers, 14.2 ± 1.7 for light users, and 19.1 ± 2.0 for heavy users. For both wives and female chairside assistants, the differ-

ences between exposed and unexposed groups were statistically significant. The rates of one or more congenital abnormalities (excluding congenital anomalies of the skin) in offspring of wives, adjusted for the same covariates, were 4.9 ± 0.3 for nonusers, 4.6 ± 0.5 for light users, and 4.8 ± 0.7 for heavy users. The rates for female chairside assistants were 3.6 ± 0.3 for nonusers, 5.7 ± 1.2 for light users, and 5.2 ± 1.2 for heavy users. Only the difference between light users and nonusers among chairside assistants was statistically significant ($p = 0.02$). Rates of musculoskeletal abnormalities were significantly increased only among children born to exposed vs unexposed chairside assistants (2.47 ± 0.61 vs 1.15 ± 0.20, $p < 0.01$). Rates of congenital abnormalities did not differ between exposed and unexposed groups for the following organ systems: cardiovascular, respiratory, digestive, nervous, and urogenital. The rates of spontaneous abortion and congenital abnormalities also were analyzed by exposure to N_2O. Among female chairside assistants exposed only to N_2O, the adjusted rates of spontaneous abortion and congenital abnormalities were 16.0 ± 1.4 and 5.5 ± 1.0, both significantly higher than the rates in the unexposed group.

Members of the Belgian Society of Anesthetics and operating theater nurses were surveyed by Lauwerys et al. (25). For comparison, the authors surveyed members of the Belgian Societies of Dermatologists and of Occupational Physicians, and social nurses and nurses working in intensive care units. Questionnaires were sent to 1305 physicians and 1715 nurses. The overall response rate was 47%. Bachelors were eliminated from the analysis, leaving 1027 respondents reporting 1910 pregnancies and 1683 children. No significant differences were found between the exposed and unexposed groups in the rate of congenital abnormalities, premature births, stillbirths, spontaneous abortions, or the sum of all abnormal pregnancies. There was an excess of boys in all groups except the control group ($p < 0.05$).

Axelsson and Rylander (26) mailed questionnaires to all women, except physicians, born 1930 or later who worked or had previously worked for at least three continuous months in departments of a Swedish hospital where the authors judged that exposure to waste anesthetics could have taken place. Unexposed controls with the same age and employment criteria were selected from personnel registers for medical wards without regular exposure to waste anesthetics. The accuracy of reported spontaneous abortion was evaluated by comparing questionnaire responses with hospital records. The overall response rates were 80.2% for cases and 78.0% for controls. The rate of spontaneous abortion was 15.8% among pregnancies in women working in high-exposure areas during the first trimester ($n = 133$), 12.4% among pregnancies in women working in high- or low-exposure areas during the first trimester, and 9.1% among pregnancies in unexposed women. The differences in the rates were not statistically significant when maternal age and smoking habits were taken into consideration. The spontaneous abortion rates for the period up to 16 weeks of gestation were 15.8% for pregnancies in women working in high-exposure areas and 8.0% for pregnancies in unexposed women ($p = 0.05$). Five children (4.4%) were born with congenital abnormalities among the 114 children whose mothers worked in high-exposure areas during the first trimester, no children whose mothers worked in low-exposure areas had congenital abnormalities, and 9 children (2.1%) were born with congenital abnormalities among the 434 unexposed children.

An important part of this study was the collection of information from hospital records on pregnancy outcomes among nonrespondents. A bias was found among the nonrespondents with respect to both place of employment during pregnancy and pregnancy outcome. All women suffering a spontaneous abortion when working in departments with exposure to waste anesthetics reported their department and spontaneous abortion, whereas one third of all spontaneous abortions occurring to women who were not exposed during pregnancy were not reported. When the 113 pregnancies among the nonrespondents were added to the data from the questionnaire, the spontaneous abortion rate became 15.1% among women working in high-exposure areas during pregnancy and 11.0% among unexposed women (still not statistically significant). For spontaneous abortions occurring up to 16 weeks of gestation, the rates were 15.1% and 9.9% (not statistically significant).

Hemminki et al. (27) studied spontaneous abortions and congenital abnormalities in the offspring of Finnish nurses working in selected departments of general hospitals who had been pregnant between the years 1973 and 1979. Cases were selected from registry data, and controls were selected from nurses who had given birth to a healthy child and who had never given birth to a malformed child nor had a spontaneous abortion during the study period. Controls were matched on maternal age (± 1.5 years) and hospital of employment. Three controls were chosen for each case. Questionnaires were sent to leading head nurses of all Finnish general hospitals to obtain exposure information for the first trimester of pregnancy for the cases and controls. Forty-eight cases and 102 controls were excluded from the analysis of spontaneous abortion because of lack of exposure or employment information or for related reasons. The odds ratio of spontaneous abortion during the first trimester was 1.2 (95% CI = 0.7–2.4), adjusted for exposure to sterilizing agents, cytostatic drugs, x-rays, hexachlorophene, telephone duty, and rotating shifts. Eight cases and 29 controls were excluded from the analysis of congenital malformations because of lack of information. The odds ratio of congenital abnormalities during the first trimester was 1.2 (95% CI = 0.3–4.6), adjusted for exposure to sterilizing agents, cytostatic drugs, X-rays, and hexachlorophene.

Johnson et al. (28) evaluated reproductive outcomes in a national sample of male and female veterinarians and female veterinary assistants exposed to waste anesthetics at concentrations near the NIOSH recommended standards. Screening questionnaires were sent to all 1914 female veterinarians and a random sample of 3000 male veterinarians who were graduated from veterinary school between 1970 and 1980, listed on the roster of the American Veterinary Medical Association, and engaged in small animal or mixed practice. A similar questionnaire was included to be given to a senior female veterinary assistant. The response rate was approximately 62% for female and 44% for male veterinarians. Cases included all spontaneous abortions, stillbirths, and live births with congenital abnormalities reported by respondents. Control pregnancies were chosen on a stratified random basis from normal births so that the distribution of pregnancy order and maternal age was approximately the same for cases and controls. A second questionnaire was sent for all study pregnancies. The response rate to this questionnaire ranged from 71% to 87%. The questionnaire gathered information on weekly use of inhaled anesthetics, type of agent, presence of scavenging equipment, and general level of anesthetic vapor. The analyses for maternal exposure included only pregnancies during which the women worked in a veterinary facility. Adjusted for use of diagnostic x-rays, the odds ratios of spontaneous abortion for maternal exposure to waste anesthetics were 2.86 (95% CI = 0.86–9.53) for veterinarians and 2.25 (95% CI = 0.92–5.52) for veterinary assistants. The adjusted odds ratios for maternal exposure to N_2O were 0.74 (95% CI = 0.36–1.52) for veterinarians and 2.18 (95% CI = 0.91–5.20) for veterinary assistants. Similar results were found when the anal-

yses were restricted to the first pregnancy. No significant dose–response trend was observed for spontaneous abortion. The adjusted odds ratio of congenital abnormalities for maternal exposure to waste anesthetics was 0.33 (95% CI = 0.12–0.90) for veterinarians. The unadjusted odds ratio for exposure to N_2O was 0.25 (95% CI = 0.06–1.06). Although the results were not shown, the authors stated that wives of male veterinarians exposed to N_2O before conception had a significant increase in the risk of spontaneous abortion. There was no significant effect resulting from exposure to waste anesthetics before conception.

Guirguis et al. (29) mailed questionnaires to 8032 personnel exposed to anesthetics in operating and recovery rooms and 2525 unexposed personnel from a representative sample of Ontario hospitals. The hospital director of OR nursing identified all persons chronically exposed to waste anesthetics. The questionnaire was based on the ASA questionnaire and asked for reproductive outcomes for the previous 20 years. The response rate was 78.8% for the exposed and 87.2% for the unexposed. A 20% random sample of the exposed personnel was identified for more intensive follow-up, and the response rate was 90.8%. The rates of spontaneous abortion, adjusted for maternal age and smoking habits at the time of pregnancy, were 15.6% for exposed women, 16.0% for women in the random sample, and 12.6% for unexposed women. Rates were 10.3% for wives of exposed men, 9.5% for wives of men in the random sample, and 8.5% for wives of unexposed men. The odds ratios, adjusted for potential confounders, were significant between exposed and unexposed workers (maternal exposure: 1.98, 95% CI = 1.53–2.56; paternal exposure: 2.30, 95% CI = 1.68–3.13). There was no significant difference in the late abortion rate between the exposed and unexposed groups, but there was a significant difference in the early abortion rate. The odds ratios of congenital abnormalities were significant between exposed and unexposed workers (maternal exposure: 2.24, 95% CI = 1.69–2.97; paternal exposure: 1.46, 95% CI = 1.04–2.05). Exposed workers reported a significantly higher proportion of minor malformations.

Rowland et al. (30) investigated the effects of occupational exposure to N_2O on the fertility of female dental assistants. Questionnaires were mailed to 7000 female dental assistants aged 18 to 39 years randomly selected from a dental assistant registry of the California Department of Consumer Affairs. The response rate was 69%. For further participation, the women had to meet the following criteria: pregnant within the past 4 years with the pregnancy not due to the failure of birth control, married at the time contraception was discontinued, employed at least 30 hours per week during the 6 months prior to unprotected intercourse, exposure to mercury did not change during this period, and provided a correct telephone number. Only 9% of women met these requirements; 91% (418) of these completed a telephone interview. Thirteen women were excluded because they did not know if their workplace scavenged N_2O. There was no association between the number of hours of exposure to scavenged N_2O and either fecundity or the mean time to conception (up to 13 menstrual cycles). An increased number of hours of exposure to unscavenged N_2O was significantly associated with decreased fecundity after adjustment for recent use of oral contraceptives, number of cigarettes smoked per day, age, history of pelvic inflammatory disease (PID), number of sexual partners, frequency of intercourse, and race. On the basis of a linear model, each hour of exposure to unscavenged N_2O per week corresponded to a 6% reduction in the probability of conception in each menstrual cycle. Reduced fecundity was found primarily in women with 5 or more hours of exposure per week ($n = 19$; adjusted fecundity ratio = 0.41, 95% CI = 0.23–0.74, $p = 0.003$). Results for the mean time to conception were similar. The mean number of menstrual cycles to conception

for women in the high unscavenged group was 32.2 ± 11.1 compared with 6.4 ± 0.8 in the unexposed group. Excluding the 93 women pregnant at the time of study, 10 of the remaining pregnancies were in women exposed to 5 or more hours of unscavenged N_2O per week. Of these, 50% ended in spontaneous abortion compared with 8% of the other 315 pregnancies.

Meta-Analysis

Meta-analysis is a method of evaluating a reported association between a potential risk factor (such as anesthetic exposure) and an event (such as an adverse reproductive or developmental outcome) by statistically pooling data from individual studies in conjunction with a systematic, qualitative review of the studies. Because of the many weaknesses in the epidemiologic studies of adverse reproductive and developmental outcomes following occupational exposure to anesthetics, a meta-analysis was not attempted for studies reviewed in this chapter. One such analysis, however, was published in 1985 by Buring et al. (10). They analyzed spontaneous abortion and congenital abnormalities among female physicians and nurses potentially exposed to waste anesthetics. Included in the quantitative analysis were the studies by Cohen et al. (13), Knill-Jones et al. (14), Rosenberg and Kirves (15), ASA Ad Hoc Committee (16), and Axelsson and Rylander (26). The summary risk ratios were 1.3 (95% CI = 1.2–1.4) for spontaneous abortion and 1.2 (95% CI = 1.0–1.4) for congenital abnormalities, both of which were statistically significant. Response or recall bias or both could explain these significant associations because most of the studies relied on voluntary responses and self-reported outcomes. In addition, all studies used OR employment as a surrogate for actual exposure to anesthetics. Buring et al. (10) concluded that they could not be certain that waste anesthetics were responsible for the observed effects, let alone assess dose–response trends and threshold levels. Further, it is not clear that the results are relevant to current ambient anesthetic gas concentrations.

SUMMARY AND CONCLUSIONS

It is difficult to draw firm conclusions from the epidemiologic studies of anesthetic exposure for pregnant nonobstetric surgical patients. These studies generally were not designed to distinguish between the reproductive and developmental effects of the underlying medical condition leading to the surgery and the anesthesia and surgery. There is evidence in some of the studies of an increased rate of spontaneous abortion and fetal and perinatal mortality. These associations appear to be dependent on a number of factors that are not uniformly related to anesthesia alone. Most studies found no association between anesthesia and congenital abnormalities. In the one study that reported an association (8), the increased rate of abnormalities was found for exposure to anesthesia and surgery during the third trimester—not a biologically plausible outcome.

The outcomes that were studied most frequently in studies of occupational exposure to waste anesthetic gases were spontaneous abortion and congenital abnormalities. Other reproductive and developmental end points were examined in relatively few studies. Although the majority of studies reported positive associations between exposure to waste anesthetics and spontaneous abortion, the study by Axelsson and Rylander (26) strongly suggests that selection bias could explain the associations. Selection bias arises from systematic differences in the characteristics of those studied from those not studied. As demonstrated by Axelsson and Rylander (26), differential nonresponse among study groups is of particular concern. It is possible that factors in the work environment other than anesthe-

sia, such as stress and other exposures, also may influence the rate of spontaneous abortion. In addition, few studies controlled for such potentially confounding factors as history of previous spontaneous abortion, maternal smoking history at conception, and other potential occupational exposures.

Approximately one half of the studies of occupational exposure to anesthetics and congenital abnormalities reported an increased rate of at least one abnormality. However, there was no pattern to the specific abnormalities reported. Most of the epidemiologic studies used a retrospective cohort study design that is subject to both selection and recall bias (for a discussion of study designs and sources of bias, see chapter by Ebi). Recall bias arises from systematic differences in accuracy or completeness of recalling and reporting prior events or experiences. Recall bias is particularly important for studies of reproductive and developmental outcomes because mothers of infants with adverse outcomes are more likely than mothers of healthy infants to recall details of possible exposures during gestation. In addition, mothers of infants with adverse outcomes may inaccurately recall events and report them as occurring following exposures when they actually occurred at other times. Another potential problem with the occupational studies is that information on the timing of anesthetic exposure in relation to gestational age generally was not verified.

One of the weakest links in the epidemiologic studies of adverse reproductive and developmental outcomes following occupational anesthetic exposure is the lack of quantification of the extent and duration of anesthetic exposure. It cannot be determined whether the reported associations are specific to an individual anesthetic or to other factors related to the work environment (e.g., other exposures) or to the study respondents (e.g., experience of degree of stress). Data generally were collected by self-administered questionnaire without verification of either exposure or outcome. In addition, the extent and duration of exposure to waste anesthetics has decreased in recent years, so it is difficult to draw conclusions on the likely adverse effects of current anesthetic exposure based on these earlier studies at higher exposure conditions.

Epidemiologic evidence alone is not sufficient to establish that exposure to anesthetics causes adverse reproductive and developmental outcomes. The following formal criteria are widely accepted to evaluate the likelihood that an association is causal: strength of the association, dose–response relationship, specificity of the association, appropriate temporal association, consistency of the association across multiple studies, biologic plausibility, and coherence of the evidence. Ideally, all criteria are fulfilled to determine that an association is causal; practically, most of the criteria have to be fulfilled.

Although the results from animal studies appear to suggest that an association between exposure to anesthetics and adverse reproductive and developmental outcomes may be biologically plausible at high, near-anesthetizing concentrations (see chapter by Rice), the epidemiologic evidence is too weak to conclude that there is a causal association between anesthetic exposure and adverse reproductive and developmental outcomes.

REFERENCES

1. Heinonen O P, Slone D, Shapiro S. Anesthetics, anticonvulsants, muscle relaxants, and stimulants. In: Kaufman D W, ed. *Birth defects and drugs in pregnancy.* Massachusetts: Publishing Sciences Group, 1977:357–365.
2. Smith B E. Fetal prognosis after anesthesia during gestation. *Anesth Analg* 1963;42:521–526.
3. Shnider S M, Webster G M. Maternal and fetal hazards of surgery during pregnancy. *Am J Obstet Gyncecol* 1965;92:891–900.
4. Brodsky J B, Cohen E N, Brown B W, Wu M L, Whitcher C. Surgery during pregnancy and fetal outcome. *Am J Obstet Gynecol* 1980;138:1165–1167.
5. Aldridge L M, Tunstall M E. Nitrous oxide and the fetus. A review and the results of a retro-
spective study of 175 cases of anaesthesia for insertion of Shirodkar suture. *Br J Anaesth* 1986; 58:1348–1356.
6. Crawford J S, Lewis M. Nitrous oxide in early human pregnancy. *Anaesthesia* 1986;41:900–905.
7. Duncan P G, Pope W D B, Cohen M M, Greer N. Fetal risk of anesthesia and surgery during pregnancy. *Anesthesiology* 1986;64;790–794.
8. Mazze R I, Kallen B. Reproductive outcome after anesthesia and operation during pregnancy: a registry study of 5405 cases. *Am J Obstet Gynecol* 1989;161:1178–1185.
9. Tannenbaum T N, Goldberg R J. Exposure to anesthetic gases and reproductive outcome. *J Occup Med* 1985;27:659–668.
10. Buring J E, Hennekens C H, Mayrent S L, Rosner B, Greenberg E R, Colton T. Health experiences of operating room personnel. *Anesthesiology* 1985;62:325–330.
11. Vaisman A I. Working conditions in surgery and their effect on the health of anesthesiologists. *Eksp Khir Anesteziol* 1967;3:44–49.
12. Askrog V, Harvald B. Teratogen effekt af inhalationsanaestetika. *Nord Med* 1970;83:498–500.
13. Cohen E N, Bellville J W, Brown B W. Anesthesia, pregnancy, and miscarriage: a study of operating room nurses and anesthetists. *Anesthesiology* 1971;35:343–347.
14. Knill-Jones R P, Moir D D, Rodrigues L V, Spence A A. Anaesthetic practice and pregnancy. Controlled survey of women anaesthetists in the United Kingdom. *Lancet* 1972;1: 1326–1328.
15. Rosenberg P, Kirves A. Miscarriages among operating theatre staff. *Acta Anaesth Scand* 1973; (suppl. 53):37–42.
16. Ad Hoc Committee. Occupational disease among operating room personnel. *Anesthesiology* 1974; 41:321–340.
17. Corbett T H, Cornell R G, Endres J L, Lieding K. Birth defects among children of nurse-anesthetists. *Anesthesiology* 1974;41:341–344.
18. Cohen E N, Brown B W, Bruce D L, et al. A survey of anesthetic health hazards among dentists. *J Am Dent Assoc* 1975;90:1291–1296.
19. Knill-Jones R P, Newman B J, Spence A A. Anaesthetic practice and pregnancy. Controlled survey of male anaesthetists in the United Kingdom. *Lancet* 1975;2:807–809.
20. Pharoah P O D, Alberman E, Doyle P, Chamberlain G. Outcome of pregnancy among women in anaesthetic practice. *Lancet* 1977;1:34–36.
21. Rosenberg P H, Vanttinen H. Occupational hazards to reproduction and health in anaesthetists and paediatricians. *Acta Anaesth Scand* 1978; 22:202–207.
22. Ericson A, Kallen B. Survey of infants born in 1973 or 1975 to Swedish women working in operating rooms during their pregnancies. *Anesth Analg* 1979;58:302–305.
23. Tomlin P J. Health problems of anaesthetists and their families in the West Midlands. *Br Med J* 1979;1:779–784.
24. Cohen E N, Brown B W, Wu M L, et al. Occupational disease in dentistry and chronic expo-

sure to trace anesthetic gases. *J Am Dent Assoc* 1980;101:21–31.

25. Lauwerys R, Siddons M, Misson C B, et al. Anaesthetic health hazards among Belgain nurses and physicians. *Int Arch Occup Environ Health* 1981;48:195–203.

26. Axelsson G, Rylander R. Exposure to anaesthetic gases and spontaneous abortion: response bias in a postal questionnaire study. *Int J Epidemiol* 1982;11:250–256.

27. Hemminki K, Kyyronen P, Lindbohm M L. Spontaneous abortions and malformations in the offspring of nurses exposed to anaesthetic gases, cytostatic drugs, and other potential hazards in hospitals, based on registered information of outcome. *J Epidemiol Community Health* 1985;39:141–147.

28. Johnson J A, Buchan R M, Reif J S. Effect of waste anesthetic gas and vapor exposure on reproductive outcome in veterinary personnel. *Am Ind Hyg Assoc* 1987;48:62–66.

29. Guirguis S S, Pelmear P L, Roy M L, Wong L. Health effects associated with exposure to anaesthetic gases in Ontario hospital personnel. *Br J Ind Med* 1990;47:490–497.

30. Rowland A S, Baird D D, Weinberg C R, Shore D L, Shy C M, Wilcox A J. Reduced fertility among women employed as dental assistants exposed to high levels of nitrous oxide. *N Engl J Med* 1992;327:993–997.

Anesthetic Toxicity, edited by
Susan A. Rice and Kevin J. Fish.
Raven Press, Ltd., New York © 1994.

11

Pharmacogenetics and Anesthetic Toxicity

Margaret Wood

*Departments of Anesthesiology and Pharmacology, Vanderbilt University School of
Medicine, Nashville, Tennessee 37232-2125*

Clinical anesthesiologists recognize that there is considerable variation in response to drugs, so that one of their principal aims is the individualization of drug therapy (1). Many factors lead to altered pharmacokinetics and pharmacodynamics and, hence, to altered drug response and, in some cases, toxicity. However, a major development in pharmacology over the last 10 years has been the application of molecular genetics to clinical problems. Pharmacogenetics is that area of genetics that examines individualization of drug response based on the presence of one or more abnormal genes leading to genetic variation in drug response. Thus, pharmacogenetics deals with the modification of drug response by hereditary or genetic influences (2).

Idle and Gonzalez have suggested that the definition of pharmacogenetics be broadened and three general areas of investigation be considered (3).

1. Molecular mechanisms of interindividual variation in expression and catalytic activities of xenobiotic-metabolizing enzymes
2. Genetic mechanisms of species differences in expression and regulation of enzymes
3. Transporters and receptors for foreign compounds and molecular mechanisms of gene control

Many drugs, including anesthetic drugs, are metabolized before elimination from the body. Pathways of drug metabolism can be divided into phase I and phase II reactions. Phase I reactions include oxidation, reduction, and hydrolysis. Examples of phase II reactions are glucuronidation, sulfation, and acetylation. Genetic variability in the pathways of acetylation and hydrolysis have been recognized for many years. Ester and amide drugs are metabolized by hydrolysis. For example, the muscle relaxant succinylcholine is hydrolyzed by plasma cholinesterase. An inherited enzyme variant of cholinesterase with a defective ability to hydrolyze succinylcholine is responsible for prolonged neuromuscular paralysis in some patients. For the drugs procainamide, hydralazine, nitrazepam, and isoniazid, acetylation is the important pathway for drug metabolism. It is well recognized that for acetylation there are two groups in the population, slow acetylators and fast acetylators (4). The proportion of fast and slow acetylators is under genetic control, and there are interethnic differences. Caucasians have about 40% to 50% fast acetylators in the population, whereas 88% to 90% of Japanese are fast acetylators. The rate of acetylation has an important effect on isoniazid, procainamide, and hydralazine toxicities.

Although polymorphism for the pathways of acetylation and hydrolysis has been recognized for over 30 years, many drugs are not metabolized by these pathways. Most drugs are metabolized by oxidation by the cytochrome P450 mixed-function oxidase system of the liver. About 20 years were to pass after the discovery of a genetic basis for the hydrolysis of succinylcholine before it was realized that genetic polymorphism for oxidative pathways also existed. The first oxidation defects to be described were for the metabolism of debrisoquine and sparteine (5,6). Debrisoquine, an adrenergic-neuron blocking agent prescribed for the management of hypertension in Europe, is metabolized by oxidation to 4-hydroxydebrisoquine. It was noted that a small number of patients became unexpectedly hypotensive following administration of the drug. This observation led to the recognition that the ability to metabolize debrisoquine by this pathway is impaired in about 8% to 10% of the population in the United States and the United Kingdom. It soon became evident that the deficient ability to metabolize sparteine was due to a deficiency of the same enzyme responsible for the metabolism of debrisoquine. Two distinct populations (polymorphism) are now recognized—the poor metabolizer (PM) phenotype and the extensive metabolizer (EM) phenotype. The worldwide importance of this enzyme lies not in its ability to metabolize debrisoquine and sparteine but in the fact that there is a large number of drugs that are metabolized by this enzyme and whose metabolism thus cosegregates with debrisoquine.

Many drugs, e.g., codeine, are not metabolized by one single route but are metabolized by a number of parallel and consecutive reactions. Codeine is metabolized by the pathways of O-demethylation, conjugation, and N-demethylation. It is the pathway of O-demethylation to morphine that is under the control of the enzyme responsible for debrisoquine metabolism. Morphine is subsequently glucuronidated to yield morphine-3-glucuronide and morphine-6-glucuronide, which are excreted in the urine. The consequences of impaired metabolism in PMs depend on the contribution that the impaired pathway makes to the drug's overall clearance and also on the pharmacologic importance of the resultant metabolites. If most of the drug's elimination is by the impaired pathway, absence of this pathway will result in decreased total drug clearance. This will lead to high parent drug concentrations, with the potential for toxicity in the PM phenotype. For some drugs, the metabolite produced is pharmacologically active and may make an important contribution to therapeutic effect. In the case of codeine, O-demethylation to morphine is principally responsible for the analgesic effect of codeine, and this is impaired in patients who are poor metabolizers of debrisoquine (7).

If enzyme activity is under the control of a single gene, alteration of drug metabolism may be seen if a defect occurs in that single gene. Monogenic inheritance implies that a characteristic is transmitted by a gene at a single locus, whereas polygenic inheritance is controlled by genes at multiple loci on the chromosomes. Thus, it is important to examine not only the clearance of the parent drug, but also the production of metabolites. Single-gene defects often produce clinically significant alterations in responses to certain drugs. Plasma cholinesterase deficiency is an example of an autosomal mendelian recessive trait that affects drug metabolism so that when the muscle relaxant succinylcholine is given, anesthetic toxicity is evident as prolonged apnea. A deficiency of acetylation is an autosomal recessive trait that leads to the slow metabolism of the antituberculosis drug, isoniazid, with consequent polyneuritis in some patients.

Malignant hyperthermia (MH) is an autosomal dominant trait in which acute hyperpyrexia, muscle rigidity, hyperkalemia, and cardiac arrest may occur due to a disturbance of muscle cell calcium regulation induced by administration of triggering agents, particularly anesthetic agents. Studies suggest that an altered ryanodine receptor due to a corresponding gene defect might cause MH. If that is the case, MH can be defined as a pharmacogenetic/pharmacodynamic disorder.

Thus, pharmacogenetic disorders of importance to the anesthesiologist that in some instances may lead to anesthetic toxicity include

1. Genetic impairment of the cytochrome P450 drug-metabolizing enzyme system
2. Malignant hyperthermia
3. Atypical plasma cholinesterase

GENETIC IMPAIRMENT OF DRUG METABOLISM BY THE CYTOCHROME P450 ENZYME SYSTEM

Cytochrome P450 is a collective term for a family of closely related enzymes that catalyze the oxidation of carcinogens, other xenobiotics, exogenously administered drugs, and many endogenous compounds, such as steroids, prostaglandins, and fatty acids. It is now recognized that many P450 enzymes exist, each encoded by a separate gene. Genetic polymorphism of the human cytochrome P450 enzyme system, resulting in enzymes being either functionally abnormal or inactive, is one of the factors responsible for the marked interindividual variation in human drug metabolism. A classification system for the P450 gene superfamily has been proposed in which genes are assigned to families and subfamilies according to the degree of similarity of the amino acid sequence of the isozymes (8,9). Genes that encode P450 proteins that are less than 40% similar in amino acid sequence are assigned as belonging to different families. Mammalian sequences within the same subfamily are >55% identical. Different families are designated by an Arabic numeral, and each subfamily is designated by a capital letter. P450 nomenclature suggests that a P450 gene be denoted by an italicized root symbol *CYP*, e.g., for the P450 gene *CYP* and for the gene product (enzyme) CYP1A1.

There are at least 221 P450 genes and 12 putative pseudogenes that have been char-

acterized in 31 eukaryotes (including 11 mammalian and 3 plant species) and in 11 prokaryotes. Of the 36 gene families described, 12 families exist in mammals. These 12 families comprise 22 mammalian subfamilies, of which 17 have been mapped in the human genome. It is interesting that genes within a defined subfamily have been shown so far to be nonsegregating and thus lie within the same gene cluster; i.e., they are located adjacent to one another on the same chromosome (8).

Each drug-metabolizing P450 enzyme can metabolize a wide range of drugs, whereas, in contrast, a specific drug may have a high affinity for one particular P450 enzyme, which catalyzes its oxidation. Many commonly administered drugs have been shown to be substrates for the subfamilies CYP1A, CYP2C and CYP2E, CYP2D6, and CYP3A3, and it is these subfamilies that have been studied extensively over the last few years. Table 1 shows the important human cyto-

TABLE 1. *Human cytochrome P450 families*

P450	Tissue	Substrate
CYP1A1	Many	Benzo(a)pyrene
CYP1A2	Liver	Aflatoxin β_1
		Caffeine
		Phenacetin
CYP2A6	Liver	Coumarin
		Diethylnitrosamine
CYP2B6	Liver	Cyclophosphamide
CYP2C	Liver	Diazepam
	Intestine	Mephenytoin
		N-Desmethyldiazepam
		S-Warfarin
		Tolbutamide
CYP2D6	Liver	Debrisoquine
	Intestine	Sparteine
	Kidney	
CYP2E1	Liver	Carbon tetrachloride
	Intestine	Ethanol
	Leukocytes	Volatile anesthetics
CYP3A	Liver	Alfentanil
	Gastrointestinal	Cyclosporine
	tract	Erythromycin
		Lidocaine
		Midazolam
		Nifedipine
		Testosterone

Adapted from Gonzalez F J. Human cytochromes P450: problems and prospects. *TIPS* 1992;13:346–352.

chrome P450 enzymes and some of the drugs metabolized by these enzymes.

The most extensively studied enzyme undoubtedly is human CYP2D6, responsible for the sparteine/debrisoquine polymorphism. This enzyme has broad substrate specificity, and its importance lies not in its ability to metabolize debrisoquine but because a large number of other drugs also are metabolized by this enzyme, including propranolol, metoprolol, and codeine (Table 2). The 8% to 10% of the U.S. population who are poor metabolizers of debrisoquine have a markedly reduced ability to oxidize debrisoquine to the metabolite, 4-hydroxy-debrisoquine. The poor metabolizer phenotype is classified by measuring the ratio of unchanged debrisoquine to 4-OH-debrisoquine in a urine sample (Fig. 1). A ratio of >12 ($\log_{10}$, 1.1) is usually used as a cutoff to identify the poor metabolizers. Thus, de-

brisoquine and sparteine oxidation have been used as probes for the activity of CPY2D6. The effect of CYP2D6 polymorphism on clinical pharmacologic response depends on the contribution of the affected pathway to overall elimination of the drug. Thus, if most of the drug's elimination is by the pathway catalyzed by CPY2D6, the absence of the pathway will result in reduced total clearance of the parent drug and increased drug concentrations, with the potential for toxicity in the poor metabolizer phenotype. Decreased enzyme activity would, therefore, result in exaggerated pharmacologic effect.

Conversely, if only a small proportion of total drug clearance is via CYP2D6, as is the case for propranolol (15%), there may be loss of the ability to form one metabolite (4-hydroxypropranolol) but little overall change in parent drug clearance and, hence, in plasma concentration and pharmacologic effect (10). If a major pathway of metabolism is reduced by polymorphism, it is possible that the parent drug may be metabolized by what are usually minor pathways, possibly leading to toxicity.

The therapeutic effect of some drugs is produced by a pharmacologically active metabolite, e.g., encainide and codeine. Encainide is metabolized by CYP2D6 to an active metabolite. Poor metabolizers form only a small amount of metabolite and, therefore, eliminate encainide very slowly.

Many commonly administered drugs are substrates for the cytochrome subfamily CYP3A (Table 3). In contrast to the two debrisoquine phenotypes, CYP3A has a broad unimodal distribution of enzyme activity, reflecting wide interindividual variability, but no distinct subgroup has been identified. The CYP3A subfamily is induced by glucocorticoids and is expressed in high amounts in human liver. The most abundant form in liver is CYP3A4. Agents that interfere with the function of CYP3A4 would be expected to markedly affect the elimination of other CYP3A4 substrates and possibly lead to drug interactions.

TABLE 2. *CYP2D6 substrates: Drugs whose metabolism is impaired in poor metabolizers of debrisoquine*

Beta-adrenergic blocking agents
Alprenolol
Propranolol
Metoprolol
Oxyprenolol
Bufaralol
Timolol
Other cardiovascular drugs
Guanoxan
Mexiletine
Debrisoquine
Sparteine
Perhexiline
Indoramin
Flecainide
Encainide
Propafenone
Psychotropic drugs
Amitriptyline
Haloperidol
Oxazepam
Temazepam
Desipramine
Clozapine
Analgesics
Codeine
Dextromethorphan
Other drugs
Phenformin

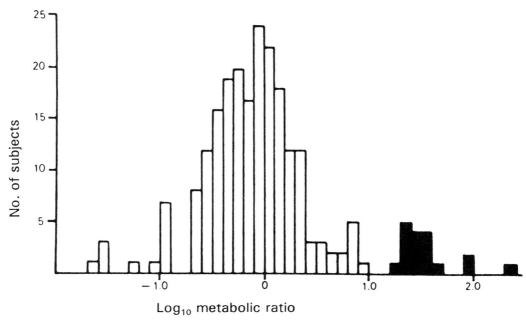

FIG. 1. Genetic polymorphism of debrisoquine metabolism. Debrisoquine metabolic ratio (ratio of unchanged debrisoquine to 4-hydroxydebrisoquine in the urine), showing the bimodal distribution. Ninety percent of the population (open bars) are extensive metabolizers with a metabolic ratio <12 ($\log_{10}$, 1.1), and 10% of the population (solid bars) are poor metabolizers with a metabolic ratio of >12. (From Woolhouse N M, Andoh B, Mahgoub A, Sloan T P, Idle J R, Smith R L. Debrisoquine hydroxylation polymorphism among Ghanians and Caucasians. *Clin Pharmacol Ther* 1979; 26:584–591.)

TABLE 3. *CYP3A substrates*

Drugs	Steroids	Carcinogens
Alfentanil	Androstenedione (6β)	Aflatoxins
Cyclosporine	17β-estradiol (2)	6-aminochrysene
Dapsone	17α-ethinylestradiol (2)	Polycyclic hydrocarbon dihydrodiols
Erthromycin	Gestodene	Pyrrolizidine alkaloids
FK506	Progesterone (6β)	
Ketoconazole	Testosterone (6β)	
Lidocaine		
Lovastatin		
Midazolam		
Nifedipine		
Quinidine		
Terfenadine		
Troleandomycin		

INDIVIDUAL CYTOCHROME P450 FAMILIES

CYP1 Family

Polymorphism exists for the enzyme CYP1A1, responsible for benzo(a)pyrene hydroxylation activity and the activation of some other polycyclic hydrocarbons (11). A tentative link among CYP1A1 activity, cigarette smoking, and lung cancer has been observed.

CYP1A2 is responsible for the metabolic activation of many potential carcinogens, including aflatoxin B_1. CYP1A2 is found in human liver. The demethylation of caffeine by CYP1A2 has been used as a specific metabolic probe for the enzyme (12,13). CYP1A2 also catalyzes the O-deethylation of phenacetin (14).

CYP2 Family

Coumarin is a substrate for CYP2A6, which is inducible by pyrazole. CYP2B6 is the major P450 enzyme induced by phenobarbital in humans (15). The CYP2C subfamily contains five genes thus far, identified by cDNA cloning. Members of this subfamily metabolize S-warfarin, tolbutamide, and S-mephenytoin (16–21). S-mephenytoin polymorphism has been identified for the stereoselective 4′-hydroxylation of S-mephenytoin. Metabolism of several drugs of anesthetic importance has been shown to cosegregate with *S*-mephenytoin metabolism, including hexobarbital hydroxylation, omeprazole hydroxylation, *N*-demethylation of diazepam, and hydroxylation of *N*-desmethyldiazepam (Table 1). The molecular biology of S-mephenytoin polymorphism has not been defined, although it is known that a CYP2C family protein must be involved. A polymorphism for tolbutamide has been described.

More information is available on the polymorphism and substrate drugs for the CYP2D6 subfamily than for any other enzyme. The human *CYP2D6* gene has been characterized and localized to chromosome 22 (22–25). Two other genes, *CYP2D7P* and *CYP2D8P,* are located near *CYP2D6* on the long arm of chromosome 22 but are not expressed in the human liver. There are four allelic variants (*CYP2D6A, CYP2D6B, CYP2D6C,* and *CYP2D6D*) containing mutations that inactivate *CYP2D6* and thus lead to the poor metabolizer phenotype (26–32). The alleles can be detected through polymerase chain reaction (PCR). Thus, there are considerable data regarding the *CYP2D6* gene that codes for debrisoquine 4-hydroxylase. In addition, there is increasing information about the basis of the PM phenotype. Several types of mutation in CYP2D6 result in lack of enzyme activity.

In 1988, four allelic variants were detected using restriction fragment length polymorphism (RFLP) analysis (33). In 1990, two new mutations in the *CYP2D6* gene were detected in poor metabolizers, in each case resulting in no active enzyme being produced (34). A randomly selected population of 73 volunteers (predominantly extensive metabolizers) and 22 previously established poor metabolizers of debrisoquine were genotyped by RFLP and polymerase chain reaction assays for two mutations (29A and 29B) (34). Ninety-five percent of the poor metabolizers could be detected as such by these techniques. A good correlation between debrisoquine 4-hydroxylation metabolic ratio and CYP2D6 genotype was observed (Fig. 2), particularly for subjects genotyped as homozygous extensive metabolizers.

The ethanol-inducible CYP2E1 enzyme metabolizes ethanol, acetone, acetaminophen, the muscle relaxant chlorzoxazone, and some anesthetics (35,36). It also is involved in the activation of a number of potential carcinogens, such as benzene, vinyl chloride, carbon tetrachloride, and chloroform.

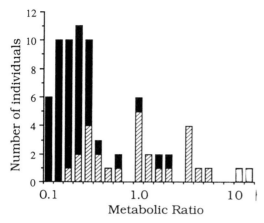

FIG. 2. P450-2D6 genotype and debrisoquine metabolism. The relationship between metabolic ratio (molar ratio of debrisoquine/4-hydroxyde-brisoquine in 0–8 hour urine) and genotype within the volunteer group. On the basis of RFLP and PCR analysis, subjects were classed as either homozygous EM (■), heterozygous EM (///), or PM (□). (From Daly A K, Armstrong M, Monkman S C, Idle M E, Idle J R. Genetic and metabolic criteria for the assignment of debrisoquine 4-hydroxylation (cytochrome P450-2D6) phenotypes. *Pharmacogenetics* 1991;1:33–41.)

CYP3A Family

The glucocorticoid-inducible CYP3A subfamily is expressed in large amounts in human liver. CYP3A3 and CYP3A4 are very similar, although the most abundant form in liver is CYP3A4. CYP3A5 is expressed in only about 10% to 20% of human liver. CYP3A7 is the major P450 found in human fetal liver. The CYP3A subfamily is responsible for the metabolism of a large number of frequently administered drugs, including the prototype nifedipine (37). At the present time, polymorphism for the CYP3A subfamily has not been identified. Considerable interindividual variability in metabolism is seen for substrates of the CYP3A family, such as alfentanil and midazolam. In addition, there is considerable potential for drug interactions to occur due to the concurrent administration of other drugs that are metabolized by CYP3A.

ETHNIC DIFFERENCES IN DRUG METABOLISM

Ethnic pharmacokinetic differences may be due to environmental or genetic factors (38). Polymorphism of acetylation was discussed earlier in this chapter. Populations can be divided into two groups, slow and fast acetylators controlled by a single gene. Slow acetylation is inherited as an autosomal homozygous recessive trait, and rapid acetylators are either heterozygotes or homozygotes. Considerable interethnic differences exist in the frequency of slow and fast acetylators (Table 4).

Polymorphism of cytochrome P450-dependent oxidation reactions has been described. The defective oxidation of debrisoquine and sparteine is controlled by a single gene *CYP2D6*, and the poor metabolizer phenotype is homozygous for an autosomal recessive allele. Considerable

TABLE 4. *Frequency of slow acetylators in populations*

Population	Number	Frequency (%)
Black		
Sudan	102	65
Nigeria	109	49
East Africa	204	55
United States	242	42–51
Caucasian		
Britain	472	55–62
Germany	524	57
Canada	102	59
United States	481	52–58
Chinese		
Taiwan	127	22
Britain	59	22
Singapore	386	22
Hong Kong	184	22
Thailand	47	34
Mainland China	108	13
Eskimo		
Canada	328	5–6
Alaska	157	21
Japanese		7–12
Japan	1990	10
United States	209	

Adapted from Wood A J J, Zhou H H. Ethnic differences in drug disposition and responsiveness. *Clin Pharmacokinet* 1991;20:350–373.

variability in the frequency of the PM phenotype has been demonstrated; 6% to 10% of Caucasians are poor metabolizers, whereas 0 to 0.5% and 0.7% of the Japanese and Chinese population, respectively, are poor metabolizers (38) (Table 5).

The metabolism of S-mephenytoin by the CYP2C subfamily also exhibits polymorphism. Hydroxylation of the S-enantiomer is deficient in about 3% of the Caucasian population but 17.4% in a Chinese population and 22.5% in Japanese (38). Hydroxylation of mephenytoin is inherited as an autosomal recessive trait. The increased frequency of the PM phenotype in the Asian population may make them particularly susceptible to drug toxicity from other

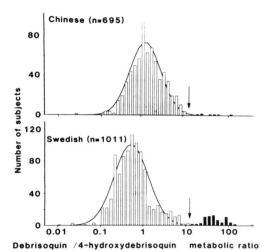

FIG. 3. Urinary debrisoquine/4-hydroxydebrisoquine metabolic ratio in a population of 687 Chinese and 938 Swedish individuals. The arrows indicate the metabolic ratio = 12.6; poor metabolizers of debrisoquine have a metabolic ratio = 12.6. (From Bertilsson L, et al. Pronounced differences between native Chinese and Swedish populations in the polymorphic hydroxylations of debrisoquine and S-mephenytoin. *Clin Pharmacol Ther* 1992;51:388–397.)

TABLE 5. *Frequency of poor metabolizers of debrisoquine-type hydroxylation in populations*

Population	Number	Frequency (%)
Native American		
Panama	51	0
Arab	102	1
Black		
Ghana	154	0.7
Nigeria	80	5
	123	8
	116	3
Caucasian		
Britain	258	9
Germany	94	3
Denmark	360	5
Switzerland	301	7
	268	9
Sweden	222	10
	226	8
	205	8.8
Finland	757	5.4
Hungary	107	6
Spain	100	10
	124	10
Canada	377	6.6
United States	83	7
Australia	156	7
Greenland	100	6
	185	3
Chinese		
China	269	0.7
	98	0
Egyptian	72	1.4
Japanese	100	0
	200	0.5

Adapted from Wood A J J, Zhou H H. Ethnic differences in drug disposition and responsiveness. *Clin Pharmacokinet* 1991;20:350–373.

drugs metabolized by CYP2C. Drugs that are of importance to anesthesiologists include diazepam and its demethyl metabolite, demethyldiazepam (Table 1).

There is evidence that in addition to the interethnic difference in the frequency of phenotypes, there may be interethnic differences in the distribution of enzyme activity within a phenotype. For example, the distribution of urinary metabolic ratio for debrisoquine (a measure of CYP2D6 activity) differs between Chinese and Swedes (Fig. 3). These data show that even in the EM phenotype, the Chinese metabolize debrisoquine more slowly than Swedes (39) and may reflect interethnic genetic differences (40,41).

An additional ethnic difference in drug metabolism occurs when substrates that cosegregate in one population do not in another population. For example, in Caucasians, sparteine and debrisoquine cosegregate, but apparently this does not happen in Ghanaians (42). In the case of CYP2C, mephenytoin and diazepam cosegregate in Caucasians but not in Chinese (43). These findings suggest that there may be subtle interethnic differences in enzyme structure that account for differences in substrate specificity.

PHARMACOGENETICS OF INHALATIONAL AND INTRAVENOUS ANESTHETICS

Inhalational Anesthetics

Enflurane, halothane, isoflurane, and methyflurane are metabolized by the mixed function oxidase system of the liver (see chapter by Waskell). Halothane is metabolized by the cytochrome P450 system and may proceed along two routes: oxidative to produce the metabolites trifluoroacetic acid and bromide and reductive to yield fluoride, bromide, and two volatile reductive metabolites. Although halothane has been used as an inhalational anesthetic for many years, and indeed it is still administered frequently in pediatric practice, its use has declined markedly because of associated liver toxicity—halothane hepatotoxicity. A description and etiology of halothane hepatotoxicity is given in the chapter by Baker and Van Dyke, and it is clear that in animal models of halothane hepatotoxicity, metabolism plays a pivotal role.

However, pharmacogenetic factors also may play a role in the etiology of halothane hepatotoxicity because species and strain differences exist for susceptibility to halothane liver toxicity in laboratory animals (44), and, in addition, halothane hepatotoxicity has been demonstrated in three pairs of closely related women (45). Gourlay et al. in 1981 showed genetic differences in reductive metabolism and hepatotoxicity in three different rat strains for halothane, and breeding studies have shown a genetic predisposition to liver damage after halo-

thane anesthesia in guinea pigs (46). Thus, speculation has arisen that halothane hepatotoxicity might be due in part to a constitutional defect (47). It has been suggested that a decreased capacity to metabolize halothane by the oxidative pathway might shunt metabolism toward the reductive pathway, leading to the production of highly reactive metabolites. As yet, the cytochrome P450(s) responsible for halothane metabolism and their contribution toward the various routes of metabolism have not been determined. However, an anesthesiologist physician who developed halothane hepatitis has been shown to be an extensive metabolizer of debrisoquine with a metabolic ratio being <12.6 (poor metabolizer >12.6) (48).

Although genetic factors may influence drug metabolism, environmental factors are important. Studies of metabolism in monozygotic and dizygotic twins have been used to distinguish between genetic and environmental factors. Cascorbi et al. studied the genetic and environmental influence on halothane metabolism in twins (49) and found that the percent differences of halothane metabolite (trifluroacetate) excreted in 24 hours for each pair varied from 2.4% to 17.3% in identical twins and from 2.9% to 70.0% in fraternal twins. This finding indicates that genetic factors probably play a role in halothane metabolism.

The role of the hepatic cytochrome enzymes in the metabolism of the volatile anesthetics is described in the chapter by Waskell. Enflurane administration rarely may result in subclinical nephrotoxicity, and a syndrome of hepatic necrosis has been described. Toxicity of the inhalational anesthetic enflurane may be related to its metabolism by hepatic cytochrome P450; enflurane oxidation results in the production of fluoride. For methoxyflurane, it is well recognized that nephrotoxicity is related to the production of inorganic fluoride, but in general, the serum levels of fluoride following enflurane anesthesia are insufficient to result in nephrotoxicity (see the chapter by Fish). In 1976, Cousins et al. reported a patient with a high serum inorganic fluoride level following enflurane anesthesia. The patient was receiving a number of medications, including the antituberculosis drug, isoniazid (50). This anecdotal case report was the stimulus to a study demonstrating isoniazid-induced enflurane defluorination in humans (51). Chronic treatment with isoniazid may result in higher than predicted fluoride concentrations and a transient urinary concentration defect following enflurane administration (51). Enflurane defluorination is probably catalyzed by CYP2E1 (52,53). Microsomal fluoride production is increased in rats that are induced by isoniazid, diabetes, and ethanol and inhibited by antibodies against the enzyme CYP2E1 (53–55). It has been shown also that CYP2E1 is the predominant enzyme catalyzing the *in vitro* defluorination of sevoflurane, isoflurane, and methoxyflurane (56).

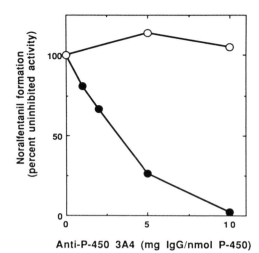

FIG. 4. Effect of anti-P450-3A4 on noralfentanil formation activity. Microsomes were preincubated with preimmune IgG (○) or P450-3A4 IgG (●). Antibody CYP3A4 nearly completely inhibited alfentanil oxidation to noralfentanil in human liver microsomes. (From Yun C H, Wood M, Wood A J J, Guengerich F P. Identification of the pharmacogenetic determinants of alfentanil metabolism: cytochrome P450-3A4. *Anesthesiology* 1992;77:467–474.)

Intravenous Anesthetics

Although the application of pharmacogenetics to hepatic drug oxidation has resulted in advances in individualization of drug therapy, the isozymes responsible for the metabolism of most of the i.v. anesthetic agents remain to be defined. Anesthesiologists recognize that among patients there is a considerable interindividual variability in plasma concentration time profiles for alfentanil, midazolam, and diazepam and that these drugs must be titrated to clinical effect.

Alfentanil is metabolized to noralfentanil by CYP3A4 *in vitro* (57) (Fig. 4). Yun et al. have shown that antibody to CYP3A4 enzyme completely inhibited alfentanil oxidation to noralfentanil, whereas the antibodies inhibitory to other cytochrome P450 enzymes (including CYP2D6) exhibited no effect (57). In addition, the selective inhibitor of CYP3A4, troleandomycin, inhibited

as much as 90% of microsomal noralfentanil formation. Henthorn et al. have shown that alfentanil clearance is not altered in poor metabolizers of debrisoquine and is thus independent of the polymorphic debrisoquine enzyme (58). In contrast to the bimodal distribution of enzyme function associated with CYP2D6, the wide interindividual activity of the enzyme CYP3A4 exhibits a broad unimodal distribution, and no distinct subgroup has been defined (59). Human CYP3A4 metabolizes many other drugs of clinical importance to the anesthesiologist (Table 3) (60–67). Therefore, the possibility exists for pharmacokinetic interaction between alfentanil and other concomitantly administered drugs that are substrates or inducers for the isozyme. Administration of the antibiotic erythromycin for 7 days increases alfentanil elimination half-life and decreases clearance, indicating that erythromycin inhibits the metabolism of alfentanil (68). Erythromycin administration does not appear to alter the pharmacokinetics of sufentanil (69). The pharmacologic effect of alfentanil may be prolonged after erythromycin administration (70), and in a study of alfentanil infusions for sedation in an intensive care unit setting, recovery from alfentanil was prolonged in a patient receiving erythromycin (71).

Midazolam, a widely used, short-acting, i.v. hypnotic and anesthetic induction agent, also exhibits wide interindividual variability when administered to anesthetized patients. Midazolam is metabolized predominantly by CYP3A4 (65). Thus, the marked interindividual variation in response to this benzodiazepine may be due to variable hepatic metabolism. A case report has described unconsciousness following midazolam and erythromycin administration to a young boy with a ventricular septal defect given erythromycin for antibiotic prophylaxis before surgery (72). The potential toxicity that may result from erythromycin and midazolam administration had been investigated by Olkkola et al. (73). Erythromycin administration increased midazolam concentrations and reduced the clearance of midazolam by 54% (Fig. 5). The authors recommended that midazolam dose should be reduced by 50% to 75% in patients receiving erythromycin.

The marked interindividual variation in the clearance of diazepam is well recognized. Although age, gender, and disease play a pivotal role in the metabolism of diazepam, pharmacogenetic factors are also important. Diazepam undergoes N-demethylation to demethyldiazepam, an active metabolite. The metabolism of diazepam (mainly demethylation) is related to the mephenytoin phenotype (74). Poor hydroxylators of mephenytoin had less than half the plasma clearance of both diazepam and demethyldiazepam compared with extensive hydroxylators of mephenytoin (Fig. 6).

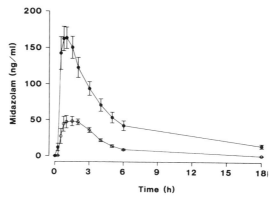

FIG. 5. Erythromycin–midazolam interaction. Concentration (mean ± SEM) of midazolam in plasma of 12 healthy volunteers after an oral dose of 15 mg following pretreatment with oral erythromycin (500 mg three times a day) or placebo for 1 week. Concentrations of midazolam after placebo (○); concentrations of midazolam after erythromycin (●). Erythromycin increased midazolam concentrations and reduced the clearance of i.v. midazolam by 54%. (From Olkkola K T, Aranko K, Luurila H, et al. A potentially hazardous interaction between erythromycin and midazolam. *Clin Pharmacol Ther* 1993;53: 298–305.)

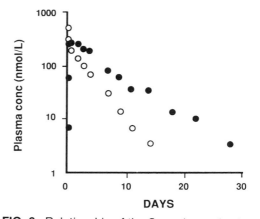

FIG. 6. Relationship of the S-mephenytoin phenotype to diazepam metabolism. Plasma concentration time curves of diazepam after a single oral dose (10 mg) of diazepam to one extensive hydroxylator (○) and one poor hydroxylator (●) of mephenytoin. (From Bertilsson L, Henthorn T K, Snaz E, Tybring G, Sawe J, Villen T. Importance of genetic factors in the regulation of diazepam metabolism: relationship to S-mephenytoin, but not debrisoquin, hydroxylation phenotype. *Clin Pharmacol Ther* 1989;45:348–355.)

Although increased drug concentrations and toxicity often are associated with deficient drug metabolism, it is important to recognize that some drugs are metabolized to active metabolites, for example, codeine. Codeine is metabolized by O- and N-demethylation and glucuronidation, but it is the O-demethylation pathway to morphine that is of importance in the production of analgesia. The pathway of morphine formation from codeine cosegregates with the debrisoquine/sparteine polymorphism, CYP2D6 (75,76). Patients who are poor metabolizers of debrisoquine do not develop an adequate analgesic response to codeine, whereas extensive metabolizers have a normal analgesic response following codeine administration (77). Thus, poor metabolizers of debrisoquine do not reliably obtain pharmacologic analgesic effects after receiving codeine. Although the clearance of the parent drug codeine may be similar in extensive and poor debrisoquine metabolizers, the partial clearance of codeine to morphine is decreased in poor metabolizers (75). Thus, anesthesiologists who administer codeine for the treatment of pain must be aware that in a small group of patients, no analgesic effect may be obtained.

PHARMACOGENETICS OF MALIGNANT HYPERTHERMIA

Malignant hyperthermia or hyperpyrexia is a syndrome triggered in genetically susceptible humans and animals by the inhalational anesthetic agents (e.g., halothane) and the depolarizing muscle relaxant succinylcholine. The syndrome (discussed in detail in the chapter by Larach) remains an important cause of perioperative morbidity and mortality. Hallmarks of the syndrome include increased metabolic rate, muscle rigidity, increased body temperature, metabolic acidosis, hyperkalemia, cardiovascular instability, and life-threatening arrhythmias, such as ventricular fibrillation. It is now well recognized that the primary MH defect probably involves an abnormality of calcium regulation in the muscle cell. Hypersensitive gating of MH-susceptible (MHS) calcium release channels of human skeletal muscle sarcoplasmic reticulum has been demonstrated, with channel opening being facilitated and closing inhibited (78–80).

Ryanodine, a natural plant alkaloid with important effects on excitation–contraction coupling in skeletal and cardiac muscle, has been shown to modify conductance and gating behavior at the calcium release channel (81,82). Ryanodine activates calcium release from the sarcoplasmic reticulum and binds with high affinity to a receptor localized to the junctional sarcoplasmic reticulum of skeletal (type 1 receptor) or cardiac (type 2 receptor) muscle, so designated because of their ability to bind ryanodine (83). Ryanodine receptors have been purified and biochemically characterized (84–89), and the two genes encoding the skeletal and cardiac receptor have been cloned (90). The *RYR1* gene encoding the skeletal muscle ryanodine receptor has been localized to human chromosome 19q13.1 (91). The effects of halothane on ryanodine receptor function have been investigated in MHS calcium release channels, and it is now believed that a defect in the ryanodine receptor may exist in MHS laboratory animals (92–95).

Susceptibility to MH is inherited as an autosomal dominant, with reduced penetrance and variable expression. The ryanodine receptor gene is a possible candidate for predisposition to MH. The *RYR1* gene encoding the skeletal muscle calcium release channel not only has been localized to human chromosome 19q13.1 but also has been linked to porcine and human MH. McCarthy et al., in an investigation of genetic linkage in several extended Irish pedigrees of MHS segregated as an autosomal dominant trait, demonstrated linkage between MHS and DNA markers from human chromosome 19 and, in particular, from the glucose phosphate isomerase (GPI) locus

(96). In another study, MacLennan et al. were able to map the ryanodine receptor gene to region q13.1 of human chromosome 19, which is in close proximity to genetic markers that have been shown to map near the MHS locus in humans (97). They also carried out genetic linkage studies to determine that the MH phenotype segregates with chromosome 19 markers, including markers in the *RYR1* gene, and concluded that MH is likely to be caused by mutations in the *RYR* gene. Healy et al., using molecular genetic linkage studies in a large MHS pedigree, demonstrated that DNA markers flanking the gene for MHS (ryanodine receptor) could be used with a high degree of accuracy (98). The authors reported that flanking markers D19S9 and D19S16 generated a lod (logarithm of the odds ratio) score of >3 (Fig. 7). It is important to recognize that this information applies to this particular well-studied pedigree and should not necessarily be extrapolated to other families.

Thus, the MH defect in some families has been tentatively located to a region on chromosome 19, and the *RYR1* gene also is encoded within this region (99). However, more than one gene may be responsible for the condition, and Levitt et al. have suggested that MH may be linked to a different chromosome (17, q11.2, q24) (100).

If a gene defect is identified, it would be an important development because a DNA-based blood test would be a simpler screening test than the laboratory diagnosis of MH using the caffeine-halothane-contracture test (101, 102, 103). However, at present, the clinical acumen of the anesthetist is still vital in the detection of susceptibility to MH.

PHARMACOGENETICS OF SUCCINYLCHOLINE METABOLISM

There are two enzymes present in humans capable of hydrolyzing esters of choline, e.g., acetylcholine (104). Acetylcholinesterase (AChE) terminates the action of acetylcholine released during cholinergic transmission at cholinoceptive sites, including the postsynaptic membrane in the neuromuscular junction. AChE is found in the region of cholinergic nerve fibers and in red cells. Butyrylcholinesterase (BChE), also known as pseudocholinesterase, plasma cholinesterase, and nonspecific cholinesterase, is a cholinesterase enzyme found in plasma and tissues. Its physiologic function is not known, but it is responsible for the degradation of succinylcholine and the ester-type local anesthetics, such as procaine.

BChE is of great importance to anesthesiologists because it is the enzyme responsible for the hydrolysis of succinylcholine,

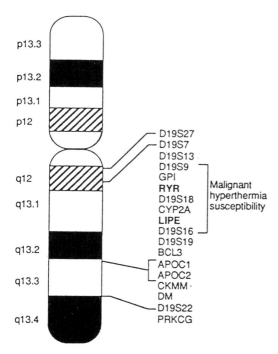

FIG. 7. Chromosome 19 and MHS. Linkage map of 18 DNA markers on the long arm of chromosome 19 showing the genetic interval to which malignant hyperthermia susceptibility locus has been mapped by linkage analysis. (From Healy J M S, Heffron J J, Lehane M, Bradley D G, Johnson K, McCarthy T V. Diagnosis of susceptibility to malignant hyperthermia with flanking DNA markers. *Br J Med* 1991;303:1225–1228.)

and some patients exhibit prolonged apnea due to slow hydrolysis of the relaxant. Slow hydrolysis is known to be related to genetic variants of the enzyme (105). BChE is synthesized in the liver and is released into the plasma. Thus, concentrations are reduced in patients suffering from liver disease and malignancy. Concentrations also are lower in the newborn and in pregnant patients, especially in the last trimester and early postpartum period. Numerous drugs, including echothiopate eyedrops, physostigmine, and neostigmine, inhibit and reduce BChE activity. Thus, plasma cholinesterase activity may be abnormal due to an acquired defect.

BChE enzyme production is controlled by two autosomal genes, and plasma cholinesterase activity may be abnormal due to genetic enzyme defects. Two varieties of BChE were first described: the common or normal type and the rare abnormal or atypical type. The common type of BChE hydrolyzes succinylcholine at therapeutic concentrations, whereas the atypical enzyme is less effective than normal BChE in hydrolyzing succinylcholine and other substrates, such as benzoylcholine. In addition, atypical BChE is more resistant to the effects of cholinesterase inhibitors, such as dibucaine. Dibucaine inhibits normal plasma cholinesterase to a much greater extent than the atypical enzyme; dibucaine inhibits the normal enzyme by 80% and atypical pseudocholinesterase by about 20%. The term dibucaine number (DN) represents the percentage inhibition of plasma cholinesterase activity by dibucaine. Normal patients have a DN of 80, and homozygotes for the atypical enzyme have a DN of 20. Heterozygote patients for the atypical enzyme have a DN of about 50% to 60%. Patients homozygous for the atypical enzyme possess only abnormal enzyme (DN = 20) and demonstrate prolonged neuromuscular blockade after succinylcholine administration. Normal homozygotes represent about 96.2% of the population, heterozygotes approximately 3.8% of the population, and about 1 in every 3000 individuals is homozygous for the atypical enzyme. The atypical enzyme is the most common form of abnormal enzyme.

Other genetic variants of cholinesterase have been described subsequently (Table 6) (106–111). The best-known include the fluoride-resistant gene and the silent gene.

TABLE 6. *Genetic variants of cholinesterase*

Activity	Genotype	Reference
Normal activity		
Usual	UU	Whittaker, 1986
Reduced activity		
Atypical	AA	Kalow and Staron, 1957
(70 Asp→Gly)		McGuire et al., 1989
Silent-1	SS	Liddell et al., 1962
(117 Gly→frameshift)		McGuire et al., 1989
Fluoride	FF	Harris and Whittaker, 1961
Quantitative variant J	JJ	Garry et al., 1966
		Evans and Wardell, 1984
Quantitative variant K	KK	Rubinstein et al., 1978
(539 Ala→Thr)		Bartels et al., 1989
Quantitative variant H	HH	Whittaker and Britten, 1987
Newfoundland		Simpson and Elliiott, 1981
Increased activity		
C_{5+}		Robson and Harris, 1966
Cynthiana variant		Neitlich, 1966
		Whittaker, 1986
Johannesburg		Krause et al., 1988

Adapted from Lockridge O. Genetic variants of human serum cholinesterase influence metabolism of the muscle relaxant succinylcholine. *Pharmacol Ther* 1990;47:35–60.

The fluoride gene is much less common than the gene for the atypical enzyme and is identified using sodium fluoride as an inhibitor in a similar manner to dibucaine identification. The fluoride-resistant variant has a reduced activity. The silent gene is very uncommon, and homozygotes for this gene exhibit no pseudocholinesterase activity. Other genetic variants of BChE exist (Table 6), some with increased activity of the cholinesterase variant C_5.

The cholinesterase gene has been characterized and cloned (106,112,113). BChE enzyme activity is encoded in a single autosomal locus (BChE) that has been assigned to chromosome 3q26. All variants arise from a single locus, and there is only one gene for human cholinesterase. Variant forms of human BChE are caused by specific mutations within the structural DNA coding for this enzyme. A point mutation in the gene for human cholinesterase has been identified for the atypical form of serum cholinesterase (111). Atypical cholinesterase has a single nucleotide substitution at nucleotide 209 that changes aspartic acid 70 to glycine (Table 6). This indicates that aspartic acid 70 is part of the anionic site because absence of the negatively charged amino acid may result in reduced affinity of atypical cholinesterase for positively charged substrates. The K variant has threonine in place of alanine 539, and the mutation for the silent gene has a frameshift at glycine 117 (107,108). The mutation for the silent gene yields no active enzyme because it prematurely terminates protein synthesis. The polymerase chain reaction has been used as a resource tool to identify persons with genetic variants of cholinesterase, but this technique has not been extended to the general population (114).

CONCLUSION

The application of pharmacogenetics to clinical pharmacology has improved individualization of drug therapy and in the future should allow the prediction of pharmacogenetic drug interactions. Genetic influence on pharmacokinetics may be either polygenetic or monogenetic (single gene type). Single gene pharmacogenetic defects may be quite common (e.g., CYP2D6 polymorphism) or rare (cholinesterase defect). DNA analysis (e.g., PCR) has become a potent pharmacokinetic tool for genotyping of both patients and study subjects (115).

REFERENCES

1. Wood M. Variability of human drug response [Editorial]. *Anesthesiology* 1989;71:631–634.
2. Kalow W. Pharmacogenetics: past and future. *Life Sci* 1990;47:1385–1397.
3. Gonzalez F J. Human cytochromes P450: problems and prospects. *TIPS* 1992;13:346–352.
4. Wood A J J, Zhou H H. Ethnic differences in drug disposition and responsiveness. *Clin Pharmacokinet* 1991;20:350–373.
5. Eichelbaum M. Defective oxidation of drugs: pharmacokinetics and therapeutic implications. *Clin Pharmacokinet* 1982;7:1–22.
6. Mahgoub A, Idle J R, Dring L G, Lancester R, Smith R L. Polymorphic hydroxylation of debrisoquine in man. *Lancet* 1977;ii:584–586.
7. Yue Q Y, Svensson J O, Alm C, Sjoqvist F, Sawe J. Codeine O-demethylation cosegregates with polymorphic debrisoquine hydroxylation. *Br J Clin Pharmacol* 1989;28:639–645.
8. Nelson D R, Kamataki T, Waxman D J, et al. The P450 superfamily: update on new sequences, gene mapping, accession numbers, early trivial names of enzymes, and nomenclature. *DNA Cell Biol* 1993;12:1–51.
9. Nebert D W, Nelson D R, Adesnik M, et al. The P450 superfamily: updated listing of all genes and recommended nomenclature for the chromosomal loci. *DNA* 1989;8:1–13.
10. Raghuram T C, Koshakji R P, Wilkinson G R, Wood A J J. Polymorphic ability to metabolize propranolol alters 4-hydroxypropranolol levels but not beta blockade. *Clin Pharmacol Ther* 1984;36:51–56.
11. Guengerich F P. The 1992 Bernard B. Brodie Award Lecture: Bioactivation and detoxification of toxic and carcinogenic chemicals. *Drug Metab Disp* 1993;21:1–6.
12. Kalow W, Tank B K. Use of caffeine metabolite ratios to explore CYP1A2 and xanthine oxidase activities. *Clin Pharmacol Ther* 1991;50:508–519.
13. Relling M V, Lin J S, Ayers G D, Evans W E. Racial and gender differences in N-acetyltransferase, xanthine oxidase, and CYP1A2* activities. *Clin Pharmacol Ther* 1992;52:643–658.

14. Distlerath L M, Reilly P E B, Martin MV, Davis G G, Wilkinson G R, Guengerich F P. Purification and characterization of the human liver cytochromes P450 involved in debrisoquine 4-hydroxylation and phenacetin O-deethylation, two prototypes for genetic polymorphism in oxidative drug metabolism. *J Biol Chem* 1985;260:9057–9067.

15. Nims R W, Lubet R A, Jones C R, Mellini D W, Thomas R E. Comparative pharmacodynamics of CYP2B induction by phenobarbital in the male and female F334/NCr rat. *Biochem Pharmacol* 1993;45:521–526.

16. Bertilsson L, Henthorn T K, Sanz E, Tybring G, Sawe J, Villen T. Importance of genetic factors in the regulation of diazepam metabolism: relationship to S-mephenytoin, but not debrisoquin, hydroxylation phenotype. *Clin Pharmacol Ther* 1989;45:348–355.

17. Shimada T, Misono K S, Guengerich F P. Human liver microsomal cytochrome P450 mephenytoin 4-hydroxylase, a prototype of genetic polymorphism in oxidative drug metabolism. *J Biol Chem* 1986;261:909–921.

18. Srivastava P K, Yun C H, Beaune P H, Ged C, Guengerich F P. Separation of human liver microsomal tolbutamide hydroxylase and (S)-mephenytoin 4'-hydroxylase. *Mol Pharmacol* 1991;40:69–79.

19. Ged C, Umbenhauer D R, Bellew T M, et al. Characterization of cDNAs, mRNAs, and proteins related to human liver microsomal cytochrome P450 (S)-mephenytoin 4'-hydroxylase. *Biochemistry* 1988;27:6929–6940.

20. Wedlund P J, Aslanian W S, McAllister C B, Wilkinson G R, Branch R A. Mephenytoin hydroxylation deficiency in Caucasians: frequency of a new oxidative drug metabolism polymorphism. *Clin Pharmacol Ther* 1984;36:773–780.

21. Andersson T, Cederberg C, Edvardsson G, Heggelund A, Lundborg P. Effect of omeprazole treatment on diazepam plasma levels in slow versus normal metabolizers of omeprazole. *Clin Pharmacol Ther* 1990;47:79–85.

22. Gonzalez F J, Meyer U A. Molecular genetics of the debrisoquin-sparteine polymorphism. *Clin Pharmacol Ther* 1991;50:233–238.

23. Eichelbaum M, Baur M P, Dengler H J. Chromosomal assignment of human cytochrome P450 (debrisoquine-sparteine type) to chromosome 22. *Br J Clin Pharmacol* 1987;23:455–458.

24. Dahl M L, Johansson I, Palmertz M P, Ingleman-Sundberg M, Sjogvist F. Analysis of the CYP2D6 gene in relation to debrisoquin and desipramine hydroxylation in a Swedish population. *Clin Pharmacol Ther* 1992;51:12–17.

25. Heim M, Meyer U A. Genotyping of poor metabolisers of debrisoquine by allele-specific PCR amplification. *Lancet* 1990;336:529–532.

26. Cholerton S, Daly A K, Idle J R. The role of individual human cytochromes P450 in drug metabolism and clinical response. *TIPS* 1992; 13:434–439.

27. Skoda R C, Gonzalez F J, Demierre A, Meyer U A. Two mutant alleles of the human cytochrome P450dbl gene *(P450-C2D1)* associated with genetically deficient metabolism of debrisoquine and other drugs. *Proc Natl Acad Sci USA* 1988;85:5240–5243.

28. Gaedigk A, Blum M, Gaedigk R, Eichembaun M, Meyer U A. Deletion of the entire cytochrome P450 *CYP2D6* gene as a cause of impaired drug metabolism in poor metabolizers of the debrisoquine/sparteine polymorphism. *Am J Hum Genet* 1991;48:943–950.

29. Kimura S, Omeno M, Skoda R C, Meyer U A, Gonzalez F J. The human debrisoquine 4-hydroxylase *(CYP2D)* locus: sequence and identification of the polymorphic *CYP2D6* gene, a related gene, and a pseudogene. *Am J Hum Genet* 1989;45:889–904.

30. Kagimoto M, Heim M, Kagimoto K, Zeugin T, Meyer U A. Multiple mutations of the human cytochrome P450-IID6 gene *(CYP2D6)* in poor metabolizers of debrisoquine. *J Biol Chem* 1990; 265:17209–17214.

31. Hanioka N, Kimura S, Meyer U A, Gonzalez F J. The human CYP2D locus associated with a common genetic defect in drug oxidation: A $G_{1934} \rightarrow A$ base change in intron 3 of a mutant *CYP-2D6* allele results in an aberrant 3'-splice recognition site. *Am J Hum Genet* 1990;47:994–1001.

32. Gough A C, Miles J S, Spurr N K, et al. Identification of the primary gene defect at the cytochrome P450 *CYP-2D* locus. *Nature* 1990; 347:773–776.

33. Skoda R C, Gonzalez F J, Demierre A, Meyer U A. Two mutant alleles of the human cytochrome P450dbl gene *(P450-C2D1)* associated with genetically deficient metabolism of debrisoquine and other drugs. *Proc Natl Acad Sci USA* 1988;85:5249–5253.

34. Daly A K, Armstrong M, Monkman S C, Idle M E, Idle J R. Genetic and metabolic criteria for the assignment of debrisoquine 4-hydroxylation (cytochrome P450-2D6) phenotypes. *Pharmacogenetics* 1991;1:33–41.

35. Kharasch E D, Thummel K E, Mhyre J, Lillibridge J H. Single-dose disulfiram inhibition of chlorzoxazone metabolism: a clinical probe for P450-2E1. *Clin Pharmacol Ther* 1993;53:643–650.

36. Koop D R. Oxidative and reductive metabolism by cytochrome P450-2E1. *FASEB J* 1992; 6:724–730.

37. Guengerich F P, Muller-Enoch D, Blair I A. Oxidation of quinidine by human liver cytochrome P450. *Mol Pharmacol* 1986;30:287–295.

38. Wood A J J, Zhou H H. Ethnic differences in drug disposition and responsiveness. *Clin Pharmacokinet* 1991;20:350–373.

39. Bertilsson L, Lou Y Q, Du Y L, et al. Pronounced differences between native Chinese and Swedish populations in the polymorphic hydroxylations of debrisoquin and S-mephenytoin. *Clin Pharmacol Ther* 1992;51:388–397.

40. Johansson I, Yue Q Y, Dahl M L, et al. Genetic analysis of the interethnic difference between Chinese and Caucasians in the polymorphic metabolism of debrisoquin and codeine. *Eur J Clin Pharmacol* 1991;40:553–556.

41. Mura C, Broyard J P, Jacqz-Aigrain E, Krishnamoorthy R. Distinct phenotypes and genotypes of debrisoquin hydroxylation among Europeans and Chinese. *Br J Clin Pharmacol* 1991;32:135–136.

42. Woolhouse N M, Eichelbaum M, Oates N S, Idle J R, Smith R L. Dissociation of coregulatory control of debrisoquin/phenformin and sparteine oxidation in Ghanaians. *Clin Pharmacol Ther* 1985;37:512–521.

43. Zhang Y, Reviriego J, Lou Y, Sjoqvist F, Bertilsson L. Diazepam metabolism in native Chinese poor and extensive hydroxylators of S-mephenytoin: interethnic differences in comparison with white subjects. *Clin Pharmacol Ther* 1990;48:496–502.

44. Gourlay G K, Adams J F, Cousins M J, Hall P. Genetic differences in reductive metabolism and hepatotoxicity of halothane in three rat strains. *Anesthesiology* 1981;55:96–103.

45. Hoft R H, Bunker J P, Goodman H I, Gregory P B. Halothane hepatitis in three pairs of closely related women. *N Engl J Med* 1981;304:1023–1024.

46. Lunam C A, Cousins M J, Hall P M. Genetic disposition to liver damage after halothane anesthesia in guinea pigs. *Anesth Analg* 1986;65:1143–1148.

47. Brown B B. Pharmacogenetics and the halothane hepatitis mystery. *Anesthesiology* 1981;55:93–94.

48. Toutoungi M, Magnenat D. Lack of defect in oxidative hydroxylation of debrisoquine in a patient with halothane hepatitis. *Eur J Clin Pharmacol* 1990;38:633–634.

49. Cascorbi H F, Vessel E S, Blade D A, Helrich M. Genetic and environmental influence of halothane metabolism in twins. *Clin Pharmacol Ther* 1971;12:50–55.

50. Cousins M J, Greenstein L R, Hitt B A, Mazze R I. Metabolism and renal effects of enflurane in man. *Anesthesiology* 1976;44:44–53.

51. Mazze R I, Woodruff R E, Heerdt M E. Isoniazid-induced enflurane defluorination in humans. *Anesthesiology* 1982;57:5–8.

52. Thummel K E, Kharasch E D, Podoll T, Kunze K. Human liver microsomal enflurane defluorination catalyzed by cytochrome P450-2E1. *Drug Metab Disp* 1993;21:350–357.

53. Hoffman J, Konopka K, Buckhorn C, Koop D R, Waskell L. Ethanol-inducible cytochrome P450 in rabbits metabolizes enflurane. *Br J Anaesth* 1989;63:103–108.

54. Pantuck E J, Pantuck C B, Conney A H. Effect of streptozotocin-induced diabetes in the rat on the metabolism of fluorinated volatile anesthetics. *Anesthesiology* 1987;66:24–28.

55. Pantuck E J, Pantuck C B, Ryan D E, Conney A H. Inhibition and stimulation of enflurane

56. metabolism in the rat following a single dose or chronic administration of ethanol. *Anesthesiology* 1985;62:255–262.

56. Kharasch E D, Thummel K E. Identification of cytochrome P450-2E1 as the predominant enzyme catalyzing human liver microsomal defluorination of sevoflurane, isoflurane, and methoxyflurane. *Anesthesiology* 1993;79:795–807.

57. Yun C H, Wood M, Wood A J J, Guengerich F P. Identification of the pharmacogenetic determinants of alfentanil metabolism: cytochrome P450-3A4. *Anesthesiology* 1992;77:467–474.

58. Henthorn T K, Avram M J, Krejcie T C. Alfentanil clearance is independent of the polymorphic debrisoquin hydroxylase. *Anesthesiology* 1989;71:635–639.

59. Schellens J H M, Soons P A, Briemer D D. Lack of bimodality in nifedipine plasma kinetics in a large population of healthy subjects. *Biochem Pharmacol* 1988;37:2507–2510.

60. Guengerich F P, Martin M V, Beaune P H, Kremers P, Wolff T, Waxman D J. Characterization of rat and human liver microsomal cytochrome P450 forms involved in nifedipine oxidation, a prototype for genetic polymorphism in oxidative drug metabolism. *J Biol Chem* 1986;261:5051–5060.

61. Kronbach T, Fischer V, Meyer U A. Cyclosporine metabolism in human liver: identification of a cytochrome P450-III gene family as the major cyclosporine-metabolizing enzyme explains interactions of cyclosporine with other drugs. *Clin Pharmacol Ther* 1988;43:630–635.

62. Combalbert J, Fabre I, Fabre G, et al. Metabolism of cyclosporin A. IV. Purification and identification of the rifampicin-inducible human liver cytochrome P450 (cyclosporin A oxidase) as a product of P450-IIIA gene subfamily. *Drug Metab Disp* 1989;17:197–207.

63. Watkins P B, Wrighton S A, Maurel P, et al. Identification of an inducible form of cytochrome P450 in human liver. *Proc Natl Acad Sci USA* 1985;82:6310–6314.

64. Brian W R, Sari M A, Iwasaki M, Shimada T, Kaminsky L S, Guengerich F P. Catalytic activities of human liver cytochrome P450-IIIA4 expressed in *Saccharomyces cerevisiae*. *Biochemistry* 1990;29:11280–11292.

65. Kronbach T, Mathys D, Umeno M, Gonzalez F J, Meyer U A. Oxidation of midazolam and triazolam by human liver cytochrome P450-IIIA4. *Mol Pharmacol* 1989;36:89–96.

66. Guengerich F P, Muller-Enoch D, Blair I A. Oxidation of quinidine by human liver cytochrome P450. *Mol Pharmacol* 1986;30:287–295.

67. Bargetzi M J, Aoyama T, Gonzalez F J, Meyer U A. Lidocaine metabolism in human liver microsomes by cytochrome P450-IIIA4. *Clin Pharmacol Ther* 1989;46:521–527.

68. Bartkowski R R, Goldberg M E, Larijano G E, Boerner T. Inhibition of alfentanil metabolism by erythromycin. *Clin Pharmacol Ther* 1989;46:99–102.

69. Bartkowski R R, Goldberg M E, Huffnagle S,

Epstein R H. Sufentanil disposition: is it affected by erythromycin administration? *Anesthesiology* 1993;78:260–265.

70. Bartkowski R R, McDonnell T E. Prolonged alfentanil effect following erythromycin administration. *Anesthesiology* 1990;73:566–568.

71. Yate P M, Thomas D, Short S M, Sebel P S, Morton J. Comparison of infusions of alfentanil or pethidine for sedation of ventilated patients on the ITU. *Br J Anaesth* 1986;58:1091–1099.

72. Hiller A, Olkkola K T, Isohanni P, Saarnivaara L. Unconsciousness associated with midazolam and erythromycin. *Br J Anaesth* 1990;65:826–828.

73. Olkkola K T, Aranko K, Luurila H, et al. A potentially hazardous interaction between erythromycin and midazolam. *Clin Pharmacol Ther* 1993;53:298–305.

74. Bertilsson L, Henthron T K, Sanz E, Tybring G, Sawe J, Villen T. Importance of genetic factors in the regulation of diazepam metabolism: relationship to S-mephenytoin, but not debrisoquin, hydroxylation phenotype. *Clin Pharmacol Ther* 1989;45:348–55.

75. Chen Z R, Somogyi A A, Reynolds G, Bochner F. Disposition and metabolism of codeine after single and chronic doses in one poor and seven extensive metabolisers. *Br J Clin Pharmacol* 1991;31:381–390.

76. Mortimer O, Persson K, Ladona M G, et al. Polymorphic formation of morphine from codeine in poor and extensive metabolizers of dextromethorphan: relationship to the presence of immunoidentified P450-IID1. *Clin Pharmacol Ther* 1990;47:27–35.

77. Sindrup S H, Brosen K, Bjerring P, et al. Codeine increases pain thresholds to copper vapor laser stimuli in extensive but not poor metabolizers of sparteine. *Clin Pharmacol Ther* 1990;47:27–35.

78. Nelson T E, Sweo T, Ca^{2+} uptake and Ca^{2+} release by skeletal muscle sarcoplasmic reticulum: differing sensitivity to inhalational anesthetics. *Anesthesiology* 1988;69:571–577.

79. Nelson T E. Abnormality in calcium release from skeletal sarcoplasmic reticulum of pigs susceptible to malignant hyperthermia. *J Clin Invest* 1983;72:862–870.

80. Mickelson J R, Ross J A, Reed B K, Louis C F. Enhanced Ca^{2+}-induced calcium release by isolated sarcoplasmic reticulum vesicles from malignant hyperthermia susceptible pig muscle. *Biochem Biophys Acta* 1986;862:318–328.

81. Rousseau E, Smith J S, Meissner G. Ryanodine modifies conductance and gating behavior of single Ca^{2+} release channel. *Am J Physiol* 1987;253:C364–C368.

82. Jenden D J, Fairhurst A S. The pharmacology of ryanodine. *Pharmacol Rev* 1969;21:1–25.

83. Sorrentino V, Volpe P. Ryanodine receptors: how many, where and why? *TIPS* 1993;14:98–103.

84. Fleischer S, Ogunbunmi E M, Dixon M C, Fleer E A M. Localization of Ca^{2+} release channels with ryanodine in junctional terminal cisternae of sarcoplasmic reticulum of fast skeletal muscle. *Proc Natl Acad Sci USA* 1985;82:7256–7259.

85. Inui M, Saito A, Fleischer S. Purification of the ryanodine receptor and identity with feet structures of junctional terminal cisternae of sarcoplasmic reticulum from fast skeletal muscle. *J Biol Chem* 1987;262:1740–1747.

86. Takeshima H, Nishimura S, Matsumoto T, et al. Primary structure and expression from complementary DNA of skeletal muscle ryanodine receptor. *Nature* 1989;399:339–445.

87. Meisner G. Ryanodine activation and inhibition of the Ca^{2+} release channel of sarcoplasmic reticulum. *J Biol Chem* 1986;261:6300–6306.

88. Imagawa T, Smith J S, Coronado R, Campbell K P. Purified ryanodine receptor from skeletal muscle sarcoplasmic reticulum is the Ca^{2+}-permeable pore of the calcium release channel. *J Biol Chem* 1987;262:16636–16643.

89. Lai F A, Erickson H P, Rousseau E, Liu Q-Y, Meissner G. Purification and reconstitution of the calcium release channel from skeletal muscle. *Nature* 1988;331:315–319.

90. Zorzato F, Fujii J, Otsu K, et al. Molecular cloning of cDNA encoding human and rabbit forms of the Ca^{2+} release channel (ryanodine receptor) of skeletal muscle sarcoplasmic reticulum. *J Biol Chem* 1990;265:2244–2256.

91. MacKenzie A E, Korneluk R G, Zorzato F, et al. The human ryanodine receptor gene: its mapping to 19q13.1, placement in a chromosome 19 linkage group, and exclusion as the gene causing myotonic dystrophy. *Am J Hum Genet* 1990;46:1082–1089.

92. Mickelson J R, Gallant E M, Litterer L A, Johnson K M, Rempel W E, Louis C F. Abnormal sarcoplasmic reticulum ryanodine receptor in malignant hyperthermia. *J Biol Chem* 1988;263:9310–9315.

93. Gallant E M, Mickelson J R, Roggow B D, Donaldson S K, Louis C F, Rempel W E. Halothane-sensitivity gene and muscle contractile properties in malignant hyperthermia. *Am J Physiol* 1989;257:C781–C786.

94. Mickelson J R, Gallant E M, Rempel W E, et al. Effects of the halothane-sensitivity gene on sarcoplasmic reticulum function. *Am J Physiol* 1989;257:C787–C794.

95. Fujii J, Otsu K, Zorzato F, et al. Identification of a mutation in porcine ryanodine receptor associated with malignant hyperthermia. *Science* 1991;253:448–451.

96. McCarthy T V, Healy J M, Heffron J J, et al. Localization of the malignant hyperthermia susceptibility locus to human chromosome 19q12-13.2. *Nature* 1990;343:562–564.

97. MacLennan D H, Duff C, Zorzato F, et al. Ryanodine receptor gene is a candidate for predisposition to malignant hyperthermia. *Nature* 1990;343:559–561.

98. Healy S J, Heffron J J, Lehane M, Bradley D G, Johnson K, McCarthy T V. Diagnosis of susceptibility to malignant hyperthermia with

flanking DNA markers. *Br Med J* 1991;303: 1225–1228.

99. MacLennan D H. The genetic basis of malignant hyperthermia. *TIPS* 1992;13:330–334.

100. Levitt R C, Nouri N, Jedlicka A E, et al. Evidence for genetic heterogenicity in malignant hyperthermia susceptibility. *Genomics* 1991; 11:543–547.

101. Ellis F R. Detecting susceptibility to malignant hyperthermia. *Br Med J* 1992;304:791–792.

102. McCarthy T V, Healy J M S, Lehane M, Heffron J J A. Recent developments in the molecular genetics of malignant hyperthermia: implications for future diagnosis at the DNA level. *Acta Anaesth Belg* 1990;41:107–112.

103. MacKenzie A E, Allen G, Lahey D, et al. A comparison of the caffeine halothane muscle contracture test with the molecular genetic diagnosis of malignant hyperthermia. *Anesthesiology* 1991;75:4–8.

104. Chatonnet A, Lockridge O. Comparison of butyrylcholinesterase and acetylcholinesterase. *Biochem J* 1989;260:625–634.

105. Whittaker M. Plasma cholinesterase variants and the anaesthetist. *Anaesthesia* 1980;35:174–197.

106. Lockridge O. Genetic variants of human serum cholinesterase influence metabolism of the muscle relaxant succinylcholine. *Pharmacol Ther* 1990;47:35–60.

107. Nogueira C P, McGuire M C, Graeser C, et al. Identification of a frameshift mutation responsible for the silent phenotype of human serum cholinesterase, Gly 117 (GCT→GGAG). *Am J Hum Genet* 1990;46:934–942.

108. Bartels C F, Jensen F S, Lockridge O, et al. DNA mutation associated with the human butyrylcholinesterase K-variant and its linkage to the atypical variant mutation and other polymorphic sites. *Am J Hum Genet* 1992;50:1086–1103.

109. Masson P, Chatonnet A, Lockridge O. Evidence for a single butyrylcholinesterase gene in individuals carrying the C_5 plasma cholinesterase variant (CHE2). *FEBS* 1990;262:115–118.

110. LaDu B N, Bartels C F, Nogueira C P, et al. Phenotypic and molecular biological analysis of human butyrylcholinesterase variants. *Clin Biochem* 1990;23:423–431.

111. McGuire M C, Nogueira C P, Bartels C F, et al. Identification of the structural mutation responsible for the dibucaine-resistant (atypical) variant form of human serum cholinesterase. *Proc Natl Acad Sci USA* 1989;86:953–957.

112. Arpagus M, Kott M, Vatsis K P, Bartels C F, LaDu B N, Lockridge O. Structure of the gene for human butyrylcholinesterase. Evidence for a single copy. *Biochemistry* 1990;29:124–131.

113. Allderdice P W, Gardner H A R, Galutira D, Lockridge O, LaDu B N, McAlpine P J. The cloned butyrylcholinesterase *(BCHE)* gene maps to a single chromosome site, 3q26. *Genomics* 1991;11:452–454.

114. LaDu B N. Identification of human serum cholinesterase variants using the polymerase chain reaction amplification technique. *Trends Pharmacol Sci* 1989;10:309–313.

115. Heim M H. Polymerase chain reaction and its potential as a pharmacokinetic tool. *Clin Pharmacokinet* 1992;23:321–327.

Anesthetic Toxicity, edited by
Susan A. Rice and Kevin J. Fish.
Raven Press, Ltd., New York © 1994.

12

Malignant Hyperthermia Triggered by Anesthetics

Marilyn Green Larach

The North American Malignant Hyperthermia Registry and Departments of Anesthesia and Pediatrics, Pennsylvania State University College of Medicine, Hershey, Pennsylvania 17033

All volatile anesthetic agents and depolarizing muscle relaxants may trigger an uncommon, but life-threatening, sustained skeletal muscle hypermetabolism called malignant hyperthermia (MH) in genetically susceptible individuals. Clinical signs of MH are variable and may include tachycardia, tachypnea, hypercarbia, respiratory acidosis, metabolic acidosis, masseter muscle rigidity, generalized muscular rigidity, myoglobinuria, rhabdomyolysis, arrhythmias, cyanosis, skin mottling, hyperkalemia, diaphoresis, rapid temperature elevation, hemodynamic instability, and coagulopathy (1–3). Acute MH events strike individuals who are usually healthy and who display no signs of disease. Abnormal susceptibility to MH-triggering anesthetic agents is most frequently inherited in an autosomal dominant fashion with variable penetrance. This chapter focuses on methods for diagnosing, treating, and predicting susceptibility to this anesthetic-induced toxicity.

BACKGROUND

Relevant Clinical and Laboratory History

In 1960, Denborough and Lovell (4) reported for the first time on a family in which anesthetic agents (ether and halothane) triggered hyperpyrexia, convulsions, and death. They suggested that the factor causing the reaction was inherited as a dominant gene. In 1962, Denborough et al. (5) expanded their earlier description of this family and reported a potentially safe anesthetic for use in affected individuals because "spinal anaesthesia produced no ill effects when used in the one member of the family who survived a reaction following a general anaesthetic."

If all volatile anesthetic agents can trigger MH in susceptible individuals, why did more than 110 years elapse between the introduction of such agents and the first MH report? Minimal monitoring and a high death rate from aspiration, infection, and hemorrhage may have obscured earlier deaths due to MH. Recently, Harrison and Isaacs (6) reported on previously unpublished letters written by physicians in 1919 that describe the deaths of a mother and son in whom "there was a tendency of abnormal rigidity coupled with a susceptibility to chloroform." These deaths occurred in a family in whom four generations are now known to have suffered death from MH. The most recent death occurred in 1987 in a 2.5-year-old child anesthetized with halothane.

In 1967, Wilson et al. (7) named the syndrome of "explosive thermal idiosyncrasy" to anesthesia malignant hyperthermia because 73% of young healthy patients affected by this syndrome died with a mean maximum temperature of 108.5°F after exposure to triggering anesthetics. Lack of an animal model impeded efforts to reduce the extremely high mortality of this syndrome. In 1966, Hall et al. (8) described death following rigidity and hyperthermia in three pig littermates anesthetized with halothane and succinylcholine. Hall et al. concluded that these pigs were genetically susceptible to an unusual reaction to succinylcholine. In 1969, Harrison et al. first described a swine model for MH investigation and made the observation that very early recognition of a developing MH reaction with discontinuation of triggering agents might prevent fatalities. Further, they concluded their article with an apt observation: "One thing is certain. If by some quirk of fate Raventós had used Landrace pigs instead [of] rats, mice, dogs, cats and monkeys on which to test his new-found anaesthetic, halothane, it would never have emerged from the laboratory to become the most widely used anaesthetic in the world. For who would dare suggest the clinical use of an agent that killed a quarter of those animals exposed to it?" (9).

Skeletal Muscle Contraction

Molecular Biology

Ionized calcium regulates skeletal muscle contraction, relaxation, and energy metabolism. To produce normal skeletal muscle excitation-contraction coupling, acetylcholine molecules must be released from a nerve ending, diffuse across the synaptic cleft, bind to the neuromuscular endplate, and trigger a muscle action potential. This action potential propagates along the muscle sarcolemma, down to the triadic structures of the transverse tubule, and to the calcium channel voltage sensors, which trigger ionized calcium release from the terminal cisternae of the sacroplasmic reticulum. The ionized calcium binds to troponin and initiates a contraction of less than 100 milliseconds. After release of ionized calcium through the sarcoplasmic reticular calcium release channels, these channels change to a predominantly closed state, and calcium uptake by the sarcoplasmic reticulum significantly exceeds calcium release, leading to skeletal muscle relaxation (10,11). In susceptible individuals exposed to MH-triggering anesthetic agents, however, inherited defects in the regulation of calcium by the sarcoplasmic reticulum impede relaxation and produce skeletal muscle contracture and hypermetabolism.

Pathophysiology

A hypersensitive gating of the calcium release channel of the sarcoplasmic reticulum (the ryanodine receptor) (12) in MH-susceptible muscle may be one underlying pathophysiologic defect in MH-susceptible individuals leading to abnormal calcium release (13,14) in response to triggering medications (15,16). The skeletal muscle calcium release channel or ryanodine receptor (*RYR1* gene) has been localized to human chromosome 19q13.1 and may be associated with MH susceptibility in selected human families (17–19).

Other pathophysiologic mechanisms that have been suggested include dihydropyridine-sensitive calcium channel abnormalities (may affect the slow calcium channel of the transverse tubule) (20), fatty acid metabolism alterations (may increase calcium-induced calcium release from the sarcoplasmic reticulum) (21,22), and inositol 1,4,5,-trisphosphate phosphatase deficiencies (may raise myoplasmic calcium concentration) (23). It is likely that excitation-contraction coupling defects may vary among different families of MH-susceptible individuals. Such differences may help explain the variable manner in which MH events occur.

The sustained elevation of myoplasmic calcium produces muscular contracture and enhanced glycolytic and aerobic metabolism. ATP, glycogen, and oxygen are consumed, and excessive carbon dioxide, lactic acid, and heat are produced during the hypermetabolic process (24–26). Sarcolemmal muscle membrane permeability increases. Calcium, potassium, and myoglobin leak into the extracellular space. If steps are not taken rapidly to decrease the elevated levels of myoplasmic calcium, the systemic consequences are severe because muscle comprises approximately 40% of body mass (27). Products of skeletal hypermetabolism initiate a cascade of secondary MH responses in the heart, brain, liver, lung, kidney, and blood. Proteins and enzymes are denatured, and cellular membranes are damaged by acidosis, hyperthermia, and loss of energy substrates. Heffron postulates that MH events become irreversible when the concentration of ATP in muscle decreases to one half of its resting concentration (28).

Anesthetic-Induced Abnormalities in Temperature Regulation

General anesthesia broadens the temperature range over which active thermoregulatory responses are absent, rendering patients poikilothermic. Under anesthesia, body temperature changes are passively determined by the difference between metabolic heat production and heat loss to the environment (29). When whole body metabolism markedly increases during an MH event, body temperature can increase precipitously (27). However, if heat loss to the environment is greater than heat production or if cardiac output drops abruptly at the beginning of an MH episode, hyperthermia may not be seen (30).

Epidemiologic Concepts

When abnormal susceptibility to MH-triggering agents can be predicted in advance of administration, toxicity can be prevented by their exclusion. In order to evaluate the utility of various tests for predicting MH susceptibility, the following epidemiologic concepts must be understood. Disease *prevalence* is defined as the number of subjects with the disease per 100,000 population. A positive diagnostic test result (true positive) should be obtained when positive controls (diseased individuals) are tested. A negative diagnostic test result (true negative) should be obtained when negative controls (healthy individuals) are tested. False negative results occur when a diseased individual has a negative test result. False positive results occur when a healthy individual has a positive test result.

Sensitivity of a test is defined as the percentage of positive test results in a diseased population. *Specificity* of a test is defined as the percentage of negative test results in a population without the disease. Sensitivity and specificity are stable properties of a test that are uninfluenced by disease prevalence.

The *predictive value of a positive test result* is defined as the percentage of positive results that are true positives, as measured by a diagnostic gold standard. The *predictive value of a negative test result* is defined as the percentage of negative results that are true negatives as measured by the gold standard. As prevalence of a disease decreases, the predictive value of a negative test result increases and the predictive value of a positive test decreases. As a consequence, for a rare disease such as MH, it is difficult to obtain a high predictive value of a positive test result. One means of increasing the predictive value of a positive test result is to increase the prevalence of MH within the test population by carefully selecting test subjects (31).

CLINICAL PRESENTATION OF MALIGNANT HYPERTHERMIA

Inheritance

Mendelian Inheritance

Data from selected Australian, North American, British, and Irish families demonstrate that MH susceptibility is inherited as an autosomal dominant trait with reduced penetrance and variable expressivity (5,18,32–34). However, several MH researchers have concluded that whereas autosomal dominant inheritance is most frequent, some cases of MH are inherited in a multifactorial manner (33,35). To date, studies of MH genetics are confounded by the variable manner in which adverse anesthetic events are classified and by nonuniform laboratory methods for diagnosing MH susceptibility in those individuals who have not personally experienced an MH event.

Molecular Genetics

Gillard et al. (19) found that a substitution of cysteine for arginine 614 in the ryanodine receptor on chromosome 19q13.1 cosegregates with MH susceptibility in 1 of 35 MH-susceptible families. Levitt et al. (36) have demonstrated that MH susceptibility in 5 of 16 families appears to be linked to a different chromosome, 17q11.2-q24. Further work by Olckers et al. (37) suggested that a gene encoding the adult muscle sodium channel α-subunit may harbor a primary mutation in certain forms of MH susceptibility. It is probable that additional mutations causative for MH will be identified in the future because several different abnormalities of excitation-contraction coupling may be present in various MH-susceptible families. α-Thalassemia (38), β-thalassemia (39), and osteogenesis imperfecta (40,41) are examples of diseases in which patients with phenotypically similar presentations are genetically dissimilar.

Prevalence

The prevalence of MH susceptibility in the United States and Canada is unknown. The incidence of acute MH events in the United States is likewise unknown because MH is not a reportable disease to the United States Centers for Disease Control or state health departments. Based on a 6-year observation period at a single children's hospital in the 1960s, an acute MH event has been estimated to take place in 1/14,000 potent inhalational anesthetics in Canada (42; Beverley A. Britt, M.D., personal communication, April 26, 1990). Since 1987, The North American Malignant Hyperthermia Registry (NAMH Registry) has asked Canadian and U.S. anesthesiologists in the field and MH diagnostic center directors to complete standardized reports of adverse metabolic responses to anesthesia.[1] As anesthesiologists have become more informed of Registry reporting procedures, the rate at which anesthesiologists are reporting MH events to the Registry is increasing but is still too low to permit an accurate determination of MH incidence or prevalence. In the last 5.5 years, approximately 86 possible MH events/year were reported to the Registry. One hundred thirty-nine of the 471 (29.6%) MH events were reported by anesthesiologists in the field. Thirteen of the 471 (2.8%) possible MH cases involved cardiac arrest, and 5 (1.2%) resulted in death despite therapy.

In 1977, the Danish Malignant Hyperthermia Register was established to collect MH event reports from Danish anesthesiologists. Over a 6.5-year period, the Danish Register reported 154 suspected MH events, or 1 of every 6,167 potent inhalation anesthetics administered (43).

---

[1]Registry report forms may be obtained by contacting The North American Malignant Hyperthermia Registry, P.O. Box 850, Hershey, PA 17033, U.S.A., phone (717)531-6936; fax (717)531-6221; INTERNET: MLARACH@anes.hmc.psu.edu.

Possible Association of MH with Other Medical Conditions

Myopathies

Central Core Disease

Central core disease is a rare, nonprogressive myopathy that usually occurs in infancy or childhood with hypotonia and mild muscle weakness (often found in the proximal muscle groups). Musculoskeletal abnormalities, such as lordosis, kyphoscoliosis, congenital hip dislocation, and foot deformities, may be present (Fig. 1). Some patients may have mitral valve prolapse, cardiomyopathy, or arrhythmias. For some patients, MH events may be the presenting sign of central core disease. Adults often are slender and short statured but do not have focal areas of muscle atrophy (44,45). Autosomal dominance is the usual mode of inheritance. Histologic and histochemical examination of muscle specimens reveals marked type 1 fiber predominance, with cores that run nearly the whole length of the muscle fiber. The cores lack oxidative enzyme and phosphorylase reactivity and on electron microscopy demonstrate an absence of mitochondria with an alteration of the myofibrillar architecture (44,46). Figure 2 shows skeletal muscle from a patient with central core disease.

Multiple reports of acute MH events as well as positive MH diagnostic laboratory tests suggest a strong association between central core disease and MH susceptibility (45,47–50). All patients with central core disease should be managed as MH susceptible unless they have had a negative MH diagnostic test.

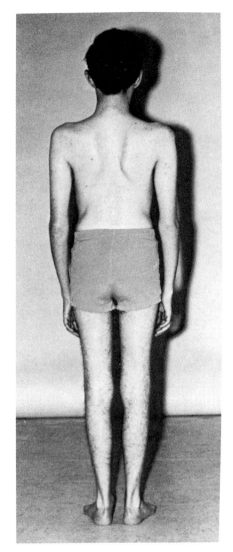

FIG. 1. A patient with central core disease who is slender, with diffuse weakness but no focal muscle wasting. (From Brooke MH. *A clinician's view of neuromuscular diseases,* 2nd ed. Baltimore: Williams and Wilkins, 1986.)

King-Denborough Syndrome

First described in 1973, the King-Denborough syndrome is a mild myopathy found predominantly in boys who are small for age, with cryptorchidism, lordosis, kyphosis, pectus carinatum, and unusual facies (small chin, low-set ears, and antimongoloid obliquity of the palpebral fissures) (51). Its incidence is unknown but is thought to be very low. Fulminant MH episodes occurred in seven children with King-Denborough syndrome. Four of the

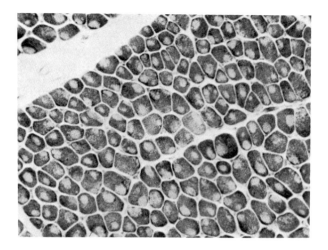

FIG. 2. Histologic examination of skeletal muscle from a patient with central core disease demonstrates that the NADH-tetrazolium reductase reaction fails to stain areas within each muscle fiber (central cores). (From Brooke MH. *A clinician's view of neuromuscular disease,* 2nd ed. Baltimore: Williams and Wilkins, 1986.)

seven children died (51,52). Two children with this syndrome had positive MH diagnostic tests (53,54). The author believes it prudent to manage all patients with the King-Denborough syndrome as MH susceptible unless they have had a negative MH diagnostic muscle biopsy.

Duchenne and Becker Muscular Dystrophy

Duchenne muscular dystrophy is a fatal X-linked recessive disease with an incidence of approximately 30 of every 100,000 male births. Patients with this disease have a deletion of the DMD locus on the X-chromosome (Xp21) (55). This deletion contributes to the agenesis of dystrophin (56), a protein associated with the triadic junctions in skeletal muscle (57), which may be vitally important for stabilizing the muscle fiber surface membrane (sarcolemma) against the stress associated with contraction and relaxation of muscle fibers. Dystrophin may help regulate skeletal muscle excitation-contraction as well (58).

Although the clinical picture is varied, patients generally become symptomatic between the ages of 2 and 6 years, with the signs of proximal muscle weakness, waddling gait, difficulty climbing stairs, Gow-

er's sign (rising from a stooped position by climbing up the legs using the hands), and calf pseudohypertrophy. These children are unable to keep up with their peers, are unable to jump, and often complain of leg pains. Between the ages of 3 and 6 years, they have frequent falls. After the age of 8 years, progressive contractures develop. By the age of 10, Duchenne patients may be unable to climb stairs or to stand up from the floor independently. Frequently by the age of 12, patients are confined to a wheelchair, and kyphoscoliosis develops (59). Eventually, striated, cardiac, and smooth muscles are progressively destroyed, leading to death in early adulthood from cardiac or respiratory failure (Fig. 3).

The clinical course of Becker muscular dystrophy closely resembles that of Duchenne dystrophy except the onset is later, and patients may survive until middle age (44). The majority of Becker patients have abnormal dystrophin, although 15% of Becker patients have normal quality but markedly reduced quantities of dystrophin (60,61).

Numerous case reports demonstrate that patients with Duchenne muscular dystrophy are uniquely vulnerable to anesthetic-induced toxicity. Clinicians report death or prolonged cardiac arrest (asystole for up to 2 hours before intrinsic cardiac rhythms are

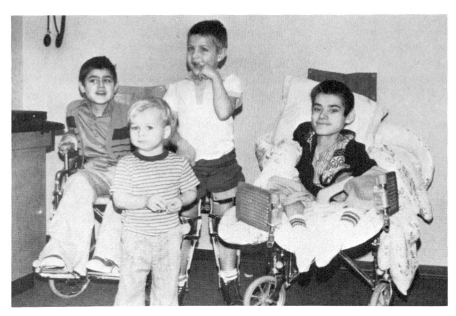

FIG. 3. A family of four brothers shown at various stages of Duchenne muscular dystrophy. (From Brooke MH. *A clinician's view of neuromuscular disease,* 2nd ed. Baltimore: Williams and Wilkins, 1986.)

restored) following the use of potent inhalational anesthetics (e.g., cyclopropane, halothane, and isoflurane) or succinylcholine in Duchenne patients. A cardiac arrest has occurred in a patient with Becker muscular dystrophy (62). Before the arrests, massive rhabdomyolysis with hyperkalemia (serum K^+ levels 7.9 to 12.6 mEq/L [62–66,69]) or fulminant MH (67–70) developed. Cardiac arrests occur at varying intervals following anesthetic exposure. Some arise shortly after succinylcholine administration (64–66,69), and others occur during recovery in the postanesthesia care unit (62,63).

Many authors emphasize that successful cardiac resuscitations with acceptable neurologic outcome may take place even after lengthy periods of asystole. Early measurement of serum potassium and vigorous treatment of hyperkalemia with hyperventilation, bicarbonate, calcium, insulin, and glucose is imperative. The NAMH Registry has received reports of successful resusci-

tations that required dialysis, pacemaker placement, or cardiopulmonary bypass. Dantrolene should be used if any signs of MH are present (e.g., masseter muscle rigidity, generalized muscular rigidity, and hypercarbia especially during cardiopulmonary resuscitation). Even if MH is severe enough to have triggered a cardiac arrest, hyperthermia may be absent due to decreased skeletal muscle perfusion and massive heat loss when the infant's or child's large surface area is exposed to a cold operating room environment during an extended resuscitation.

Frequently, cardiac arrests strike young boys [aged 3 months (66,71) to 8 years (62)] undergoing minor elective surgery. Cardiac arrest may be the first sign of dystrophy in a patient regarded as healthy by both family and physicians (64,66–69,71–74). Rosenberg and Gronert report a series of four deaths in 1 year following cardiac arrests in boys thought to be healthy whose probable Duchenne muscular dystrophy diagnosis was revealed postmortem (75). Even after death, frozen muscle tissues may be analyzed to confirm absent or severely diminished dystrophin levels in Duchenne muscular dystrophy or the presence of abnormal or decreased levels of dystrophin in Becker muscular dystrophy.[2]

The strength of the association between MH susceptibility and Duchenne muscular dystrophy is not known. Several patients with Duchenne muscular dystrophy have experienced fulminant MH (67–70). Others have had reliable laboratory investigations that indicate MH susceptibility (76). One patient had both survived a fulminant MH episode and had a positive MH diagnostic test (64). The percentage of Duchenne muscular dystrophy patients who will develop fulminant MH when they are exposed to MH-triggering anesthetic agents is unknown. Retrospective chart reviews document only 1 fulminant MH event in 123 Duchenne muscular dystrophy patients who received 211 general anesthetics with MH-triggering anesthetic agents. Only 23 of these patients received succinylcholine (77–79). It is not known whether relatives of a patient with Duchenne muscular dystrophy and MH are MH susceptible if they do not also suffer from Duchenne muscular dystrophy. Until family members undergo MH diagnostic testing, they also must be considered MH susceptible (80). The author believes that potent inhalational anesthetics or succinylcholine or both should be avoided in patients who are known to have Becker or Duchenne muscular dystrophy because they may trigger life-threatening cardiac arrests and MH.

Myotonia Congenita

Myotonia congenita is a rarely occurring condition that may be inherited in either an autosomal dominant (Thomsen) or autosomal recessive (Becker) fashion. Patients usually experience in the first decade of life painless myotonia or muscle stiffness that is improved by exercise. Muscular hypertrophy may occur even though they lack type 2B fibers. Those with the more common autosomal recessive variant also may display transient muscle weakness. The clinical course is usually nonprogressive, with more severe myotonia noted in those patients with autosomal recessive inheritance (44,81). A decreased chloride conductance across muscle membranes is the underlying molecular defect. In the autosomal dominant form, the genetic defect has been linked to an abnormal portion of chromosome 7q (81).

The relationship between myotonia congenita and the occurrence of MH is unclear. There are two well-described case reports of fatal reactions following general anesthesia—halothane/ether in a 12-year-old girl (82) and pentothal/dextroramide/nitrous oxide in a 5-year-old boy (83)—that are compatible with an MH reaction. Results of MH diagnostic testing on patients with myotonia congenita are mixed. A total of nine patients with myotonia congenita have undergone standardized MH diagnostic testing. Only two sisters with a history of an adverse reaction to anesthesia (succinylcholine-induced generalized muscular rigidity) had a test outcome indicating MH susceptibility (84–86). It is not known what percentage of myotonia congenita patients would have a positive MH diagnostic test if a large prospective study were conducted. Clearly, succinylcholine is contraindicated in all patients with myotonia congenita because it will provoke sustained myotonia (muscular rigidity). Potent inhalational anesthetics carry some risk of triggering MH. This risk must be weighed against the potential benefits rendered to the patient.

Minor Muscular or Temperature-Regulating Problems

Retrospective reviews of patients who have experienced possible MH events have indicated that such individuals may have a

---

[2]Frozen muscle tissues may be sent for analysis to Genica Pharmaceuticals, Two Biotech Park, 373 Plantation Street, Worcester, MA 01605, U.S.A.; phone: 1(800)394-4493.

more frequent occurrence of minor muscular defects (hernia, strabismus, ptosis, kyphoscoliosis, patellar laxity), muscle cramps, fevers, and heat stroke (42, 123). In a survey completed by 171 MH-susceptible members of an MH organization, 8% had a muscle abnormality, 60% complained of muscle cramps, 43% complained of muscle weakness, 14% to 39% reported unexplained high fevers, and 12% to 47% said that they had experienced heat stroke. The survey was flawed by lack of an appropriate control group and a possible bias toward reporting muscular and temperature-regulating abnormalities (87). Ranklev et al. (88) investigated the incidence of neuromuscular symptoms found in 50 MH-susceptible, 83 MH-nonsusceptible, and 19 control patients referred to their laboratory for MH diagnostic testing and found no difference in complaints of inguinal hernia, strabismus, kyphoscoliosis, patellar laxity, muscle cramps, or muscle weakness between MH-susceptible, MH-nonsusceptible, and control groups. The NAMH Registry is conducting a large-scale prospective epidemiologic study of whether minor muscular abnormalities or temperature-regulating difficulties occur more frequently in the MH-susceptible as compared to the nonsusceptible surgical population.

Neurolept Malignant Syndrome

Neurolept malignant syndrome is an idiosyncratic disorder marked by hyperthermia, skeletal muscle hypertonicity, fluctuating consciousness, and autonomic nervous system instability. Clinical signs also include pallor, diaphoresis, blood pressure instability, tachycardia, arrhythmias, tachypnea, and rhabdomyolysis. Administration of phenothiazines, butyrophenones, thioxanthenes, lithium, or tricyclics or discontinuation of antiparkinsonian drugs may trigger neurolept malignant syndrome. This syndrome typically develops over 24 to 72 hours and lasts from 5 to 10 days after oral neuroleptics are discontinued. If a depot form of the neurolept drug has been used, the syndrome may last two to three times longer. Mortality rates of 8% to 20% persist even with dantrolene, bromocriptine, amantadine, and supportive treatment (89–91).

Whether patients who experience neurolept malignant syndrome are also susceptible to MH is unknown. The issue has been raised because many of the clinical signs of both syndromes are similar, and patients respond well to dantrolene even though neurolept malignant syndrome is thought to be due to excessive central and peripheral nervous system dopaminergic blockade rather than to abnormal calcium regulation within skeletal muscle sarcoplasmic reticulum. Hermesh et al. (92) retrospectively reviewed the anesthetic records of 20 patients who experienced neurolept malignant syndrome. They found that no MH episodes were triggered even though these patients with a history of neurolept malignant syndrome were exposed to 159 MH-triggering anesthetics. Succinylcholine was given to 5 patients without adverse effects during a neurolept malignant event. There are conflicting outcomes from two small, well-designed prospective studies comparing MH diagnostic test results for three groups of individuals: (a) those with no suspicion of neurolept malignant or MH syndromes, (b) those with MH susceptibility only, and (c) those with a history of neurolept malignant syndrome only. In one MH diagnostic laboratory, 5 of 7 neurolept malignant syndrome patients had positive MH diagnostic tests (93). In another diagnostic laboratory, 0 of 8 neurolept malignant syndrome patients had positive MH diagnostic tests (94). The author believes that until further studies are completed, MH-triggering anesthetic agents should be avoided during neurolept malignant episodes, since such agents may trigger further rhabdomyolysis.

Sudden Infant Death Syndrome and Sudden Death

Although most investigators generally believe that MH-susceptible individuals are asymptomatic unless they receive MH-triggering anesthetic agents, some have questioned whether those susceptible to MH may also be susceptible to a generalized human stress syndrome producing sudden death in the absence of triggering anesthetic agents (95,96). If so, humans would more closely resemble MH-susceptible swine, who frequently die from MH episodes triggered by the stress of breeding, farrowing, fighting, mild exercise, restraint, transport, and ambient temperature increases [porcine stress syndrome (97–100)].

Sudden infant death syndrome (SIDS) is defined as "the sudden death of any infant or young child which is unexpected by history, and in which a thorough post-mortem examination fails to demonstrate an adequate cause for death" (101). In 1981, Denborough (102) first questioned whether there was a possible association between SIDS and MH syndromes when he performed MH diagnostic tests on a father with unexplained anesthetic-induced cardiac arrests whose son had died from SIDS. He subsequently performed MH diagnostic testing on an additional 14 parents of 12 children who had died from SIDS. He concluded that there was an association between these two syndromes because 38% of families with a history of SIDS had a parent with a positive MH diagnostic test (103). However, selection bias may have occurred because testing was preferentially performed on those families with a history of both SIDS and prior anesthetic difficulties (104). In 1988, Ellis et al. (104) queried their MH-susceptible population concerning their experience with SIDS and found that the incidence of SIDS did not differ significantly from that of the general population. Also, parents of 106 SIDS infants reported no personally experienced episodes of MH. Finally, 14 parents of SIDS victims had negative MH diagnostic test results in their laboratory. Thus, the association between a commonly occurring (sudden infant death) and a rarely occurring (MH) syndrome is questioned.

Evidence of an association between MH and unexplained sudden death in older children is scant. Ranklev et al. (105) report the unexplained sudden deaths of two brothers, aged 16 and 19 years, whose father had a positive MH diagnostic test. Britt (106) reports the sudden deaths of two MH-susceptible siblings. However, the deaths are not entirely unexplained because one sibling was suffering from acute cocaine intoxication, and the other sibling had a lower respiratory infection.

Triggers

All known potent inhalational anesthetic agents may trigger MH, including the older anesthetics (e.g., chloroform, diethyl ether, ethylene, cyclopropane, and methoxyflurane) as well as the modern potent inhalational anesthetics (e.g., halothane, isoflurane, enflurane, sevoflurane, and desflurane). The depolarizing muscle relaxants, succinylcholine and decamethonium, also trigger MH (6,7,42,107–110). To date, there is no convincing evidence to implicate any other medication as an MH trigger. Specifically, amide local anesthetics (111–115), anticholinergic and anticholinesterase medications (1,116), and calcium salts (117, 118) may be used safely in MH-susceptible individuals.

Although most MH researchers believe that MH-triggering anesthetic exposure is a necessary precondition for the development of an acute MH event, it is clear that other, as yet unidentified factors, also contribute. MH-susceptible humans do not consistently develop MH after each anesthetic exposure. One child received 44 anesthetics with halothane or succinylcholine or both before his MH susceptibility was discovered (1).

Clinical and Laboratory Signs of MH

As noted earlier, the clinical and laboratory signs of an acute MH episode are multiple and variable in their presentation, intensity, and time course. The abnormal signs are related to skeletal muscle hypermetabolism and ischemia and their systemic sequelae. These signs may include tachycardia, masseter muscle rigidity, generalized muscle rigidity, myoglobinuria, increased creatine kinase, tachypnea, hypercarbia, respiratory acidosis, metabolic acidosis, skin mottling, cyanosis, hyperkalemia, arrhythmias including ventricular tachycardia and fibrillation, cardiac arrest, hypertension, diaphoresis, rapid temperature rise, and excessive bleeding (1–3).

Table 1 lists the clinical signs observed most frequently during possible MH events that were reported to the NAMH Registry. Although masseter rigidity represents the most frequently reported clinical sign in this series, several studies show that masseter rigidity is a nonspecific sign of MH susceptibility because 39% to 75% of patients experiencing masseter rigidity have a negative MH diagnostic test (1,2,119–122). On the other hand, masseter rigidity should not be ignored because it is the presenting sign of many acute MH episodes. Generalized muscular rigidity is a more specific sign of MH. Its presence is associated with a significant 18- to 20-fold increase in the risk of a patient's being MH susceptible (as

measured by a positive MH diagnostic test) (1,2).

In a series of 337 patients reported by Britt et al. (123), tachycardia or other rapid arrhythmia was the sign most frequently observed during the first 30 minutes of an undefined MH event. Anesthesiologists ranked the order in which clinical signs of a probable MH event occur and reported these data to the NAMH Registry. In this series of 83 patients, anesthesiologists observed that masseter spasm was the first sign in 46%, inappropriate tachycardia was the first sign in 29%, and inappropriate hypercarbia was the first sign in 25% of probable MH events.

The clinical signs of a possible MH episode are nonspecific. Before confirming a diagnosis of MH susceptibility, the following alternate explanations for adverse anesthetic reactions should be considered: insufficient anesthetic depth, local anesthetic and vasoconstrictor toxicity, anaphylaxis, hypoxia, hypercarbia, temporomandibular joint dysfunction, iatrogenic hyperthermia, heat stroke, sepsis, radiologic contrast material within the central nervous system (124), thyrotoxicosis (125,126), pheochromocytoma (127,128), and neurolept malignant syndrome. If a patient is critically ill, treatment for MH and other life-threatening disorders should be instituted before a diagnostic workup is completed.

TABLE 1. *Possible signs of malignant hyperthermia observed in 738 patients reported to the Registry*

Clinical sign	Number of patients	Frequency (percentile)
Masseter rigidity	364	49.3
Rapid temperature increase	267	36.2
Hypercarbia	165	22.4
Generalized rigidity	120	16.3
Tachypnea	73	9.9
Cola-colored urine	64	8.7
Sinus tachycardia	63	8.5
Elevated temperature	63	8.5
Cyanosis	33	4.5
Sweating	28	3.8
Ventricular tachycardia	7	0.9
Ventricular fibrillation	4	0.5
Excessive bleeding	3	0.4

MH Toxicity

Morbidity

The morbidity of a fulminant MH episode may be considerable because the sustained skeletal muscle contracture and hypermetabolism produce multisystem derangement (28,129). Skeletal muscle destruction as evidenced by massive elevation in serum creatine kinase, potassium, and myoglobin may lead to muscle edema, compartment syndrome, muscle weakness, and wasting (123). Rhabdomyolysis with subsequent myoglobinuria may produce acute renal failure (130). Hyperkalemia and acidosis may generate severe arrhythmias, depressed cardiac contractility, pulmonary edema, and cardiac arrest (30,42). Hyperthermia, acidosis, hyperkalemia, and hypoxia may lead to seizures, cerebral edema, coma, and brain death (7). Acidosis, hyperthermia, and hyperkalemia may result in the release of tissue thomboplastins, with resultant disseminated intravascular coagulopathy (27). The NAMH Registry is studying the frequency with which these complications occur and the extent to which dantrolene therapy prevents or ameliorates them.

Mortality

In 1967, before the introduction of dantrolene, the mortality rate from an MH episode was reported to be 73% (7). Today, the mortality rate is very low, perhaps less than 5% for those experiencing a full-blown MH event. In the 1990s, uncontrollable coagulopathy or untreatable cardiac arrhythmias secondary to hyperkalemia are the terminal events in patients suffering from fulminant MH. The marked decline in MH mortality rates in the past decade is due to earlier recognition of developing MH events (as continuous expired CO_2 and temperature monitoring have become standard practice for all patients receiving a general anesthetic) and the widespread availability of a specific and highly effective therapy, dantrolene (131). It is hoped that universal application of expired CO_2 and temperature monitoring and immediate availability of adequate amounts of dantrolene in all anesthetizing locations will further decrease MH morbidity and mortality.

TREATMENT OF MH

Dantrolene

Dantrolene is a highly lipid, soluble hydantoin analogue that was synthesized originally for use as a muscle relaxant. Dantrolene depresses the rate and amount of calcium release from the sarcoplasmic reticulum, decreases myoplasmic calcium levels, modifies contractile activity in skeletal muscle, and thereby terminates MH episodes (16,132–136).

Dantrolene's therapeutic effect was first reported by Harrison in 1975. He demonstrated that dantrolene aborted fulminant MH episodes in seven of eight susceptible swine (137). In 1982, Kolb et al. (129) demonstrated dantrolene's efficacy in aborting unequivocal or probable MH in 11 human patients. In 1984, Britt (138) reported retrospectively that 12 patients who received at least 6.0 mg/kg of dantrolene for MH events survived.

In a recent NAMH Registry study of outcome following dantrolene treatment for probable or certain MH episodes, 70 (95.9%) of the 73 treated patients survived. Fifteen (24.6%) of the treated patients recrudesced following an initial 2.3 mg/kg mean dose of dantrolene. In contrast to Britt's series, 3 (4.1%) patients who received high-dose dantrolene still succumbed in spite of total dantrolene doses of 10.3 to 20 mg/kg. The total dose of dantrolene used to treat a probable MH episode ranged from 0.9 to 33.9 mg/kg, with a mean of 5.6 mg/kg. Five (5.9%) patients receiving dantrolene experienced respiratory failure, which appeared to be unrelated to the severity of the MH episode (139).

Supportive Therapy

The administration of all MH-triggering agents must be terminated immediately on suspicion of an acute MH event. Supportive therapy for the multisystem disorders induced by MH includes: hyperventilation with 100% oxygen for treatment of respiratory acidosis and ischemia; sodium bicarbonate therapy for metabolic acidosis; glucose, insulin, and calcium chloride administration for hyperkalemia; fluids, mannitol, and furosemide to ensure a diuresis that helps

TABLE 2. *Malignant hyperthermia treatment regimen*

1. Call for **help.**

2. Notify the surgeon to **rapidly terminate the procedure.**

3. **Stop all triggering anesthetic agents.**
   Administer *dantrolene sodium* 2.5 mg/kg i.v. and titrate to effect (total dose may exceed 10 mg/kg).

4. **Intubate and hyperventilate** with 100% oxygen and high gas flows of at least 10 L/minute.

5. Insert arterial, central venous, and urinary **catheters.**

6. Obtain **blood samples** (arterial and venous blood gases, potassium, ionized calcium, myoglobin, creatine kinase, PT, PTT, platelet count, fibrinogen).

7. **Cool** with i.v. fluid infusion, body cavity lavage, and surface cooling.
8. Promote a **diuresis** with i.v. normal saline, mannitol (0.25 g/kg), and furosemide (1 mg/kg). Ensure urine output of greater than 2 mL/kg/hour.

9. **Treat hyperkalemia** with glucose and insulin. (Add 10 units of regular insulin to 50 ml of 50% glucose and titrate to effect.) Calcium chloride (2–5 mg/kg) may be helpful.

10. **Treat acidosis** with sodium bicarbonate (1–2 mEq/kg increments guided by arterial pH and P_{CO_2}).

11. **Treat arrhythmias** with antiarrhythmics as needed but avoid calcium channel blockers. Boys <9 years of age who experience sudden cardiac arrest after succinylcholine in the absence of hypoxemia should be treated for acute hyperkalemia first. (See 9 above.)

12. Call the MH **Hotline** Consultant—(209) 634-4917, Index Zero—for expert help.

13. When the patient has been stabilized **transfer** the patient to an intensive care or postanesthesia care unit. An anesthesiologist should monitor the patient for a possible MH recurrence. Continue dantrolene 1 mg/kg i.v. q6h for 24–48 hours post-MH event.

14. Report the event to The North American Malignant Hyperthermia **Registry** (717) 531-6936.

15. Refer the patient for diagnostic MH muscle biopsy.

16. Inform the **family** of possible MH susceptibility and refer the patient and family to MH patient support organizations, MHAUS in the U.S. (203) 847-0407 or MHA in Canada (416) 222-0150.

17. Instruct the patient to obtain a **Medic-Alert** bracelet.

Adapted from Larach MG. Advances in understanding malignant hyperthermia. *Oral Maxillofac Surg Clin North Am* 1992;4:851–861.

eliminate myoglobin and potassium; cool intravenous fluids, surface cooling, and body cavity lavage to achieve normothermia; and appropriate clotting factor and blood product administration to treat coagulopathy. Although supportive therapy is helpful, early dantrolene administration (initial dose of 2.5 mg/kg titrated to 10 mg/kg or greater to control MH signs) is essential for the successful treatment of MH events. Table 2 outlines an MH treatment regimen.

PREDICTING MH SUSCEPTIBILITY

The MH Clinical Grading Scale

Prior to 1994, a clinical case definition for MH events or MH susceptibility did not exist. Lack of a clinical case definition interferes with efforts to predict a patient's MH susceptibility. The tasks of appropriately managing future anesthetics in patients who have experienced adverse anesthetic events that might have represented early MH episodes, and of providing genetic counseling for these patients' relatives, are made more difficult if the probability of the patient's being MH susceptible is unknown. Also, research into improved means for diagnosing MH is hindered by the absence of a standardized means for estimating the likelihood of MH in a given patient.

For these reasons, a panel of 11 international MH experts used the Delphi method for achieving a group consensus to develop a multi-factor MH clinical grading scale. This MH grading scale contains standardized clinical diagnostic criteria that can classify existing anesthetic records and also can be applied to new patients (140).

The MH clinical grading scale ranks the likelihood that an adverse anesthetic event represents MH or that, with further investigation of family history, an individual patient will be diagnosed as being susceptible to MH. The rank assigned to the individual patient represents the lower limit of the likelihood of MH in that patient. Several factors, including aborting an anesthetic early in the course of a reaction or use of inadequate patient monitoring, may lead to an underestimation, but rarely an overestimation, of the likelihood of an MH event or an individual's MH susceptibility.

The clinical grading scale requires the anesthesiologist to judge whether or not specific clinical signs are appropriate when considered in the context of the patient's medical problems, anesthetic, and surgical operation. Points are assigned for each clinical indicator present. These points then are summed to produce a likelihood score that a MH event took place or that an individual is MH susceptible.

TABLE 3. *Scoring rules for the MH clinical grading scale*

1. **MH Indicators**
   Review the list of clinical indicators. If any indicator is present, add the points applicable for each indicator while observing the double counting rule below which applies to multiple indicators representing a single process.
   If no indicator is present, the patient's MH score is zero.

2. **Double-counting**
   If more than one indicator represents a single process, count only the indicator with the highest score. Application of this rule prevents double counting when one clinical process has more than one clinical manifestation.
   Exception: the score for any relevant indicators in the final category of Table 4 ("other indicators") should be added to the total score without regard to double counting.

3. **MH Susceptibility Indicators**
   The *italicized* indicators listed below apply only to MH susceptibility. Do not use these indicators to score a MH event. To calculate the score for MH susceptibility, add the score of the *italicized* indicators below to the score for the highest ranking MH event.
   Positive family history of MH in relative of 1st degree
   Positive family history of MH in relative not of 1st degree
   Resting elevated serum creatine kinase
   Positive family history of MH together with another indicator
      from the patient's own anesthetic experience
      other than elevated serum creatine kinase

4. **Interpreting the raw score: MH rank and qualitative likelihood**

Raw score range	MH rank	Description of likelihood
0	1	Almost never
3–9	2	Unlikely
10–19	3	Somewhat less than likely
20–34	4	Somewhat greater than likely
35–49	5	Very likely
50+	6	Almost certain

Reprinted with permission, from Larach M G, Localio A R, Allen G C et al. A clinical grading scale to predict malignant hyperthermia susceptibility. *Anesthesiology* 1994;80:771–779.

TABLE 4. *Clinical indicators for use in determining the MH raw score*

Process I: Rigidity

Indicator	Points
Generalized muscular rigidity (in absence of shivering due to hypothermia, or during or immediately following emergence from inhalational general anesthesia)	15
Masseter spasm shortly following succinylcholine administration	15

Process II: Muscle Breakdown

Indicator	Points
Elevated creatine kinase >20,000 IU after anesthetic that included succinylcholine	15
Elevated creatine kinase >10,000 IU after anesthetic without succinylcholine	15
Cola colored urine in perioperative period	10
Myoglobin in urine >60 μg/L	5
Myoglobin in serum >170 μg/L	5
Blood/plasma/serum K^+ > 6 mEq/L (in absence of renal failure)	3

Process III: Respiratory Acidosis

Indicator	Points
$P_{ET}CO_2$ >55 mmHg with appropriately controlled ventilation	15
Arterial P_aCO_2 >60 mmHg with appropriately controlled ventilation	15
$P_{ET}CO_2$ >60 mmHg with spontaneous ventilation	15
Arterial P_aCO_2 >65 mmHg with spontaneous ventilation	15
Inappropriate hypercarbia (in anesthesiologist's judgment)	15
Inappropriate tachypnea	10

Process IV: Temperature Increase

Indicator	Points
Inappropriately rapid increase in temperature (in anesthesiologist's judgment)	15
Inappropriately increased temperature > 38.8°C (101.8°F) in the perioperative period (in anesthesiologist's judgment)	10

Process V: Cardiac Involvement

Indicator	Points
Inappropriate sinus tachycardia	3
Ventricular tachycardia or ventricular fibrillation	3

Process VI: Family History (Use to determine MH Susceptibility Only)

Indicator	Points
Positive MH family history in relative of 1st degree[a]	15
Positive MH family history in relative not of 1st degree[a]	5

Other indicators that are not part of a single process
(Note: these should be added without regard to double counting)

Indicator	Points
Arterial base excess more negative than −8 mEq/L	10
Arterial pH <7.25	10
Rapid reversal of MH signs of metabolic and/or respiratory acidosis with i.v. dantrolene	5
Positive MH family history together with another indicator from the patient's own anesthetic experience other than elevated resting serum creatine kinase[a]	10
Resting elevated serum creatine kinase (in patient with a family history of MH)[a]	10

[a]Indicators in *italics* should be used only for determining MH susceptibility.
Reprinted with permission, from Larach M G, Localio A R, Allen G C et al. A clinical grading scale to predict malignant hyperthermia susceptibility. *Anesthesiology* 1994;80:771–779.

The likelihood that an adverse anesthetic event represents MH is derived from points assigned to specific abnormal signs and laboratory findings (clinical indicators) observed during an acute anesthetic reaction. Additional points for family history are added to the raw score to determine an individual's MH susceptibility. The raw score is designed to be converted to an MH rank designating the risk with which MH could occur from 1 (almost never) to 6 (almost certain). Table 3 shows the scoring rules created by the MH experts for the MH clinical grading scale. The clinical indicators used to determine the MH raw scores are listed in Table 4. The MH clinical grading scale should be used as a comprehensive clinical case definition for the MH syndrome (140).

Laboratory Diagnosis

Invasive: Caffeine Halothane Contracture Testing

The caffeine halothane contracture test is the only laboratory test used to diagnose MH susceptibility. This invasive diagnostic test was developed in the early 1970s following the observations of Kalow et al. and Ellis et al. of abnormal skeletal muscle contracture responses to caffeine (141) and halothane (142) in survivors of fulminant MH events. The test is performed by placing replicate samples of fresh skeletal muscle in a 37°C tissue bath of Krebs-Ringer solution buffered with carbogen. Replicate samples of muscle are used, since it is not possible to repeat the test on each individual fascicle, and each individual subject usually undergoes caffeine halothane contracture testing only once. Each muscle fascicle is electrically stimulated. In North America, the threshold contracture responses to the test agents, 3% (v/v) halothane and caffeine (administered incrementally), are then measured. All testing is completed within 5 hours of muscle excision (143).

If the North American caffeine halothane contracture test were modified so that a patient would be diagnosed as MH susceptible when a 3% halothane contracture ≥0.5 g or a 2 mM caffeine contracture ≥0.3 g is measured, preliminary Registry studies indicate that test sensitivity would be 100% (one-sided 95% confidence interval of 88.3%) and test specificity would be 78% (one-sided 95% confidence interval of 70.9%) (144). To compare the caffeine halothane contracture test with a commonly used clinical test for diagnosis of myocardial infarction, elevated creatine phosphokinase-MB enzyme values are equivalent in sensitivity (100%) but

higher in specificity (85%) for the diagnosis of acute myocardial infarction (145).

The caffeine halothane contracture test should not be used to screen for MH susceptibility because it is invasive and disfiguring (3 g of muscle must be excised under general or regional anesthesia), expensive ($2700 per test), not readily available, and cannot be performed on children <20 kg.

Less Invasive: Spin Resonance, Magnetic Resonance Spectroscopy, Molecular Genetic Tests

Is the development of an MH screening test likely in the next decade? If the genetic heterogeneity underlying the MH syndrome is extensive, molecular genetics may not ever provide anesthesiologists with a preoperative screening test for MH susceptibility. In this case, genetic testing may be restricted to selected, well-characterized families. Other noninvasive techniques that have failed to discriminate between MH-susceptible and MH-nonsusceptible individuals include measurement of cytosolic free calcium concentrations in lymphocytes (146), spin resonance spectroscopy of red blood cell membranes (147), and phosphorus magnetic resonance spectroscopy of muscle (148). In this author's judgment, the caffeine halothane contracture test will likely remain the sole clinically useful MH diagnostic test for the next decade.

CONCLUSION

MH is a potentially fatal syndrome induced by the administration of anesthetic agents. In individuals with inherited skeletal muscle excitation-contracture coupling defects, potent inhalational anesthetics and succinylcholine produce elevated myoplasmic calcium concentrations that trigger sustained skeletal muscle contracture and hypermetabolism, which may initiate multisystem derangement. Although most MH-susceptible individuals are otherwise healthy, those patients with central core disease, King-Denborough syndrome, myotonia congenita, Duchenne's and Becker's muscular dystrophy are at increased risk for MH events. In humans, MH is genetically heterogeneous, which decreases the probability that a noninvasive MH screening test will be developed in the next decade. The recent creation of an MH clinical grading scale will facilitate prediction of MH susceptibility and will promote research into improved diagnostic and treatment methods for this anesthetic-induced disease.

ACKNOWLEDGMENTS

This work was supported in part by the American Society of Anesthesiologists, Department of Anesthesia, Pennsylvania State University College of Medicine, the Foundation for Anesthesia Education and Research, the Malignant Hyperthermia Association, the Malignant Hyperthermia Association of the United States, and Proctor and Gamble Pharmaceuticals, Inc.

The author thanks Linda J. Fuhrman, B.A., for her assistance with Registry database inquiries, Laura J. Simon, M.A., for statistical analysis of dantrolene data, Michele E. McKee, B.A., for retrieval of references, and Gregory C. Allen, M.D., and David R. Larach, M.D., Ph.D., for helpful suggestions.

REFERENCES

1. Larach M G, Rosenberg H, Larach D R, Broennle A M. Prediction of malignant hyperthermia susceptibility by clinical signs. *Anesthesiology* 1987;66:547–550.
2. Hackl W, Mauritz W, Schemper M, Winkler M, Sporn P, Steinbereithner K. Prediction of malignant hyperthermia susceptibility: statistical evaluation of clinical signs. *Br J Anaesth* 1990; 64:425–429.
3. Rosenberg H. Clinical presentation of malignant hyperthermia. *Br J Anaesth* 1988;60:268–273.
4. Denborough M A, Lovell R R H. Anaesthetic deaths in a family [Letter]. *Lancet* 1960;ii:45.
5. Denborough M A, Forster J F A, Lovell R R H, Maplestone P A, Villiers J D. Anaesthetic deaths in a family. *Br J Anaesth* 1962;34:395–396.
6. Harrison G G, Isaacs H. Malignant hyperthermia: an historical vignette. *Anaesthesia* 1992; 47:54–56.
7. Wilson R D, Dent T E, Traber D L, McCoy N R, Allen C R. Malignant hyperpyrexia with anesthesia. *JAMA* 1967;202:183–186.
8. Hall L W, Woolf N, Bradley J W P, Jolly D W. Unusual reaction to suxamethonium chloride. *Br Med J* 1966;2:1305.
9. Harrison G G, Saunders S J, Biebuyck J F, et al. Anaesthetic-induced malignant hyperpyrexia and a method for its prediction. *Br J Anaesth* 1969;41:844–855.
10. Nelson T E. SR function in malignant hyperthermia. *Cell Calcium* 1988;9:257–265.
11. MacLennan D H, Phillips M S. Malignant hyperthermia. *Science* 1992;256:789–794.
12. Fill M, Coronado R, Mickelson J R, et al. Abnormal ryanodine receptor channels in malignant hyperthermia. *Biophys J* 1990;50:471–475.
13. Ohta T, Endo M, Nakano T, Morohoshi Y, Wanikawa K, Ohga A. Ca-induced Ca release in malignant hyperthermia-susceptible pig skeletal muscle. *Am J Physiol* 1989;256:C358–C367.
14. Carrier L, Villaz M, Dupont Y. Abnormal rapid Ca^{2+} release from sarcoplasmic reticulum of malignant hyperthermia susceptible pigs. *Biochim Biophys Acta* 1991;1064:175–183.
15. Lopez J R, Allen P D, Alamo L, Jones D, Streter F A. Myoplasmic free $[Ca^{2+}]$ during a malignant hyperthermia episode in swine. *Muscle Nerve* 1988;11:82–88.
16. Ohnishi S T. Effects of halothane, caffeine, dantrolene and tetracaine on the calcium permeability of skeletal sarcoplasmic reticulum of malignant hyperthermic pigs. *Biochim Biophys Acta* 1987;897:261–268.
17. MacLennan D H, Duff C, Zorzato F, et al. Ryanodine receptor gene is a candidate for predisposition to malignant hyperthermia [Letter]. *Nature* 1990;343:559–561.
18. McCarthy T V, Healy J M S, Heffron J J A, et al. Localization of the malignant hyperthermia susceptibility locus to human chromosome 19q12-13.2 [Letter]. *Nature* 1990;343:562–564.
19. Gillard E F, Otsu K, Fujii J, et al. A substitution of cysteine for arginine 614 in the ryanodine receptor is potentially causative of human malignant hyperthermia. *Genomics* 1991;11: 751–755.
20. Ervasti J M, Claessens M T, Mickelson J R, Louis C F. Altered transverse tubule dihydropyridine receptor binding in malignant hyperthermia. *J Biol Chem* 1989;264:2711–2717.
21. Fletcher J E, Tripolitis L, Erwin K, et al. Fatty acids modulate calcium-induced calcium release from skeletal muscle heavy sarcoplasmic reticulum fractions: implications for malignant hyperthermia. *Biochem Cell Biol* 1990;68:1195–1201.

22. Seewald M J, Eichinger H M, Iaizzo P A. Malignant hyperthermia: an altered phospholipid and fatty acid composition in muscle membranes. *Acta Anaesthesiol Scand* 1991;35:380–386.

23. Foster P S, Gesini E, Claudianos C, Hopkinson K C, Denborough M A. Inositol 1,4,5, trisphosphate phosphatase deficiency and malignant hyperpyrexia in swine. *Lancet* 1989; ii:124–127.

24. Berman M C, Harrison G G, Bull A B, Kench J E. Changes underlying halothane-induced malignant hyperpyrexia in landrace pigs [Letter]. *Nature* 1970;225:653–655.

25. Lucke J N, Hall G M, Lister D. Porcine malignant hyperthermia. I: Metabolic and physiologic changes. *Br J Anaesth* 1976;48:297–304.

26. MacLennan D H. The genetic basis of malignant hyperthermia. *TIPS* 1992;13:330–334.

27. Gronert G A, Mott J, Lee J. Aetiology of malignant hyperthermia. *Br J Anaesth* 1988;60:253–267.

28. Heffron J J A. Malignant hyperthermia: Biochemical aspects of the acute episode. *Br J Anaesth* 1988;60:274–278.

29. Sessler D I. Temperature monitoring. In: Miller RD, ed. *Anesthesia*, 3rd ed. New York: Churchill Livingstone, 1990:1227–1242.

30. Gronert G A, Schulman S R, Mott J. Malignant hyperthermia. In: Miller R D, ed. *Anesthesia*, 3rd ed. New York: Churchill Livingstone, 1990: 935–956.

31. Galen R S, Gambino S R. *Beyond normality: the predictive value and efficiency of medical diagnoses.* New York: Wiley, 1975.

32. Britt B A, Locher W G, Kalow W. Hereditary aspects of malignant hyperthermia. *Can Anaesth Soc J* 1969;16:89–98.

33. Kalow W. Inheritance of malignant hyperthermia—a review of published data. In: Britt B A, ed. *Malignant hyperthermia.* Boston: Martinus Nijhoff, 1987:155–180.

34. Ellis F R, Halsall P J, Harriman D G F. The work of the Leeds Malignant Hyperpyrexia Unit, 1971–84. *Anaesthesia* 1986;41:809–815.

35. McPherson E, Taylor C A Jr. The genetics of malignant hyperthermia: evidence for heterogeneity. *Am J Med Gen* 1982;11:273–285.

36. Levitt R C, Olckers A, Meyers S, et al. Evidence for the localization of a malignant hyperthermia susceptibility locus (MHS2) to human chromosome 17q. *Genomics* 1992;14:562–566.

37. Olckers A, Meyers D A, Meyers S, et al. Adult muscle sodium channel α-subunit is a gene candidate for malignant hyperthermia susceptibility. *Genomics* 1992;14:829–831.

38. Higgs D R, Vickers M A, Wilkie A O M, Pretorius I-M, Jarman A P, Weatherall D J. A review of the molecular genetics of the human α-globin gene cluster. *Blood* 1989;73:1081–1104.

39. Kazazian H H, Dowling C E, Boehm C D, et al. Gene defects in β-thalassemia and their prenatal diagnoses. *Ann NY Acad Sci* 1990;612:1–14.

40. Byers P H, Bonadio J F, Cohn D H, Starman B J, Wenstrup R J, Willing M C. Osteogenesis imperfecta: the molecular basis of clinical heterogeneity. *Ann NY Acad Sci* 1988;543:117–128.

41. Prockop D J, Baldwin C T, Constantinou C D. Mutations in type 1 procollagen genes that cause osteogenesis imperfecta. *Adv Hum Genet* 1990;19:105–132.

42. Britt B A, Kalow W. Malignant hyperthermia: a statistical review. *Can Anaesth Soc J* 1970; 17:293–315.

43. Ørding H. Incidence of malignant hyperthermia in Denmark. *Anesth Analg* 1985;64:700–704.

44. Brooke M H. *A clinician's view of neuromuscular diseases,* 2nd ed. Baltimore: Williams & Wilkins, 1986.

45. Shuaib A, Paasuke R T, Brownell A K W. Central core disease: clinical features in 13 patients. *Medicine* 1987;66:389–396.

46. Dubowitz V, Pearse A G E. Oxidative enzymes and phosphorylase in central-core disease of muscle. *Lancet* 1960;ii:23–24.

47. Denborough M A, Dennett X, Anderson R McD. Central-core disease and malignant hyperthermia. *Br Med J* 1973;1:272–273.

48. Isaacs H, Barlow M B. Central core disease associated with elevated creatine phosphokinase levels—two members of a family known to be susceptible to malignant hyperpyrexia. *S African Med J* 1974;48:640–642.

49. Eng G D, Epstein B S, Engel W K, McKay D W, McKay R. Malignant hyperthermia and central core disease in a child with congenital dislocating hips. *Arch Neurol* 1978;35:189–197.

50. Frank J P, Harati Y, Butler I J, Nelson T E, Scott C I. Central core disease and malignant hyperthermia syndrome. *Ann Neurol* 1980;7:11–17.

51. King J O, Denborough M A. Anesthetic-induced malignant hyperpyrexia in children. *J Pediatr* 1973;83:37–40.

52. McPherson E W, Taylor C A. The King syndrome: malignant hyperthermia, myopathy, and multiple anomalies. *Am J Med Genet* 1981;8:159–165.

53. Heiman-Patterson T D, Rosenberg H R, Binning C P S, Tahmoush A J. King-Denborough syndrome: contracture testing and literature review. *Pediatr Neurol* 1986;2:175–177.

54. Isaacs H, Badenhorst M E. Dominantly inherited malignant hyperthermia (MH) in the King-Denborough syndrome. *Muscle Nerve* 1992; 15:740–742.

55. Monaco A P, Neve R L, Colletti-Feener C, Bertelson C J, Kurnit D M, Kunkel L M. Isolation of candidate cDNAs for portions of the Duchenne muscular dystrophy gene [Letter]. *Nature* 1986;323:646–650.

56. Hoffman E P, Brown R H, Kunkel L M. Dystrophin: the protein product of the Duchenne muscular dystrophy locus. *Cell* 1987;51:919–928.

57. Hoffman E P, Knudson C M, Campbell K P, Kunkel L M. Subcellular fractionation of dystrophin to the triads of skeletal muscle [Letter]. *Nature* 1987;330:754–758.

58. Arahata K, Sugita H. Dystrophin and the membrane hypothesis of muscular dystrophy. *TIPS* 1989;10:437–439.

59. Brooke M H, Fenichel G M, Griggs R C, et al. Clinical investigation in Duchenne dystrophy: 2. Determination of the "power" of therapeutic trials based on the natural history. *Muscle Nerve* 1983;6:91–103.

60. Hoffman E P, Kunkel L M, Angelini C, Clarke A, Johnson M, Harris J B. Improved diagnosis of Becker muscular dystrophy by dystrophin testing. *Neurology* 1989;39:1011–1017.

61. Beggs A H, Kunkel L M. Improved diagnosis of Duchenne/Becker muscular dystrophy. *J Clin Invest* 1990;85:613–619.

62. Chalkiadis G A, Branch K G. Cardiac arrest after isoflurane anaesthesia in a patient with Duchenne's muscular dystrophy. *Anaesthesia* 1990;45:22–25.

63. Kelfer H M, Singer W D, Reynolds R N. Malignant hyperthermia in a child with Duchenne muscular dystrophy. *Pediatrics* 1983;71:118–119.

64. Brownell A K W, Paasuke R T, Elash A, et al. Malignant hyperthermia in Duchenne muscular dystrophy. *Anesthesiology* 1983;58:180–182.

65. Henderson W A V. Succinylcholine-induced cardiac arrest in unsuspected Duchenne muscular dystrophy. *Can Anaesth Soc J* 1984;31:444–446.

66. Delphin E, Jackson D, Rothstein P. Use of succinylcholine during elective pediatric anesthesia should be reevaluated. *Anesth Analg* 1987;66:1190–1192.

67. Boltshauser E, Steinmann B, Meyer A, Jerusalem F. Anaesthesia-induced rhabdomyolysis in Duchenne muscular dystrophy [Letter]. *Br J Anaesth* 1980;52:559.

68. Linter S P K, Thomas P R, Withington P S, Hall M G. Suxamethonium associated hypertonicity and cardiac arrest in unsuspected pseudohypertrophic muscular dystrophy. *Br J Anaesth* 1982;54:1331–1332.

69. Wang J M, Stanley T H. Duchenne muscular dystrophy and malignant hyperthermia—two case reports. *Can Anaesth Soc J* 1986;33:492–497.

70. Sethna N F, Rockoff M A. Cardiac arrest following inhalation induction of anaesthesia in a child with Duchenne's muscular dystrophy. *Can Anaesth Soc J* 1986;33:799–802.

71. Solares G, Herranz J L, Sanz M D. Suxamethonium-induced cardiac arrest as an initial manifestation of Duchenne muscular dystrophy [Letter]. *Br J Anaesth* 1986;58:576.

72. Seay A R, Ziter F A, Thompson J A. Cardiac arrest during induction of anesthesia in Duchenne muscular dystrophy. *J Pediatr* 1978;93:88–90.

73. Oka S, Igarashi Y, Takagi A, et al. Malignant hyperpyrexia and Duchenne muscular dystrophy: a case report. *Can Anaesth Soc J* 1982;29:627–629.

74. Tang T T, Oechler H W, Siker D, Segura A D, Franciosi RA. Anesthesia-induced rhabdomyolysis in infants with unsuspected Duchenne dystrophy. *Acta Paediatr* 1992;81:716–719.

75. Rosenberg H, Gronert G A. Intractable cardiac arrest in children given succinylcholine [Letter]. *Anesthesiology* 1992;77:1054.

76. Heiman-Patterson T D, Natter H M, Rosenberg H, Fletcher J E, Tahmoush A J. Malignant hyperthermia susceptibility in X-linked muscle dystrophies. *Pediatr Neurol* 1986;2:356–358.

77. Richards W C. Anaesthesia and serum creatine phosphokinase levels in patients with Duchenne's pseudohypertrophic muscular dystrophy. *Anaesth Intens Care* 1972;1:150–153.

78. Larsen U T, Juhl B, Hein-Sørensen O, Olivarius B D F. Complications during anaesthesia in patients with Duchenne's muscular dystrophy (a retrospective study). *Can J Anaesth* 1989;36:418–422.

79. Peluso A, Bianchini A. Malignant hyperthermia susceptibility in patients with Duchenne's muscular dystrophy [Letter]. *Can J Anaesth* 1992;39:1117–1118.

80. Brownell A K W. Malignant hyperthermia: relationship to other diseases. *Br J Anaesth* 1988;60:303–308.

81. Ptacek L J, Johnson K J, Griggs R C. Genetics and physiology of the myotonic muscle disorders. *N Engl J Med* 1993;328:482–489.

82. Saidman L J, Havard E S, Eger E I II. Hyperthermia during anesthesia. *JAMA* 1964;190:73–76.

83. Haberer J-P, Fabre F, Rose E. Malignant hyperthermia and myotonia congenita (Thomsen's disease) [Letter]. *Anaesthesia* 1989;44:166.

84. Heiman-Patterson T D, Martino C, Rosenberg H, Fletcher J, Tahmoush A. Malignant hyperthermia in myotonia congenita. *Neurology* 1988;38:810–812.

85. Heiman-Patterson T D, Rosenberg H, Fletcher J E, Tahmoush A J. Halothane-caffeine contracture testing in neuromuscular diseases. *Muscle Nerve* 1988;11:453–457.

86. Lehmann-Horn F, Iaizzo P A. Are myotonias and periodic paralyses associated with susceptibility to malignant hyperthermia? *Br J Anaesth* 1990;65:692–697.

87. Larach M G, The Professional Advisory Council of MHAUS. Report of the MHAUS malignant hyperthermia survey. *Communicator* 1988;6:1–6.

88. Ranklev E, Henriksson K G, Fletcher R, Germundsson K, Oldfors A, Kalimo H. Clinical and muscle biopsy findings in malignant hyperthermia susceptibility. *Acta Neurol Scand* 1986;74:452–459.

89. Guze B H, Baxter L R. Neuroleptic malignant syndrome. *N Engl J Med* 1985;313:163–166.

90. Levinson D F, Simpson G M. Neuroleptic-induced extrapyramidal symptoms with fever: heterogeneity of the "neuroleptic malignant syndrome." *Arch Gen Psychiatry* 1986;43:839–848.

91. Heiman-Patterson T D. Neuroleptic malignant syndrome and malignant hyperthermia. *Med Clin North Am* 1993;77:477–492.

92. Hermesh H, Aizenberg D, Lapidot M, Munitz H. Risk of malignant hyperthermia among patients with neuroleptic malignant syndrome and their families. *Am J Psychiatry* 1988;145:1431–1434.

93. Caroff S N, Rosenberg H, Fletcher J E, Heiman-Patterson T D, Mann S C. Malignant hyperthermia susceptibility in neuroleptic malignant syndrome. *Anesthesiology* 1987;67:20–25.

94. Adnet P J, Krivosic-Horber R M, Adamantidis M M, et al. The association between the neuroleptic malignant syndrome and malignant hyperthermia. *Acta Anaesthesiol Scand* 1989;33:676–680.

95. Wingard D W. Malignant hyperthermia—acute stress syndrome of man? In: Henschel E O, ed. *Malignant hyperthermia: current concepts.* New York: Appleton-Century-Crofts, 1977:79–95.

96. Britt B A. Malignant hyperthermia. *Can Anaesth Soc J* 1985;32:666–677.

97. Topel D G, Bicknell E J, Preston K S, Christian L L, Matsushima C Y. Porcine stress syndrome. *Mod Vet Pract* 1968;49:40–60.

98. Jones E W, Nelson T E, Anderson I L, Kerr D D, Burnap T K. Malignant hyperthermia of swine. *Anesthesiology* 1972;36:42–51.

99. Denborough M A. The pathopharmacology of malignant hyperpyrexia. *Pharm Ther* 1980;9:357–365.

100. McGrath C J. Malignant hyperthermia. *Semin Vet Med Surg (Small Animal)* 1986;1:238–244.

101. *Sudden infant death syndrome: Proceedings of the second international conference on causes of sudden death in infants.* Seattle: University of Washington, 1970.

102. Denborough M A. Sudden infant death syndrome and malignant hyperpyrexia [Letter]. *Med J Aust* 1981;1:649–650.

103. Denborough M A, Galloway G J, Hopkinson K C. Malignant hyperpyrexia and sudden infant death. *Lancet* 1982;2:1068–1069.

104. Ellis F R, Halsall P J, Harriman D G F. Malignant hyperpyrexia and sudden infant death syndrome. *Br J Anaesth* 1988;60:28–30.

105. Ranklev E, Fletcher R, Krantz P. Malignant hyperpyrexia and sudden death. *Am J Forensic Med Pathol* 1985;6:149–150.

106. Britt B A. Combined anesthetic- and stress-induced malignant hyperthermia in two offspring of malignant hyperthermic-susceptible parents. *Anesth Analg* 1988;67:393–399.

107. Thomas D W, Dev V J, Whitehead M J. Malignant hyperpyrexia and isoflurane. *Br J Anaesth* 1987;59:1196–1198.

108. Sainsbury D A, Osborne G A. A case of malignant hyperthermia. *Anaesth Intens Care* 1988;16:218–221.

109. Wedel D J, Iaizzo P A, Milde J H. Desflurane is a trigger of malignant hyperthermia in susceptible swine. *Anesthesiology* 1991;74:508–512.

110. Ochiai R, Toyoda Y, Nishio I, et al. Possible association of malignant hyperthermia with sevoflurane anesthesia. *Anesth Analg* 1992;74:616–618.

111. Wingard D W, Bobko S. Failure of lidocaine to trigger porcine malignant hyperthermia. *Anesth Analg* 1979;58:99–103.

112. Harrison G G, Morrell D F. Response of MHS swine to i.v. infusion of lignocaine and bupivicaine. *Br J Anaesth* 1980;52:385–387.

113. Berkowitz A, Rosenberg H. Femoral block with mepivacaine for muscle biopsy in malignant hyperthermia patients. *Anesthesiology* 1985;62:651–652.

114. Minasian A, Yagiela J A. The use of amide local anesthetics in patients susceptible to malignant hyperthermia. *Oral Surg* 1988;66:405–415.

115. Dershwitz M, Ryan J F, Guralnick W. Safety of amide local anesthetics in patients susceptible to malignant hyperthermia. *J Am Dent Assoc* 1989;118:276–280.

116. Ørding H, Nielsen V G. Atracurium and its antagonism by neostigmine (plus glycopyrrolate) in patients susceptible to malignant hyperthermia. *Br J Anaesth* 1986;58:1001–1004.

117. Gronert G A, Ahern C P, Milde J H, White R D. Effects of CO_2, calcium, digoxin, and potassium on cardiac and skeletal muscle metabolism in malignant hyperthermia susceptible swine. *Anesthesiology* 1986;64:24–28.

118. Harrison G G, Morrell D F, Brain V, Jaros G G. Acute calcium homeostasis in MHS swine. *Can J Anaesth* 1987;34:377–379.

119. Flewellen E H, Nelson TE. Halothane–succinylcholine-induced masseter spasm: indicative of malignant hyperthermia susceptibility? *Anesth Analg* 1984;63:693–697.

120. Rosenberg H, Fletcher J E. Masseter muscle rigidity and malignant hyperthermia susceptibility. *Anesth Analg* 1986;65:161–164.

121. Christian A S, Ellis F R, Halsall P J. Is there a relationship between masseteric muscle spasm and malignant hyperpyrexia? *Br J Anaesth* 1989;62:540–544.

122. Allen G C, Rosenberg H. Malignant hyperthermia susceptibility in adult patients with masseter muscle rigidity. *Can J Anaesth* 1990;37:31–35.

123. Britt B A, Kwong F H F, Endrenyi L. The clinical and laboratory features of malignant hyperthermia management—a review. In: Henschel EO, ed. *Malignant hyperthermia: current concepts.* New York: Appleton-Century-Crofts, 1977:9–45.

124. Ong R O, Rosenberg H. Malignant hyperthermia-like syndrome associated with metrizamide myelography. *Anesth Analg* 1989;68:795–797.

125. Stevens J J. A case of thyrotoxic crisis that mimicked malignant hyperthermia [Letter]. *Anesthesiology* 1983;59:263.

126. Bennett M H, Wainwright A P. Acute thyroid crisis on induction of anaesthesia. *Anaesthesia* 1989;44:28–30.

127. Crowley K J, Cunningham A J, Conroy B, O'Connell P R, Collins P G. Phaeochromocytoma—a presentation mimicking malignant hyperthermia. *Anaesthesia* 1988;43:1031–1032.

128. Allen G C, Rosenberg H. Phaeochromocytoma presenting as acute malignant hyperthermia—a

diagnostic challenge. *Can J Anaesth* 1990; 37:593–595.

129. Kolb M E, Horne M L, Martz R. Dantrolene in human malignant hyperthermia: a multicenter study. *Anesthesiology* 1982;56:254–262.

130. Jones D E, Ryan J F. Treatment of acute hyperthermia crises. In: Britt BA, ed. *Malignant hyperthermia.* Boston: Martinus Nijhoff, 1987: 393–406.

131. Larach M G. Malignant hyperthermia [Letter]. *Science* 1992;257:11–12.

132. Van Winkle W B. Calcium release from skeletal muscle sarcoplasmic reticulum: site of action of dantrolene sodium? *Science* 1976;193:1130–1131.

133. Desmedt J E, Hainaut K. Inhibition of the intracellular release of calcium by dantrolene in barnacle giant muscle fibres. *J Physiol* 1977; 265:565–585.

134. Lopez J R, Allen P, Alamo L, Ryan J F, Jones D E, Streter F. Dantrolene prevents the malignant hyperthermic syndrome by reducing free intracellular calcium concentration in skeletal muscle of susceptible swine. *Cell Calcium* 1987;8:385–396.

135. Foster P S, Denborough M A. The effect of calcium channel antagonists and BAY K 8644 on calcium fluxes of malignant hyperpyrexia-susceptible muscle. *Int J Biochem* 1993;25: 495–504.

136. Harrison G G. Dantrolene—dynamics and kinetics. *Br J Anaesth* 1988;60:279–286.

137. Harrison G G. Control of the malignant hyperpyrexic syndrome in MHS swine by dantrolene sodium. *Br J Anaesth* 1975;47:62–65.

138. Britt B A. Dantrolene. *Can Anaesth Soc J* 1984;31:61–75.

139. Larach M G, Simon L J, Allen G C, The North American Malignant Hyperthermia Registry. Safety and efficacy of dantrolene sodium for the treatment of malignant hyperthermia

events [abstract]. *Anesthesiology* 1993;77: A 1079.

140. Larach M G, Localio A R, Allen G C, et al. A clinical grading scale to predict malignant hyperthermia susceptibility. Anesthesiology, 1994; 80:771–779.

141. Kalow W, Britt B A, Terreau M E, Haist C. Metabolic error of muscle metabolism after recovery from malignant hyperthermia. *Lancet* 1970;2:895–898.

142. Ellis F R, Harriman D G F, Keaney N P, Kyei-Mensah K, Tyrrell J H. Halothane-induced muscle contracture as a cause of hyperpyrexia. *Br J Anaesth* 1971;43:721–722.

143. Larach M G, For the North American Malignant Hyperthermia Group. Standardization of the caffeine halothane muscle contracture test. *Anesth Analg* 1989;69:511–515.

144. Larach M G, Landis J R, Shirk S J, Diaz M, The North American Malignant Hyperthermia Registry. Prediction of malignant hyperthermia susceptibility in man: improving sensitivity of the caffeine halothane contracture test [Abstract]. *Anesthesiology* 1992;77:A1052.

145. Galen R S, Reiffel J A, Gambino S R. Diagnosis of acute myocardial infarction. *JAMA* 1975; 232:145–147.

146. Ørding H, Foder B, Scharff O. Cytosolic free calcium concentrations in lymphocytes from malignant hyperthermia susceptible patients. *Br J Anaesth* 1990;64:341–345.

147. Halsall P J, Ellis F R, Knowles P F. Evaluation of spin resonance spectroscopy of red blood cell membranes to detect malignant hyperthermia susceptibility. *Br J Anaesth* 1992;69:471–473.

148. Allen G C, Cameron I, Avruch L, Rutter A, Ashley A, Saunders J. Detection of malignant hyperthermia susceptibility using 31P magnetic resonance spectroscopy [Abstract]. *Anesthesiology* 1992;77:A1054.

Anesthetic Toxicity, edited by
Susan A. Rice and Kevin J. Fish.
Raven Press, Ltd., New York © 1994.

13

Immunosuppression in the Postoperative Period

Girish C. Moudgil

*Department of Anesthesiology, Tulane University School of Medicine,
New Orleans, Louisiana 70112*

> An anesthetic is not a special poison for the nervous system. It anesthetizes all cells, benumbing all the tissues and stopping their irritability. . . .
> —C. Bernard, 1875

The possibility that anesthesia may alter the course of an infection has been under consideration for more than a century (1). As early as 1903, Snel reported that ether, chloroform, and chloral hydrate enhanced the mortality from anthrax in guinea pigs (2). Rubin made similar observations in rabbits infected with streptococci or pneumococci and exposed to ether or chloroform (3). Since then, several other investigators have shown similar deleterious effects (4–7) of anesthesia in experimental animal models. Although a wide variety of factors, such as age, sex, race, nutrition, metabolic and electrolyte imbalance, cardiovascular and respiratory disturbances, and duration and urgency of surgery, are important in the pathogenesis of infections, in the ultimate analysis it is depression of the host defense system that allows the invading organisms to become established.

Despite continued advances in medical, surgical, and anesthetic skills, infection in the perioperative period remains a significant problem and is a major source of enhanced morbidity and mortality in surgical patients (8,9). It has been estimated that in-fections develop in one quarter to one half of the patients in surgical intensive care units (ICU), and the mortality among these patients may be has high as 70% (10,11). Therefore, it is important that we acquire a better understanding of the host defense system and the ways and means whereby it may be compromised in the perioperative period. Although trauma, hemorrhage, and metabolic and nutritional factors do influence the immune response, an understanding of anesthesia-induced immunosuppression is desirable. An appreciation of anesthesia-induced immunosuppression should help curtail the incidence of infection, tumor growth, and metastatic dispersal in the postoperative period.

THE IMMUNE SYSTEM

The human body has to contend with a bewildering array of harmful organisms and agents of diverse shapes and sizes. The ability of the body to distinguish self from nonself, along with a memory and specificity of earlier encounters and exposures, formulates the essentials of the immune response. There are two functional divisions of the immune system—an innate or nonspecific and an adapative or specific component of immunity.

Nonspecific or Innate Immunity

Nonspecific immunity is the first line of defense against foreign organisms, and it functions without a prior memory of an earlier encounter with the infectious agent, antigen, or foreign molecule. A ready ingress of microbes into the body is circumvented by an intact epithelial barrier, mucous membranes and their secretions, ciliary action of the tracheobronchial lining, the lavaging action of antibacterial fluids, and acidity of the gastric juices. If penetration occurs, bacteria are destroyed by soluble factors (e.g., lysozyme) and phagocytosis with intracellular digestion. Besides the mechanical integrity of the epithelial and mucosal barriers, most bacteria fail to survive on skin because of the direct inhibitory effects of lactic acid and fatty acids in sweat and sebaceous secretions. Likewise, mucus secreted by membranes lining the inner surfaces of the body acts as a protective barrier by hindering bacterial adherence. Ciliary locomotion along with coughing and sneezing provide protection against airborne pathogens. The washing actions of the tears, saliva, and urine are equally beneficial in eliminating invading organisms. The epithelial and mucosal barriers along with other physical and biochemical barriers formulate the essential components of nonspecific immunity.

Both specific and nonspecific immunity are composed of cellular and humoral components. The cellular components of nonspecific immunity involve mononuclear phagocytes, polymorphonuclear granulocytes, and natural killer (NK) lymphocytes (12), whereas the humoral elements refer to the activation of properdin and complement systems along with the liberation of lysozymes, the enzymes that mediate the demise of the offending organisms. Additionally, polypeptides released by various subsets of cellular elements, termed biologic response modifiers (BRM), further modulate the different aspects of the immune response.

Nonspecific Cell-Mediated Immunity

The cellular arm of nonspecific immunity is comprised of phagocytic leukocytes, which include neutrophils, eosinophils, basophils, mononuclear phagocytes, and tissue macrophages. Polymorphonuclear neutrophils form the first line of defense against pathogenic microorganisms (13,14). These cells are derived from the stem cells in the bone marrow, and about 10^{11} cells enter into the circulation every day after maturation for 2 weeks (15,16). The neutrophils are nondividing and short-lived, with a half-life of 6 to 20 hours in the peripheral circulation. Within minutes after tissue damage or following injury, neutrophils migrate along the endothelium of the vessel walls and penetrate into the tissue planes along the gradients of different chemotactic signals. The bactericidal capability of neutrophils is similar to that of monocytes. However, fewer BRMs are released by the neutrophils. Monocytes are released from the bone marrow into the peripheral circulation at an immature stage. Their half-life in the circulation is approximately 1 day. They subsequently differentiate into macrophages and migrate into adjoining tissues, thus forming the mononuclear phagocyte system. They are present throughout the connective tissues and around the basement membrane of small blood vessels and are particularly concentrated in the lung (alveolar macrophages), liver (Kupffer cells), spleen sinusoids, and lymph node medullary sinuses. Whereas polymorphonuclear leukocytes are best at destroying pyogenic bacteria, macrophages are best at combating bacteria, viruses, and protozoa that are capable of living within the cells of the host. Monocytes can capture bacteria in the circulation, and their killing capabilities are markedly enhanced following exposure to γ-interferon. In addition to their phagocytic functions, monocytes secrete several BRMs, coagulation proteins, complement components, prostaglandins, and fibronectin, which are associated with the inflammatory response.

Besides neutrophils and monocytes, NK cells also belong to the cellular component of the nonspecific arm of immune response. NK cells recognize structures on high molecular weight glycoproteins that appear on the surface cells infected with viruses. This recognition occurs through receptors on the NK cell surface that bring killer and target into close apposition. These cells have the capability to bind and kill target cells without antibody coating or complement activation. The precise lineage of NK cells is yet to be resolved. They express surface markers that are normally restricted to the T cells. They have interleukin 2 (IL-2) receptors and undergo lymphoproliferation by IL-2 and also can produce γ-interferon. The tumor-killing capabilities of NK cells are greatly enhanced by soluble factors, such as α-interferon. In addition, NK cells also secrete several other BRMs that modulate the functioning of other components of the immune response. More than 100 such BRMs have been identified, and they modulate both specific and nonspecific functions of the immune response (17) (Table 1).

TABLE 1. *Principal activities of biologic response modifiers (BRM)*

Cell type source	BRM		Principal activities
B lymphocyte	Ig	(immunoglobulin)	
T lymphocyte	IL-2	(interleukin 2; T cell growth factor)	Promotes activation of B, T, and NK lymphocytes; promotes proliferation and killing function of T and NK lymphoctyes
	IL-3	(interleukin 3; multi-CSF)	Promotes differentiation of platelets, eosinophils, basophils, neutrophils, monocytes, and red blood cells
	IL-4	(interleukin 4; B cell stimulating factor)	Stimulates B lymphocyte and cytotoxic T lymphocyte activation
	IL-5	(interleukin 5; T cell replacing factor)	Promotes B lymphocytes differentiation and immunoglobulin secretion
	GM-CSF	(granulocyte-monocyte colony-stimulating factor)	Stimulates granulocyte-monocyte production
	IFN-γ	(gamma interferon)	Inhibits viral replication; inhibits growth of certain tumor cells; activates T lymphocytes
	TNF-α	(lymphotoxin)	Can directly kill certain types of tumor cells; activates NK lymphocytes
Natural killer (NK) cell	NKCF	(Natural killer cell factor)	Can directly kill certain types of tumor cells
	IFN-α	(alpha interferon)	Activates NK lymphocytes
Monocyte	IL-1	(interleukin 1; lymphocyte-activation factor)	Promotes early phases of the B and T lymphocyte activation processes
	TNF-β	(tumour necrosis factor)	Can directly kill certain types of tumor cells
	IL-6	(B_2 interferon)	Promotes B lymphoctye differentiation
	G-CSF	(granulocyte colony-stimulating factor)	Stimulates granulocyte differentiation
	M-CSF	(monocyte colony-stimulating factor)	Stimulates monocyte production; activates monocyte cytotoxicity
	C	(complement components)	Activated form directly kills target cells

From Stevenson GW, Hall SC, Rudnick S, Seleny FL, Stevenson HS. The effect of anesthetic agents on the human immune response. *Anesthesiology* 1990;72:542–552.

Nonspecific Humoral Immunity
Complement System

The complement system is the principal element of nonspecific humoral immunity. This system is comprised of some 20 proteins that, along with blood clotting, fibrinolysis, and kinin formation, produce an amplified response to a triggering stimulus in a cascade fashion. The most abundant and most important component is C3, which has a molecular weight of 195 kDa and is present in plasma at concentrations around 1.2 mg/ml. The key step in distinguishing the self from nonself by complement is the covalent binding of C3 to foreign particles and membranes. Complement C3 becomes activated at a slow rate under normal circumstances by a process of hydrolysis. Complement has a range of biologic activities that can be grouped under the following three headings.

Adherence Reactions

Phagocytic cells have receptors for C3b that facilitate the adherence of complement-coated organisms to the cell surfaces.

Biologically Active Fragments

During complement activation, peptide split products C3a and C5a are produced, which are anaphylatoxins and have strong chemotactic properties. Both act directly on phagocytes and stimulate the production of oxygen metabolites and enhance the expression of surface receptors for C3b. Besides chemotactic properties, C5a acts directly on capillary endothelium to produce vasodilation and increased permeability.

Membrane Lesions

The plasma membranes of cells, viruses, and other microorganisms are damaged by insertion of the membrane attach complex, which subsequently brings about cell destruction. Following complement activation, there is an insertion of hydrophobic plug into the membrane bilayers that allows an osmotic disruption of offending cells.

Acute Phase Proteins

These plasma proteins are increased dramatically following injury or infection. The acute phase proteins include C-reactive protein (CRP), serum amyloid A protein, α_1-antitrypsin, α_2-macroglobulin, fibrinogen, ceruloplasmin, C9, and factor β. During an infection, endotoxins stimulate the production of pyrogens, such as IL-1, in addition to other BRMs. Additionally, interferons that are a family of broad-spectrum antiviral agents also formulate another line of defense. There are at least 14 different α-interferons produced by leukocytes, and probably all cell types synthesize β-interferon. γ-Interferon and other macrophage-activating factors switch on microbicidal mechanisms that bring about the death of intracellular microorganisms.

Specific or Adaptive Cellular Immunity

Memory of an earlier exposure to an antigen specificity and the recognition of the nonself are the key components of specific or adaptive immunity, which always requires previous exposure to an antigen. In all vertebrates, the small lymphocyte is the basic unit of immune response because it specifically recognizes the foreign antigen. On an anatomic and functional basis, immunocompetent lymphocytes can be classified into either thymus-dependent T lymphocytes or bursa-dependent B lymphocytes (18). On exposure to an appropriate antigen, T lymphocytes transform themselves into large cells known as lymphoblasts, which undergo proliferation and perform functions that depend on their subclass. Thus, we have the dichotomy of the immune response into cellular and humoral components.

Specific Cellular Immunity

T lymphocytes are critical in the development of cell-mediated immune reactions. However, most T lymphocytes are unable to recognize free antigens circulating in the blood or the lymph. These cells only recognize antigen when it is on the surface of a cell and is displayed in conjunction with one of the cell's own proteins. Therefore, surface receptors on the T lymphocytes are different from the antibody molecules used by B lymphocytes, and T lymphocytes recognize an antigen plus a surface marker. These cell markers belong to an important group of molecules known as the major histocompatibility complex (MHC). The functional differences between different subsets of T cell populations are reflected in the different ways by which they recognize antigen plus MHC. Typically, cytotoxic T cells recognize an antigen in association with class I MHC products, whereas helper T cells and the lymphocytes responding to antigens by lymphoproliferation recognize an antigen in association with class II MHC products that are expressed mostly on antigen-presenting cells. On the basis of the cell membraneglycoproteins, two major subsets of T cells may be defined through monoclonal antibodies. The CD4+ subset expresses a 62 kDa glycoprotein, and the CD8+ subset expresses a 76 kDa protein. It appears that CD4+ and CD8+ possess receptors for class II and class I glycopeptides, respectively.

Once an antigen enters the body, it is processed by the cells of the monocyte/macrophage series and is presented to the T cells (19). The monocytes secrete IL-1, which activates the T cells along with the induction of receptors for IL-2, which is a T cell-derived lymphokine (20). IL-2 facilitates lymphoproliferation and differentiation into subsets of cells with helper, inducer, suppressor, and cytotoxic functions. T cells also secrete γ-interferon, which augments the tumoricidal and microbicidal activities of K cells, monocytes, and macrophages (21). Additionally, it may augment B cell-mediated antibody synthesis (22).

Four subsets of T lymphocytes have been recognized. However, on the basis of their biochemical surface markers, two main subsets are T4 or CD4+ lymphocytes with helper and inducer roles and T8 or CD8+ cells with suppressor/cytotoxic functions.

T4 (CD4+) Helper Cells

These cells recognize antigen presented in association with class II MHC proteins, which are found mainly on the surfaces of antigen-presenting cells. On recognition of specific antigen, they facilitate T cell-mediated cytotoxic activity and B cell antibody production. They also help in mounting a delayed hypersensitivity response and release IL-4 and IL-5, which result in B cell lymphoproliferation and expansion of B cell clones.

T4 (CD4+) Inducer Cells

The inducer lymphocytes help in the maturation of precursor forms into functionally distinct and competent lymphocytes. These cells, although dormant, may be activated readily for initiation of secondary immune responses.

T8 (CD8+) Cytotoxic Cells

These cells are professional defenders and can lyse foreign cells, infected cells, or malignant cells. They possess T8 surface markers and may recognize the antigen only in combination with class I MHC proteins. T4-liberated γ-interferon enhances their cytotoxic activity.

T8 (CD8 +) Suppressor Cells

These cells finetune the immune response by exerting an inhibitory influence on the activities of both the T and the B lymphocytes. They also secrete suppressor factor (SF-Ig), which decreases synthesis and release of immunoglobulins.

Killer (K) Cells

Unlike the four subsets described previously, these lymphocytes do not bear specific cell surface markers but can destroy cells coated with specific antibodies. One of the mechanisms for dstruction of target cells is mediated through the liberation of lymphotoxin.

Specific Humoral Antibody Immunity

B cells are concerned mainly with the synthesis of circulating antibodies and are fundamental to the humoral immune response. Following appropriate antigenic stimulation, B cells transform themselves into large cells that have a great amount of rough endoplasmic reticulum and are known as plasma cells. Plasma cells are capable of producing various types of immunoglobulins against circulating antigens. These circulating antibodies confer humoral immunity that can be transferred passively from one individual to another. Although the T and B lymphocytes specifically participate in either the cellular or the humoral components of the immune response, their activities are always interrelated with each other and with other cell types, which allows amplification and regulation of the different aspects of the host defense system.

ANESTHESIA AND THE IMMUNE RESPONSE

It has long been known that anesthetic agents can adversely affect different aspects of cellular function. It would appear, however, that the cell has a pivotal role in body defenses and could be susceptible to anesthetic actions. The evidence in the literature supports the concept that anesthetics adversely affect the host defense systems (23–28). However, because of a multiplicity of factors that may affect the host defense systems in the perioperative period, the direct effects of anesthetic agents and techniques need to be delineated further and with clarity.

Anesthesia and the Cell

The cytoplasm of the sea urchin eggs becomes less viscous following exposure to ether, chloroform, paraldehyde, chloral hydrate, and urethane (29). Chloroform and cyclopropane reversibly stop cytoplasmic streaming in the slime mold *Physarum polycephalum* (30). A tight crosslinking of colloidal constituents of plasma gel resulting in cessation of movement and amoebae was thought to be due to the effects of exposure to different anesthetic agents (31,32). An interaction between anesthetic agents and proteins was postulated and later revealed by a demonstration of Van der Waal's bonding between xenon and cyclopropane and the proteins myoglobin and hemoglobin (33,34). It also was shown that general anesthetic agents in clinically used concentrations caused a 0.49% expansion of the erythrocyte membranes (35). Local anesthetic agents, such as procaine, decreased the permeability of alkali metal cations in a lipid bilayer membrane system, whereas volatile inhalation anesthetics caused an increase (36–38). In view of these interactions with cell membranes and cellular proteins, it seems likely that anesthetic agents may modulate several of the cellular functions, including receptor sites, molecule synthesis, recognition, and interactions, along with locomotion and cellular replication.

Anesthesia and Cell Division

The effects of anesthetics on cell division have been studied for as long as their narcotic properties have been known. Davy (1800) was unsuccessful in demonstrating an inhibition of growth of peas by nitrous oxide (39). However, Bernard (1878) demonstrated that higher concentrations of ether could inhibit plant growth and cell division in seedlings (40). Exposure of seeds to 88% nitrous oxide and 12% oxygen doubled their germination time (41). Östergen demonstrated that nitrous oxide, chloroform, trichloroethylene, and diethyl ether caused an arrest of mitosis in metaphase with an appearance identical to that produced by colchicine mitosis (42).

Studies with mammalian cell cultures and inhalation anesthetics have demonstrated a dose-dependent inhibition of growth of mouse heteroploid cells, mouse sarcoma 1 cells, mouse hepatoma cells, and Chinese hamster fibroblasts (43–46). This effect may be due either to an effect on metaphase mitosis (47), a reversible depolymerization of mitotic spindle microtubules (48), an inhibition of DNA synthesis (49), an interference with prometaphase movement (50), or a prolongation of the G_2 postsynthetic phase, causing an increase in cell cycle time (46). Administration of certain anesthetics also results in production of abnormal products of mitosis (50). Halothane and nitrous oxide exert a synergistic effect, resulting in production of cells with abnormal nuclei (51). Patients receiving long-term therapy with nitrous oxide for treatment of tetanus developed a depression of cell growth in the bone marrow with granulocytopenia and thrombocytopenia (52). Likewise, toxic effects in bone marrow cells, accompanied by a decrease in peripheral white cell counts, was observed in rats chronically exposed to nitrous oxide (53).

Thus, it seems that anesthetic agents act on all the different phases of cell cycle, culminating in a prolongation of cell cycle time and an inhibition of cell division. Since proliferation of sensitized cells of lymphoid tissue on contact with an appropriate antigen is a key event in the immune response, anesthesia may result in depression of immune response by suppressing cell replication of the immunocompetent cells.

Anesthesia and Leukocyte Migration

The migration of granulocytes, macrophages, and lymphocytes toward the inflamed or injured tissues is one of the earliest events in the body's defense against infection. Any depression of this migration may allow the invading organisms to become established and enhance the incidence of infection.

Following exposure to halothane, a reversible dose-dependent inhibition of random locomotion of *Tetrahymena pyriformis* and peripheral blood human lymphocytes has been observed (54,55). Similarly, a dose-dependent depression of monocyte and neutrophil migration *in vitro* following exposure to local anesthetics and i.v. induction agents, such as thiopentone, methohexitone, ketamine, and alfathesin, has been reported (56). Some volatile anesthetics caused a short-lived, reversible severe depression of leukocyte chemotactic migration at clinical concentrations. Etomidate and thiopentone also caused depression leukocyte migration (57), but enflurane either had no effect or enhanced the migration (58). An inhibition of leukocyte migration in the postoperative period following surgery under general anesthesia has been reported (59,60). In patients undergoing major orthopedic surgery, peripheral blood neutrophils during spinal anesthesia and surgery migrated farther toward complement-derived chemoattractant than did neutrophils obtained from patients undergoing surgery under either halothane or isoflurane anesthesia (61). Contradictory data showing no depression under the influence of thiopentone or 2% halothane have been reported (62,63).

To clarify these contradictory findings, Moudgil et al. investigated the effects of equipotent concentrations of 1 MAC (MAC 1) of different volatile anesthetic agents and 70% nitrous oxide on polymorphonuclear leukocyte and monocyte chemotactic migration (64). These investigations revealed that exposure to MAC 1 of various anesthetic agents produced varied degrees of depression of chemotactic migration that paralleled the lipid solubility of the anesthetic agent, with the exception of nitrous oxide. Neutrophil and monocyte chemotactic migrations were least affected by isoflurane and most affected by methoxyflurane and 70% nitrous oxide (Figs. 1 and 2). Nitrous oxide, such narcotics as morphine, fentanyl, and meperidine, and the agonist-antagonist narcotic agents, nalbuphine and butorphanol, also have been shown to decrease the chemotactic migration of human neutrophils *in vitro* (65–67). It has been suggested that pancuronium and curare may adversely affect leukocyte locomotion, whereas gallamine and succinylcholine may increase the movement. However, the ef-

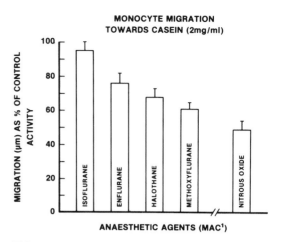

FIG. 2. Effect of equipotent concentrations of volatile anaesthetics (MAC-1) and 70% nitrous oxide on monocyte migration toward casein (2 mg/kg). Distance migrated is expressed as percent of control activity ± SE. (From Moudgil GC, Gordon J, Forrest JB. Comparative effects of volatile anaesthetic agents and nitrous oxide on human leukocyte chemotaxis *in vitro*. *Can Anaesth Soc J* 1984;31:631–637.)

fects were seen at generally higher than clinical concentrations (58).

The combined effects of surgery and anesthesia typically produce a leukocytosis with increased proportions of neutrophils and monocytes and decreased proportions of eosinophils and lymphocytes (68). Neutrophil adherence is decreased immediately after surgery and increased thereafter (69–71). Although a depression of chemotactic migration and spontaneous leukocyte locomotion ranging from a few hours to some days is associated with surgery and anesthesia (72,73), this depression is particularly obvious in patients with postoperative sepsis (74).

In summary, many anesthetic agents, either alone or in combination with surgery, have been shown to interfere with both random and chemotactic locomotion. This depression of locomotion is short-lived and reversible. The pros and cons of anesthesia-induced suppression of leukocyte locomotion have been addressed (75). However,

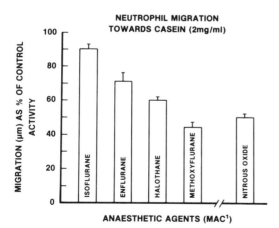

FIG. 1. Effect of equipotent concentrations of volatile anaesthetics (MAC-1) and 70% nitrous oxide on neutrophil migration toward casein (2 mg/kg). Distance migrated is expressed as percent of control activity ± SE. (From Moudgil GC, Gordon J, Forrest JB. Comparative effects of volatile anaesthetic agents and nitrous oxide on human leukocyte chemotaxis *in vitro*. *Can Anaesth Soc J* 1984;31:631–637.)

any depression of chemotactic migration could be clinically relevant and germane to postoperative infection.

Anesthesia and Phagocytosis

Intact phagocytic function is essential for host defense. At the turn of the century, animal studies demonstrated that ether and chloroform inhibited phagocytosis in a dose-dependent manner (76). Similarly, a decrease in the number of *Salmonella* bacteria ingested by peritoneal neutrophils was observed in mice exposed to halothane anesthesia (4). Although anesthesia with halothane or with nitrous oxide/narcotic technique without any surgical intervention caused a significant decrease in the phagocytosis of latex particles in one instance, only minimal inhibition was observed after anesthesia with 0.5% to 2.5% halothane or 80% nitrous oxide (77). The phagocytic capacity was depressed in a dose-dependent manner after halothane and enflurane both *in vivo* and *in vitro* (78).

Surgery under halothane anesthesia, but not with neurolept or regional anesthesia, decreases the metabolic activity of phagocytic cells for several days postoperatively (79). A depression of oxygen-dependent microbicidal mechanisms along with superoxide-generating ability has been observed following general anesthesia (80–83). High-dose fentanyl anesthesia for coronary artery bypass surgery resulted in depression of phagocytic activity up to the fourth postoperative day (84). *In vitro* exposure of neutrophils to premedicants, induction agents, narcotics, and local anesthetics produced a dose-dependent inhibition of phagocytosis (85). The inhibitory effects of induction agents, narcotics, and local anesthetics on human leukocyte phagocytic activity are shown in Figures 3, 4 and 5, respectively. Depression of phagocytosis is augmented by surgical stress in animals and humans (86). However, contradictory data showing

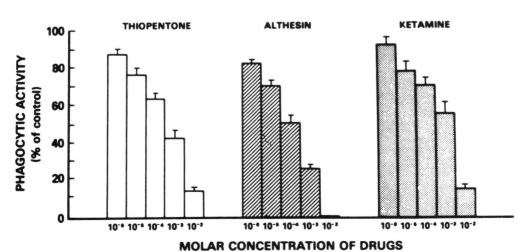

PHAGOCYTIC ACTIVITY (± S.E.)

FIG. 3. Dose-dependent inhibitory effect on the leukocyte phagocytic activity produced by i.v. anesthetic agents. The phagocytic activity is expressed as percentage of the control activity. (From Moudgil GC. Effect of premedicant, intravenous anaesthetic agents and local anaesthetics on phagocytosis *in vitro. Can Anaesth Soc J* 1981;28:597–602.)

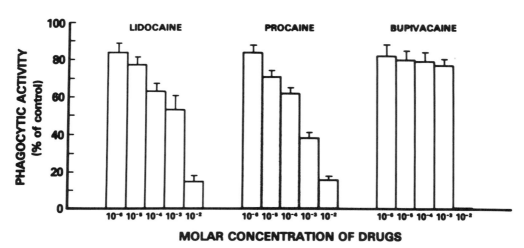

FIG. 4. Dose-dependent inhibitory effect on the leukocyte phagocytic activity produced by three local anesthetic agents. The phagocytic activity is expressed as a percentage of the control activity. (From Moudgil GC. Effect of premedicant, intravenous anaesthetic agents and local anaesthetics on phagocytosis *in vitro. Can Anaesth Soc J* 1981;28:597–602.)

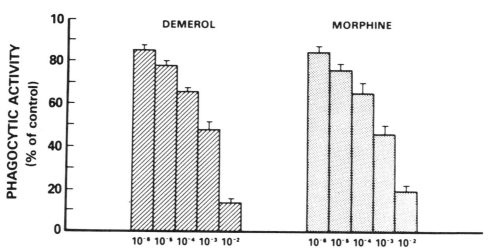

FIG. 5. Dose-dependent inhibitory effect on the leukocyte phagocytic activity produced by meperidine (Demerol) and morphine. The phagocytic activity is expressed as percentage of the control activity. (From Moudgil GC. Effect of premedicant, intravenous anaesthetic agents and local anaesthetics on phagocytosis *in vitro. Can Anaesth Soc J* 1981;28:597–602.)

no change in the leukocyte functions also has been reported (87,88).

Serum opsonic activity also is decreased after major surgery (89,90), although this appears not to be the case after cardiopulmonary bypass surgery (91,92). Several parameters of neutrophil phagocytic function are decreased following surgery and anesthesia (73,84,93–95). Phagocytosis by monocytes and macrophages, an important step in antigen processing, is adversely affected by surgery and anesthesia. Although an initial increase in numbers of circulating cells, ingestive capacity, chemiluminescence responses, and lysozyme production may occur immediately, a decrease of these values occurs following major surgery (96–98). However, the results are not consistent and may vary in patients with malignancy (99). The decrease in monocyte phagocytic capacity has been associated with decreases in plasma concentrations of fibronectin (100), an opsonin for nonbacterial particles. The serum concentration of fibronectin is decreased after surgery (101–105) and after major trauma (106). Administration of fibronectin to patients with this deficiency does not decrease the numbers of infectious complications (107).

Because of a wide array of factors that contribute to perioperative infections, the effects of anesthesia alone or in combination with surgery need further clarification. The current knowledge suggests that anesthetic agents do contribute toward decreased phagocytic activity.

Anesthesia and Bactericidal Activity

To combat an invading organism effectively, the leukocytes not only must have the ability to migrate and phagocytose but also should possess the ability to destroy the ingested organisms. Both phagocytic and bactericidal activities are associated with the generation of highly reactive radicals, such as superoxide, hydrogen peroxide (H_2O_2), and single oxygen ($\dot{O}$), that can

be measured by chemiluminescence. Several investigators have studied the ability of anesthetic agents to impair neutrophil microbicidal activity *in vitro* and *in vivo* (108). Earlier investigations used reduction of nitroblue tetrazolium (NBT) as an index of microbicidal activity, but more recent studies have used the technique of chemiluminescence, which is a highly sensitive indicator of neutrophil oxidative microbicidal activity. This technique evaluates the emission of light generated by the highly reactive oxygen radical species produced during the process of bactericidal activity (109). Using this technique, it was shown that the bactericidal activity of human neutrophils for *Escherichia coli, Kelbsiella pneumoniae,* and *Staphylococcus aureus* was decreased *in vitro* even at clinical concentrations of halothane (110). Similarly, it was reported that only enflurane inhibited the bactericidal activity (111). The production of H_2O_2, another oxidative radical species necessary for cidal activity, was reported to have decreased following monocyte exposure to halothane, although simultaneous exposure to γ-interferon had a protective effect (112).

Nakagawara et al. demonstrated a reversible inhibition of superoxide radical production by human neutrophils following exposure to halothane and to a lesser degree to enflurane, whereas isoflurane had minimal effect at clinically relevant concentrations (113). These authors further observed that neutrophils exposed to halothane, enflurane, and isoflurane have a decreased entry of extracellular Ca^{2+}, with a resultant decrease in intracellular Ca^{2+} that may have resulted in an anesthesia-induced decrease in superoxide-generating ability. A dose-dependent depression of bactericidal activity was observed with thiopentone and alfathesin, although methohexitone, morphine, diazepam, and lidocaine failed to produce similar effects (114). Likewise, a dose-dependent *in vitro* inhibition of superoxide-releasing activity of granulocytes on exposure to phenobarbital, ketamine, mepivacaine, lidocaine, diazepam, and droperidol also has been reported (115). These investigations have shown that anesthetic agents may adversely modulate the host defense systems by an inhibition of neutrophil oxidative functions and bactericidal activity. Therefore, patients requiring prolonged periods of surgery and anesthesia may have a depression of host defenses commensurate with the severity of anesthetic and surgical stresses.

Anesthesia and Lymphocyte Function

In addition to affecting nonspecific immunity adversely, anesthetic agents and surgery have been shown to affect specific or cell-mediated immunity. Lymphocyte number, the relative proportions of different subsets of lymphocytes, and their proliferative functions in response to antigenic challenges may all be affected by anesthesia and surgery. The absolute numbers of lymphocytes may remain unchanged during minor to moderate surgery. However, a decrease in numbers is observed during major surgical interventions under anesthesia, returning to original preoperative values within a few days of surgery (116,117). Depending on the extent of surgery, the numbers of T and B lymphocytes tend to decrease, and their proportions change in favor of B cells (117–119). T4 helper/inducer CD4+ and T8 suppressor CD8+ cell numbers also are decreased. However, with increasing severity of surgery and trauma, the proportions change in favor of CD8+ cells (117–124). The number of NK cells is also decreased in the postoperative period (123).

In addition to changes in lymphocyte numbers, lymphocyte proliferative functions also are adversely affected. The ability of the peripheral blood lymphocytes to proliferate in response to a mitogen (e.g., phytohemagglutinin, PHA) or an alloantigen is a recognized *in vitro* correlate of an *in vivo* intact cell-mediated immune response. Similarly, lymphocyte cytotoxicity, T4 helper/T8 suppressor cell ratios (HSR) are used to assess the immunocompetence of cell-mediated immunity. Because of their ability to destroy malignant cells, the NK cells are thought to form a primary defense against the development of tumors. Several studies have shown that anesthesia and surgery depress the overall lymphocyte function (125), and the severity of this depression may be further correlated with the degree of surgical stress (126).

Experimental evidence regarding the effects of inhalation anesthetic agents on lymphocyte function is not conclusive. *In vitro*, lymphocyte exposure to halothane produced a decrease in mitogen-induced lymphoproliferation at concentrations found in clinical anesthesia. However, a prolonged exposure was required to produce this effect (127). Similarly, lymphocyte cytotoxicity against malignant cells was inhibited following *in vitro* exposure to 1% or 2.5% halothane (128). The addition of several different anesthetics to lymphocyte cultures produced additive effects. One percent halothane and thiopentone (14 μg/ml) separately inhibited the cytotoxicity reaction by 20% but together caused a 45% inhibition (129).

A dose-dependent, reversible *in vitro* inhibition of NK cell cytotoxicity following exposure to halothane, enflurane, and nitrous oxide has been reported (130,131). Depression of mitogen-induced lymphoproliferation under the influence of different anesthetic agents has been reported by several investigators (132–136). Thiopentane inhibited lymphocytotoxicity at peak concentrations achieved during induction of anesthesia and also depressed PHA-induced lymphoproliferation at higher concentrations of the drug (137). Ketamine, droperidol, and lidocaine were unable to affect lymphocyte transformation at clinical concentrations, but higher levels did result in a depression of lymphoproliferation (138). Thus, it appears that *in vitro* anesthetic agents may cause a depression of lymphoproliferation and cytotoxicity reactions.

Studies of the effects of clinical anesthesia on lymphocyte functions have produced divergent opinions. In healthy volunteers, halothane and enflurane anesthesia for 5 to 7 hours failed to produce an effect on lymphoproliferation, but a significant proliferative depression after only 3 hours' exposure to halothane/nitrous oxide anesthesia was observed (139). In contrast to the depression observed with halothane, balanced anesthesia using a narcotic/relaxant technique did not produce depression of PHA-induced lymphoproliferation (134, 140). In a recent study of a randomized surgical population, Moudgil et al. observed that halothane, but not isoflurane, inhibited PHA-induced lymphoproliferation in the postoperative period (141).

The effects of regional vs general anesthesia on the immune response also have been investigated. A significant reduction of mitogen and alloantigen-induced lymphoproliferation was observed in patients having prostatic resection under general anesthesia, whereas only minimal changes were seen when surgery was performed under spinal anesthesia (133). Similarly, NK cell activity was significantly depressed in mothers having cesarean section under general anesthesia but not under epidural anesthesia (142). Only the sera obtained from patients having surgery under general anesthesia, but not epidural, caused a depression of monocyte-mediated cytolysis and mitogen-induced lymphocyte proliferation (143).

Anesthesia and Immune Mediators

In addition to depression of cell-mediated immunity, anesthesia and surgery are known to initiate alterations in secretion of cytokines, such as interleukins, tumor necrosis factor (TNF), platelet-activating factor (PAF), interferons (IFN), eicosanoids,

and the expression of cytokine receptors, all of these being important in the determination of postoperative immunomodulation (144–146).

Interleukins

IL-1 is secreted mainly by monocytes and macrophages, and it activates acute phase response, protein catabolism, induction by fever, the fibrinolytic system, and trace metal distribution (147). The levels of IL-1 and IL-6, another inflammatory cytokine, have been shown to be increased immediately after surgery and anesthesia. However, these levels return to preoperative values in about 5 days after surgical intervention (148–151).

IL-2 is released from lymphocytes following their stimulation by IL-1. IL-2 stimulates rapid proliferation of lymphocytes, and this response decreases following all major surgery (152). Furthermore, there appears to be a correlation between the severity of injury and depression of IL-2 production. Although a slight increase in the expression of IL-2 surface receptors on T lymphocytes (IL-2R) after cholecystectomy has been reported (150), other studies have shown a depressed expression of these receptors after surgery (153) and trauma (154,155). A decrease or removal of adherent monocytes or administration of a cyclooxygenase inhibitor can circumvent the decrease in IL-2 and IL-2 receptor expression. In contrast, the levels of the soluble form of IL-2 receptors are increased after surgery (156).

IL-3 and IL-5 levels are decreased after hemorrhage in mice (157). To date, there are no data on the levels of IL-7 through IL-11 during anesthesia and surgery.

Eicosanoids

Immunosuppressive eicosanoids, particularly prostaglandins (e.g., PGE_2), play a major role in perioperative immunosuppression (158,159). Indomethacin-mediated inhibition of prostaglandin and IL-2 production has been shown to improve outcome in patients after trauma and thermal injury (160,161). TNF is not measurable in blood after uncomplicated surgery, and no reports have been published on the effects of anesthesia and surgery on PAF in humans. In contrast, γ-interferon production is decreased after accidental injury (162). Recently, it has been shown that halothane and isoflurane inhibit α-interferon and β-inducible cytotoxicity (163). Although some of the investigations suggest an anesthetic-mediated suppression of immune mediators, there is no definitive evidence.

Anesthesia and Humoral Immunity

Reports on the effects of anesthesia on humoral immunity in humans are relatively sparse, with inconclusive results. B lymphocyte numbers are decreased in the peripheral blood, and lymphoproliferative responses to mitogens are depressed following surgery under general anesthesia (164). The number of immunoglobulin-synthesizing and secreting cells is decreased after open heart surgery, and their capacity to produce polyclonal immunoglobulin, IgG, IgM, and IgA, in response to pockweed mitogen is also depressed in cultures (165). Although a slight decrease of immunoglobulin concentrations in the postoperative period has been reported (166), there is no firm evidence that anesthesia alters the production, functional activity, or immunoglobulin levels in the perioperative period. The serum immunoglobulin decreases reported after surgery (167,168) are possibly the result of hemodilution, loss of protein into extravascular tissues, and immunoglobulin consumption. A temporary decrease in Ig synthesis cannot result in decreased immunoglobulin concentration in the immediate postoperative period because the biologic half-lives of IgG, IgA, and IgM are, respectively, 28, 6, and 5 days.

It is generally accepted that specific antibody response is better maintained during surgery. Following exposure to 4% halothane for 8 hours *in vitro,* no significant change from controls in B cell lymphoproliferation was observed (169). Animal studies, however, have shown increased (170–172), decreased (173), or unaltered (174) antibody responses after surgery. When evaluating the effects of anesthetic agents, one must consider the effect of surgical stress on immunoglobulin production. Depression of antibody production correlates well with the severity of surgical trauma (165–167).

The capping of surface immunoglobulins after exposure of lymphocytes to 1% halothane has been investigated. The capping phenomenon is a cell surface antigen-antibody reaction believed to be the initial step in lymphocyte activation. Following exposure to halothane *in vitro,* capping was observed to be decreased (175) or unchanged (169). Thus, there is conflicting evidence about the effects of anesthesia on immunoglobulin levels and B lymphocyte antibody synthesizing capabilities. The postoperative decreases may well be dilutional and not the result of direct anesthetic effects.

Anesthesia and Infection

The precise role of anesthesia in the pathogenesis of perioperative infection is difficult to ascertain because several factors may contribute. Furthermore, anesthetic intervention is seldom indicated on its own, and one must take into consideration the effects of surgical stress and trauma in the pathogenesis of perioperative infections. However, animal studies appear to indicate that anesthetic intervention alone may alter the course of infection. Halothane anesthesia alone increased the mortality from *Salmonella* infection in mice (4) and doubled the mortality from fecal peritonitis in another study (6). Halothane anesthesia was shown to increase the mortality from murine hepatitis virus (MHV₃) infection in newly weaned mice. This mortality was significantly enhanced when anesthesia was given immediately before and up to 24 hours after infection (7) (Fig. 6). A more recent investigation, using the cecal ligation and puncture model, has revealed that the i.v. induction agents ketamine and pentobarbital or the inhalation agents halothane, enflurane, and isoflurane produced significantly enhanced mortality from sepsis in mice (176). All these agents significantly depressed the helper/suppressor lymphocyte ratio, and this effect persisted for 72 hours following anesthetic intervention. Morphine also decreased the resistance to infection in mice by drastically suppressing the reticuloendothelial system activity, phagocyte count, phagocytic index, and superoxide generation by polymorphonuclear leukocytes and macrophages (177). A similar depression of alveolar macrophage counts, phagocytosis, and bactericidal activities was observed in rabbits, thus suggesting a lack of species specificity (177).

Other animal experiments have shown depressed immune response and infections with anesthesia and surgery (178,179). The correlation between postoperative depression of immune response, frequency of infection, and mortality in humans is best documented by delayed hypersensitivity skin testing. Patients who are anergic or acquire anergy postoperatively (180–182), and patients with severe suppression of T cell lymphoproliferative responses are at the greatest risk of mortality from sepsis (183). In trauma patients, it was shown that depression of complement below 50% of normal levels for about 1 week resulted in bacteremia in all patients (184). The infectious outcome largely depends on the magnitude of changes, whether they are simple physiologic events or have pathologic sequelae. Also, changes in the immune response are not entirely responsible for postoperative infections because alterations also occur in the outer host defenses, microbial flora, and the varying degrees of bacterial contamination (185).

Alterations in mucosal integrity, decreased gastrointestinal motility, and decreased mucous secretions all may contribute to postoperative infections. Anesthetic and surgically induced suppression of the immune response contributes to enhanced postoperative infections, particularly if the disturbance is severe and prolonged or if the patient was immunocompromised in the preoperative period. In patients with AIDS or with preoperative immunosuppression, the incidence of postoperative septic complications is high after intraabdominal surgery (186). Surgery may also cause recurrence of latent infections, such as malaria (187).

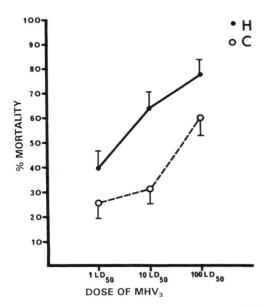

FIG. 6. Percentage differences in mortality ($\pm$ SE) in control and anesthetized groups of animals infected with 0.1 ml of 1, 10, and 100 LD₅₀ dose of MHV₃.

Anesthesia and Malignancy

Neoplastic cells appear to be antigenic in nature, and cell-mediated responses of the host are stimulated on exposure to tumor antigens. Studies of the effects of anesthesia on tumor takes are contradictory. Both enhanced pulmonary metastasis (188) and no significant effect by anesthesia (189) have been reported. Administration of equipotent concentrations of halothane and isoflurane resulted in significantly higher numbers of pulmonary metastases from B16 melanoma tumors in C57 B1/6J mice compared with controls (190) (Fig. 7). Besides general tests of overall immunity, tumor-specific responses have been evaluated in the perioperative period. The ability of host leukocytes to kill tumor cells (tumor type-specific leukocytotoxicity) was depressed up to 7 days after mastectomy under halothane anesthesia for carcinoma of the breast (191) and after surgery for Wilms' tumor (192).

Tumor cell killing by cytotoxic cells *in vitro* was decreased by local anesthetics (193), barbital (194), and halothane (136). Different studies have reported a rapid dissemination of malignancy after surgery (195), as well as an exacerbation of cancer

after unrelated surgery (196). Evidence indicates that immunosurveillance mechanisms are not only important in defense against primary malignancy but also may be equally important in eliminating microscopic residual tumors postoperatively (197). Any suppression of immune response, anesthetically or surgically induced, is clearly detrimental to the patient. Further data are necessary to clearly define the implications of anesthesia-induced immunosuppression in malignancy.

TRAUMA, HEMORRHAGE, BLOOD TRANSFUSION, AND IMMUNE RESPONSE

Trauma

Trauma and surgery are generally considered to have a deleterious effect on the host defense system. The ability of a patient to mount an inflammatory response to an antigenic challenge is an index of immune surveillance. There appears to be a correlation between the extent of the trauma and changes in leukocyte and differential counts, lymphocyte and subtype counts, mitogen and antigen-induced lymphocyte proliferative responses, plasma volume necessary for halving of tuberculin (PPD)-induced lymphocytic responses (198–200), and in IL-6 responses (201). Delayed hypersensitivity skin testing with recall antigens has been shown to be reduced after surgical trauma (202) and hypovolemic shock (203). Depression of chemotactic migration and bactericidal activity was observed following trauma and thermal injury (204). Substantial alterations in the release of several lymphokines have been observed following accidental trauma, hemorrhage, and burns (205,206). Changes during open heart surgery are somewhat greater than those during a major operation, possibly as a result of additional effects of the extracorporeal circulation (207–210).

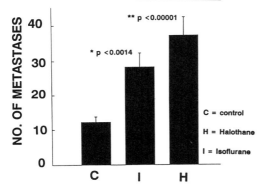

FIG. 7. Diagram showing number of metastases/mouse in control and anesthetized animals following challenge with B$_{16}$ melanoma tumor cells. (From Moudgil GC, Frame B, Blajchman, MA, Singal DP. Effects of anaesthesia on tumour metastasis. *Can Anaesth Soc J* 1990; 38:A127.)

Hemorrhage

Hemorrhage of approximately 30% of the blood volume produces multiple abnormalities in the immune response. Serum immunoglobulin levels (211), intestinal antibody-producing cells (212), T cell lymphoproliferation, and lymphokine production (157) are all decreased. Hypoperfusion and tissue ischemia, particularly of intestinal mucosa, result in intestinal mucosal barrier dysfunction, with subsequent translocation of intestinal endotoxins and microorganisms (213). In surgical patients who are already immunocompromised, this may result in systemic infection and multiple organ failure (214). Hypovolemic shock in experimental animals was shown to impair T cell lymphoproliferation, antigen presentation by macrophages, and IL-2 generation, thus resulting in enhanced susceptibility to infection and sepsis (215).

Transfusion

Homologous blood transfusions containing leukocytes have immunosuppressive effects (216). Blood transfusions appear to enhance graft survival after organ transplantation (217) but also result in increased cancer recurrence and decreased survival (216). Transfused patients also show an increased incidence of postoperative infections (218,219) and increased susceptibility to multiple organ failure (220). Laboratory investigations support the concept of immunosuppression resulting from blood transfusion (221–226). In a study of 500 patients requiring colorectal surgery, a poorer prognosis was observed among patients who had blood transfusion compared to the nontransfused patients (227). However, in another study of 1000 patients with gastric cancer, factors other than blood transfusion were deemed to be responsible for immunosuppression (228). In patients undergoing abdominal surgery, the frequency of infection and sepsis was increased when the patients were transfused with more than three units of blood (229). Thus, the issue of transfusion-induced immunosuppression and its clinical sequelae remains a controversial issue.

Drug-Induced Immunosuppression in the ICU

Infection and sepsis are the major determinants of enhanced morbidity and mortality in ICU patients. Nosocomial infections develop in up to 50% of the patients in critical care units, and mortality from these infections may occur in up to 70% of the patients (10,11). Although these infections are multifactorial in origin, depression of the host defense systems plays a pivotal role in their pathogenesis.

The immune response of a patient can be adversely affected at several stages. Host defense abnormalities are likely to occur after initial trauma, hemorrhage, and thermal injury. The immune system may be further compromised by surgical and anesthetic interventions before admission to the ICU. The physical environment of the ICU and the mental state of the traumatized patient further suppress the host defenses. Invasive monitoring breaks the natural barriers against infection. The use of immunosuppressant drugs in patient management favors the invading organisms. This sequence of events subsequently results in enhanced morbidity and mortality from infection.

Antibiotics and Immune Response

A large number of investigators have shown that antibiotics can adversely affect the cellular and humoral components of the immune response. Chemotaxis, lymphocyte transformation, delayed hypersensitivity, and antibody production are depressed *in vivo* and *in vitro* by several commonly used antibiotics (230). These investigations underscore the necessity for intelligence and restraint in prescribing antibiotics, especially for immunosuppressed patients. The management of infection in the immunosuppressed patient requires a critical understanding of the relationship among clinical infection, antibiotics, and the immune response. Although such antibiotics as gentamicin are active against most strains of *Pseudomonas,* gentamicin is largely ineffective in neutropenic patients with bacteremia (231). Likewise, antibiotic therapy in agammaglobulinemia is rarely successful. Failure of antimicrobial therapy may be due to depressed immune function rather than to an inability to reach effective drug concentrations at the site of infection.

Narcotics, Sedatives, and Immune Response

Many patients require narcotics and sedatives, such as morphine and diazepam, for prolonged periods of time to alleviate pain and stress and to gain control of the ventilatory parameters. Although the effects of these drugs on the cardiovascular, respiratory, and other organ systems are well documented, their effects on the host defenses are largely unknown. In an *in vitro* study, endogenous opiate β endorphin, dynorphin, and methionine-enkephalin caused a reduction of NK cell activity as well as antigen-specific cytolysis (232). These immunosuppressive effects of morphine appear to be mediated by opiate receptors in the brain, since NK cell activity was unaffected by administration of n-methylmorphine, a morphine analog that does not cross blood–brain barrier (233). These direct effects of opiates on the cytolytic T cell and NK cell function may provide a link between stress and disease susceptibility.

In addition to adverse effects on the NK cell activity, suppression of mitogen-induced lymphoproliferation and marked atrophy of immune organs following a morphine pellet implant in animals have been reported (234). Both cellular and humoral components of the immune response may be compromised after opiate therapy (235).

Well-controlled clinical studies are needed to substantiate further the observations made in *in vitro* and in animal models.

Steroids and Immune Response

In ICUs, steroids are used widely, but unfortunately they often are prescribed with no clear indication and no recognized dosage schedule. They have become an essential part of our therapeutic armamentarium to combat shock, adult respiratory distress syndrome (ARDS), acute liver failure, and brain edema following head injury. However, controversy continues about their safety and effectiveness in these disorders.

Although the beneficial effects of steroid therapy are far from established, there is evidence that they exert potent harmful and suppressive effects on the immune response. Corticosteroids exert their immunosuppressive effects by modifying several aspects of the cellular and humoral arms of the host defense system (236). The effects of corticosteroids on B lymphocytes are less pronounced than those on T lymphocytes. Serum IgG, IgA, and IgM levels are suppressed by corticosteroid therapy (237). A trial of high-dose methylprednisolone failed to elicit a significant difference in the prevention or reversal of septic shock (238). However, in the subgroup of patients with elevated serum creatinine levels at enrollment, the mortality was significantly increased among those receiving methylprednisolone. Likewise, a trial of early, short-term, high-dose methylprednisolone for treatment of systemic sepsis failed to demonstrate a significant reduction in mortality (239). Dexamethasone and barbiturate therapy has been used routinely for the management of patients with head injury. Different concentrations of barbiturates and dexamethasone alone and in combination with each other have been shown to produce a dose-dependent inhibition of chemotaxis, as well as mitogen- and allo-antigen-induced lymphoproliferation (240).

These and other studies would suggest that steroid and barbiturate administration may enhance morbidity and mortality from infections.

Bronchodilators and Immune Response

Bronchodilator therapy is commonly employed in the treatment of bronchial asthma and chronic obstructive pulmonary disease. Several clinical situations in the ICU may warrant the use of such therapy. Experimental data suggest that bronchodilator drugs cause a dose-dependent inhibition of both PHA-induced lymphocyte proliferation and IL-2 and γ-interferon production. However, T cell proliferation *in vivo* was unaffected after drug administration (241).

Stress, Antacids, and Immune Response

Stress ulcer syndrome occurs in up to 74% of ICU patients (242). Cimetidine and ranitidine are used routinely in patients on mechanical ventilatory support to maintain intragastric pH>4 and decrease gastric bleeding. It has been shown that cimetidine at low doses stimulates the immune response by enhancing mitogen-induced lymphoproliferation. An enhancement of IgG and IgM immunoglobulins also was observed following cimetidine administration in animals (243). Higher doses of cimetidine have been shown to cause immunosuppression (244). Prolonged use of these modulators may enhance the incidence of pneumonia by altering the bacterial flora through change of gastric pH toward alkalinity.

CONCLUSIONS

The effects of anesthesia, surgery, and other therapy are difficult to define in surgical patients. The available evidence supports the concept that anesthetic agents influence a wide variety of specific and nonspecific components of the host defense system, but the precise role of anesthesia alone in the pathogenesis of perioperative infection remains to be defined with clarity. Patients with anergy, trauma, hemorrhage, and hypoperfusion, preexisting immunologic defects, and nutritional and metabolic defects all have an additive suppressive effect on the immune function. Typically, the sicker the patient, the greater the propensity for significant immunosuppression even with an otherwise benign stress, such as anesthesia alone. By understanding the nature and mechanisms of anesthesia-induced immunosuppression, one may be able to reduce the incidence of morbidity and mortality due to anesthesia and other drug-induced defects of the host defense systems.

REFERENCES

1. Bernard C. *Anesthésiques et l'asphyxie,* Paris: Ballière, 1875.
2. Snel J J. Immunität und Narkose. *Berl Klin Wochenschr* 1903;40:212.
3. Rubin G. The influence of alcohol, ether and chloroform on natural immunity in its relation to leukocytosis and phagocytosis. *J Infect Dis* 1904;1:425.
4. Bruce D L. Effect of halothane anesthesia on experimental salmonella peritonitis in mice. *J Surg Res* 1967;7:180–185.
5. Goldstein E, Munson E S, Eagle C, Martucci R W, Hoeprich P D. The effects of anesthetic agents on murine pulmonary bactericidal activity. *Anesthesiology* 1971;34:344–352.
6. Duncan P G, Cullen B F, Pearsall N. Anesthesia and the modification of the response to infection in mice. *Anesth Analg* 1976;55:776–781.
7. Moudgil G C. Proceedings: influence of halothane on mortality from murine hepatitis virus (MHV₃). *Br J Anaesth* 1973;45:1236.
8. Pollock A V. Laparotomy. *J R Soc Med* 1981; 74:480–484.
9. Pruitt B A Jr. Host–opportunist interactions in surgical infection. *Arch Surg* 1986;121:13–22.
10. Larson E. Infection control issues in critical care: an update. *Heart Lung* 1985;14:149–155.
11. Preston G A, Larson E L, Stamm W E. The effect of private isolation rooms on patient care practices, colonization and infection in an intensive care unit. *Am J Med* 1981;70:641–645.
12. Huffer T, Kanapa D, Stevenson G W. Mononuclear phagocyte, polymorphonuclear granulocyte, and natural killer lymphocyte function. In: Stevenson H D, Miseil R, eds. *Introduction to human immunology.* Boston: Jones and Bartlett Publishers, Inc, 1986:113–117.

13. Densen P, Mandell G L. Phagocyte strategy vs microbial tactics. *Rev Infect Dis* 1980;2: 817–838.
14. Van Furth R. Phagocytic cells in the defence against infection: introduction. *Rev Infect Dis* 1980;2:No.1:104.
15. Cartwright G E, Athens J W, Wintrobe M M. The kinetics of granulopoiesis in normal man. *Blood* 1964;24:780–803.
16. Dancey J T, Deubelbeiss K A, Harker L A, Funch C A. Neutrophil kinetics in man. *J Clin Invest* 1976;58:705–715.
17. Barth N M, Galazka A R, Rudnick S A. Lymphokines and cytokines. In: Oldham R K, ed. *Principles of cancer biotherapy.* New York: Raven Press, 1987:273.
18. Roitt I, Brostoff J, Male D. *Immunology,* 2nd ed. London: Gower Medical Publishing, 1989.
19. Cantor H T. Lymphocytes. In: Paul W E, ed. *Fundamental immunology.* New York: Raven Press, 1984:57.
20. Dinarello C A. Interleukin 1. *Rev Infect Dis* 1984;6:51–95.
21. Griffin F M Jr. Mononuclear cell phagocytic mechanisms and host defense. In: Gallin J I, Fauci A S, eds. *Advances in host defense mechanisms. Vol 1, Phagocytic cells.* New York: Raven Press, 1982:13.
22. Le thi Bich-Thuy, Fauci A S. Recombinant interleukin 2 and gamma-interferon act synergistically on distinct steps of *in vitro* terminal human B cell maturation. *J Clin Invest* 1986; 77:1173.
23. Moudgil G C, Wade A G. Anaesthesia and immunocompetence. *Br J Anaesth* 1976;48:31–39.
24. Duncan P G, Cullen B F. Anesthesiology and immunology. *Anesthesiology* 1976;45:522–538.
25. Walton B. Anaesthesia, surgery and immunology. *Anaesthesia* 1978;33:322–348.
26. Kehlet H, Wandall J H, Hjortso N C. Influence of anesthesia and surgery on immunocompetence. *Reg Anesth* 1982;7(4S):S68–S74.
27. Ryhanen P. *Effects of anesthesia and operative surgery on the immune response of patients of different ages* (Thesis). Oulu, Finland: Oulu University, 1977.
28. Stevenson G W, Hall S C, Rudnick S, Seleny F L, Stevenson H S. The effect of anesthetic agents on the human immune response. *Anesthesiology* 1990;72:542–552.
29. Heilbrunn L V. The physical effect of anesthetics upon living protoplasm. *Biol Bull Marine Biol Lab Woods Hole* 1920;39:307–315.
30. Seifriz W. A theory of anesthesia based on protoplasmic behavior. *Anesthesiology* 1941;2: 300–309.
31. Goldacre R J. The action of general anaesthetics on amoebae and the mechanism of the response to touch. In: *Structural aspects of cell physiology.* Symposia of the Society of Experimental Biology, No. 6. London: Cambridge University Press, 1952;128–144.
32. Bruce D L, Christiansen R. Morphologic changes in the giant amoeba. Chaos induced by halothane and ether. *Exp Cell Res* 1965;40:544–553.
33. Schoenborn B P, Watson H C, Kendrew J C. Binding of xenon to sperm whale myoglobin. *Nature (Lond)* 1965;207:28–30.
34. Schoenborn B P. Binding of anesthetics to protein: an x-ray crystallographic investigation. *Fed Proc* 1968;27:888–894.
35. Seeman P, Roth S. General anaesthetics expand cell membranes at surgical concentrations. *Biochim Biophys Acta* 1972;255:171–177.
36. Bangham A D, Standish M M, Miller N. Cation permeability of phospholipid model membranes: effect of narcotics. *Nature (Lond)* 1965;208: 1295–1297.
37. Johnson S M, Bangham A D. The action of anaesthetics on phospholipid membranes. *Biochim Biophys Acta* 1969;193:92–104.
38. Johnson S M, Miller K W, Bangham A D. The opposing effects of pressure and general anaesthetics on the cation permeability of liposomes of varying lipid composition. *Biochim Biophys Acta* 1973;307:42–57.
39. In: Davy, H, ed. *Researches, chemical and philosophical; chiefly concerning nitrous oxide, or dephologisticated nitrous air and its respiration.* London: J. Johnson, 1800.
40. In: Bernard C, ed. *Lecons sur les phenomenes de la vie communs aux animaux et vegetaux.* Paris: J B Ballière, 1878:259.
41. Martin M C. In: Delahaye A, Lecrosnier E, Georg H, eds. *De l'anesthesie par le protoxyde d'azote avec ou sans tension.* Paris, Lyons: Compt. Rend. Ac. Sci., 1888:106,290–291.
42. Östergren G. Colchicine mitosis, chromosome contractions, narcosis, and protein chain folding. *Hereditas (Lund)* 1944;30:429.
43. Anderson N B. The effects of CNS depressants on mitosis. *Acta Anaesth Scand* 1966;22(suppl): 1–36.
44. Fink B R, Kenny G E. Metabolic effects of volatile anesthetics in cell culture. *Anesthesiology* 1968;29:505–516.
45. Jackson S H. The metabolic effects of halothane on mammalian hepatoma cells *in vitro*. II. Inhibition of DNA synthesis. *Anesthesiology* 1973;39:405–409.
46. Sturrock J E, Nunn J F. Mitosis in mammalian cells during exposure to anesthetics. *Anesthesiology* 1975;43:21–33.
47. Nunn J F, Sturrock J E, Howell A. Effect of inhalation anaesthetics on division of bone marrow cells *in vitro*. *Br J Anaesth* 1976;48:75–81.
48. Allison A C, Nunn J F. Effects of general anesthetics on micro-tubules: a possible mechanism of anesthesia. *Lancet* 1968;ii:1329–1396.
49. Bruce D L, Traurig H. The effect of halothane on the cell cycle in rat small intestine. *Anesthesiology* 1969;30:401–405.
50. Brinkley B R, Rao P N. Nitrous oxide: effects on the mitotic apparatus and chromosome movement in HeLa cells. *J Cell Biol* 1973;58: 96–106.
51. Sturrock J E, Nunn J F. Effects of halothane on DNA synthesis and the presynthetic phase (G_1) in dividing fibroblasts. *Anesthesiology* 1976;45:413–420.

52. Lassen H C A, Henriksen E, Neukirch F, et al. Treatment of tetanus: severe bone marrow depression after prolonged nitrous oxide anesthesia. *Lancet* 1956;1:527–530.

53. Green C D, Eastwood D W. Effects of nitrous oxide inhalation on hemopoiesis in rats. *Anesthesiology* 1963;24:341–345.

54. Nunn J F, Dixon K L, Moore J R. Effect of halothane on *Tetrahymena pyriformis. Br J Anaesth* 1968;40:145.

55. Nunn J F, Sharp J A, Kimball K L. Reversible effects of an inhalational anaesthetic on lymphocyte motility. *Nature (Lond)* 1970;226: 85–86.

56. Moudgil G C, Allan R B, Russell R J, Wilkinson P C. Inhibition, by anaesthetic agents, of human leucocyte locomotion towards chemical attractants. *Br J Anaesth* 1977;49:97–104.

57. Knudsen F, Klausen N O, Ferguson A H, Pederson J O. *In vitro* effect of etomidate and thiopental on granulocyte migration. *Acta Anaesth Scand* 1987;31:93–95.

58. Mathieu A, Mathieu D. Effects of volatile anesthetics and neuromuscular blocking agents in PMN chemotaxis. *Anesthesiology* 1980;53:560.

59. Stanley T H, Hill G E, Portas M R, Hogan N A, Hill H R. Neutrophil chemotaxis during and after general anesthesia and operation. *Anesth Analg* 1976;55:668–673.

60. Moudgil G C, Pandya A R, Ludlow D J. Influence of anaesthesia and surgery on neutrophil chemotaxis. *Can Anaesth Soc J* 1981;28: 232–238.

61. Erskine R, Janicki P K, Ellis P, James M F M. Neutrophils from patients undergoing hip surgery exhibit enhanced movement under spinal anaesthesia compared with general anaesthesia. *Can J Anaesth* 1992;39:905–910.

62. Duncan P G, Cullen B F. Neutrophil chemotaxis and anaesthesia. *Br J Anaesth* 1977;49: 345–349.

63. Nunn J F, Sturrock J E, Jones A J, et al. Halothane does not inhibit human neutrophil function *in vitro. Br J Anaesth* 1979;51:1101–1108.

64. Moudgil G C, Gordon J, Forrest J B. Comparative effects of volatile anaesthetic agents and nitrous oxide on human leucocyte chemotaxis *in vitro. Can Anaesth Soc J* 1984;31:631–637.

65. Nunn J F, O'Morain C. Nitrous oxide decreases mobility of human neutrophils *in vitro. Anesthesiology* 1982;56:45–48.

66. Mathieu A, Mathieu D, Hyslop N. Effect of induction agents and non-volatile anesthetics on chemotaxis of polymorphonuclear leukocytes. *Anesthesiology* 1979;51:556.

67. Mathieu A, Mathieu D, Kahan D B. Effects of nalbuphine and butorphanol, two new narcotic analgesics, on chemotaxis of polymorphonuclear leukocytes. *Fed Proc* 1980;39:879.

68. Salo M. Effects of anaesthesia and surgery on the immune response. In: Watkins J, Salo M, eds. *Trauma, stress and immunity in anaesthesia and surgery.* London: Butterworths, 1982:211–253.

69. Bowers T K, O'Flaherty J, Simmons R L, Jacobs H S. Postsurgical granulocyte dysfunction: studies in healthy kidney donors. *J Lab Clin Med* 1977;90:720–727.

70. Palmblad J. Activation of the bactericidal capacity of polymorphonuclear granulocytes after surgery, measured with a new *in vitro* assay. *Scand J Haematol* 1979;23:10–16.

71. Morris J S, Meakins J L, Christou N V. *In vivo* neutrophil delivery to inflammatory sites in surgical patients. Correlation with *in vitro* neutrophil chemotaxis and adherence. *Arch Surg* 1985;120:205–209.

72. Solomkin J S, Bauman M P, Nelson R D, Simmons R L. Neutrophils dysfunction during the course of intra-abdominal infection. *Ann Surg* 1981;194:9–17.

73. Wandall J H. Leucocyte mobilization and function *in vitro* of blood and exudative leucocytes after inguinal herniotomy. *Br J Surg* 1982;69: 669–672.

74. Duignan J P, Collins P B, Johnson A H, Bouchier-Hayes D. The association of impaired neutrophil chemotaxis with postoperative surgical sepsis. *Br J Surg* 1986;73:238–240.

75. Moudgil G C. Anaesthesia and leucocyte locomotion [Editorial]. *Can J Anaesth* 1992;39: 899–904.

76. Hamburger H J. Researches on phagocytosis. *Br Med J* 1916;1:37.

77. Cullen B F. The effect of halothane and nitrous oxide on phagocytosis and human leukocyte metabolism. *Anesth Analg* 1974;53:531–536.

78. Lippa S, De Sole P, Meucci E, Littarru G P, De Francisci G, Magalini S I. Effect of general anesthetics on human granulocyte chemiluminescence. *Experientia* 1983;39:1386–1388.

79. Bardosi L, Tekeres M. Impaired metabolic activity of phagocytic cells after anaesthesia and surgery. *Br J Anaesth* 1985;57:520–523.

80. Barth J, Petermann W, Entzian P, Wustrow C, Wustrow J, Ohnhaus E E. Modulation of oxygen-free radicals from human leukocytes during halothane- and enflurane-induced general anesthesia. *Acta Anaesth Scand* 1987;31: 740–743.

81. Busoni P, Sarti A, De Martino M, Graziani E, Santoro S. The effect of general and regional anesthesia on oxygen-dependent microbicidal mechanisms of polymorphonuclear leukocytes in children. *Anesth Analg* 1988;67:453–456.

82. Mealy K, O'Farrelly C, Stephens R, Feighery C. Impaired neutrophil function during anesthesia and surgery is due to serum factors. *J Surg Res* 1987;43:393–397.

83. Solomkin J S, Bauman M P, Nelson R D, Simmons R L. Neutrophils dysfunction during the course of intra-abdominal infection. *Ann Surg* 1981;194:9–17.

84. Perttila J, Lehtonen O-P, Salo M, Tertti R. Effects of coronary bypass surgery under high-dose fentanyl anaesthesia on granulocyte chemiluminescence. *Br J Anaesth* 1986;58: 1027–1030.

85. Moudgil G C. Effect of premedicant, intravenous anaesthetic agents and local anaesthetics

on phagocytosis *in vitro. Can Anaesth Soc J* 1981;28:597–602.

86. Hole A. Peri- and postoperative monocyte and lymphocyte functions: effects of sera from patients operated under general or epidural anaesthesia. *Acta Anaesth Scand* 1984;28:287–291.

87. Herberer M, Zbinden A M, Ernst M, Durig M, Harder F. The effect of surgery and anesthetic agents on granulocyte-chemiluminescence in whole blood. *Experientia* 1985;41:342–346.

88. Perttila J, Salo M, Rajamaki A. Granulocyte microbicidal function in patients undergoing major abdominal surgery under balanced anaesthesia. *Acta Anaesth Scand* 1987;31:100–103.

89. van Dijk W, Verbrugh H, Rijswijk R E N, Vos A, Verhoef J. Neutrophil function, serum opsonic activity, and delayed hypersensitivity in surgical patients. *Surgery* 1982;92:21–29.

90. Perttila J, Lilius E-M, Salo M. Effects of anaesthesia and surgery on serum opsonic capacity. *Acta Anaesth Scand* 1986;30:173–176.

91. van Oeveren W, Kazatchkine M D, Descamps-Latscha B, et al. Deleterious effects of cardiopulmonary bypass. A prospective study of bubble versus membrane oxygenation. *J Thorac Cardiovasc Surg* 1985;89:888–899.

92. Burrows F A, Steele R W, Marmer D J, Van Devanter S H, Westerman G R. Influence of operations with cardiopulmonary bypass on polymorphonuclear leukocyte function in infants. *J Thorac Cardiovasc Surg* 1987;93:253–260.

93. Semb A G, Vaage J, Lie M, Sorlie D, Mjos O D. Leucocytes and cardiopulmonary bypass: *in vitro* production of oxygen free radicals and trapping in the reperfused myocardium. *Perfusion* 1990;5:169–180.

94. El-Maallem H, Fletcher J. Effects of surgery on neutrophil granulocyte function. *Infect Immun* 1981;32:38–41.

95. Konn G, Himal H S. Leukocyte lysosomal function in sepsis. *Surg Gynecol Obstet* 1984;159:457–460.

96. Oladimeji M, Grimshaw A D, Baum M, Patterson K G, Goldstone A H. Effect of surgery on monocyte function. *Br J Surg* 1982;69:145–146.

97. Everson N W, Neoptolemos J P, Scott D J A, Wood R F M. The effect of surgical operation upon monocytes. *Br J Surg* 1981;68:257–260.

98. Neoptolemos J P, Wood P, Everson N W, Bell P R F. Monocyte function following surgery in man. Increased numbers and stimulation of migration, phagocytosis and chemiluminescence following abdominal surgery. *Eur Surg Res* 1985;17:215–220.

99. Neoptolemos J P, Wood P, Everson N W, Bell P R F. The effect of surgical procedures on monocyte function in patients with carcinoma of the colon and rectum. *Surg Gynecol Obstet* 1986;163:235–242.

100. Saba T M, Cho E. Reticuloendothelial systemic response to operative trauma as influenced by cryoprecipitate or cold-insoluble

globulin therapy. *J Reticuloendothel Soc* 1979;26:171–186.

101. Richards W O, Scovill W A, Shin B. Opsonic fibronectin deficiency in patients with intraabdominal infection. *Surgery* 1983;94:210–217.

102. Högström H, Borgström A, Haglund U. Plasma fibronectin in relation to surgical trauma. *Scand J Clin Lab Invest* 1985;45:87–89.

103. Powell J T, Poskitt K R, Irwin J T, Attanoos R L, McCollum C N. Opsonic dysfunction secondary to plasma fibronectin depletion after aortic surgery. *Br J Surg* 1986;73:38–40.

104. Perttila J, Salo M, Peltola O. Effects of different plasma substitutes on plasma fibronectin concentration in patients undergoing abdominal surgery. *Acta Anaesth Scand* 1990;34:304–307.

105. Vedrinne J M, Hoen J P, Bussery D, Veyssere C, Richard M, Motin J. Plasma fibronectin and complement following infusion of colloidal solutions after spinal anaesthesia. *Intensive Care Med* 1991;17:83–86.

106. Perttila J, Salo M, Peltola O, Irjala K. Changes in granulocyte chemiluminescence and plasma fibronectin concentrations following major blunt trauma. *Eur Surg Res* 1988;20:211–219.

107. Powell F S, Doran J E. Current status of fibronectin in transfusion medicine: focus on clinical studies. *Vox Sang* 1991;60:193–202.

108. Welch WD. Inhibition of neutrophil cidal activity by volatile anesthetics. *Anesthesiology* 1986;64:1–3.

109. Welch W D. Correlation between measurements of the luminol-dependent chemiluminescence response and bacterial susceptibility to phagocytosis. *Infect Immun* 1980;30:370–374.

110. Welch W D. Halothane reversibly inhibits human neutrophil bacterial killing. *Anesthesiology* 1981;55:650–654.

111. Welch W D. Effect of enflurane, isoflurane, and nitrous oxide on the microbicidal activity of human polymorphonuclear leukocytes. *Anesthesiology* 1984;61:188–192.

112. Stevenson G W, Hall S, Rudnick S J, et al. Halothane anesthesia decreases human monocyte hydrogen peroxide generation. Protection of monocytes by activation with gamma interferon. *Immunopharmacol Immunotoxicol* 1987;9:489–510.

113. Nakagawara M, Takeshige K, Takamatsu J, Takahashi S, Moshitake J, Minakami S. Inhibition of superoxide production and Ca_{2+} mobilization in human neutrophils by halothane, enflurane, and isoflurane. *Anesthesiology* 1986;64:4–12.

114. White I W C, Gelb A W, Wexler H R, Stiller C R, Keowa P A. The effects of intravenous anaesthetic agents on human neutrophil chemiluminescence. *Can Anaesth Soc J* 1983;30:506–511.

115. Nakagawara M, Hirokata Y, Yoshitake J-I. Effects of anesthetics on superoxide releasing activity in human polymorphonuclear leukocytes. *Jpn Anaesth J Rev* 1986;1:215.

116. Salo M. Effect of anaesthesia and surgery on

the number of and mitogen-induced transformation of T- and B-lymphocytes. *Ann Clin Res* 1978;10:1–13.

117. Fosse E, Opdahl H, Aakvaag A, Svennevig J-L, Sunde S. White blood cell populations in patients undergoing major vascular surgery. *Scand J Thorac Cardiovasc Surg* 1985;19:247–252.

118. Hansbrough J F, Bender E M, Zapata-Sirvent R, Anderson J. Altered helper and suppressor lymphocyte populations in surgical patients. *Am J Surg* 1984;148:303–307.

119. Hole A, Bakke O. T-lymphocytes and the subpopulations of T-helper and T-suppressor cells measured by monoclonal antibodies (T11, T4 and T8) in relation to surgery under epidural and general anaesthesia. *Acta Anaesth Scand* 1984;28:296–300.

120. Lennard T W J, Shenton B K, Borzotta A, et al. The influence of surgical operations on components of the human immune system. *Br J Surg* 1985;72:771–776.

121. Hansbrough J F, Zapata-Sirvent R L, Bender E M. Prevention of alterations in postoperative lymphocyte subpopulations by cimetidine and ibuprofen. *Am J Surg* 1986;151:249–255.

122. Madsbad S, Buschard K, Siemssen O, Ropke C. Changes in T lymphocyte subsets after elective surgery. *Acta Chir Scand* 1986;152:81–84.

123. Tonnesen E, Brinklov M M, Christensen N J, Olesen A S, Madsen T. Natural killer cell activity and lymphocyte function during and after coronary artery bypass grafting in relation to the endocrine stress response. *Anesthesiology* 1987;67:526–533.

124. Hisatomi K, Isomura T, Kawara T, et al. Changes in lymphocyte subsets, mitogen responsiveness, and interleukin 2 production after cardiac operations. *J Thorac Cardiovasc Surg* 1989;98:580–591.

125. Riddle P R. Disturbed immune reactions following surgery. *Br J Surg* 1967;54:882.

126. Cullen B F, Duncan P G, Ray-Keil L. Inhibition of cell-mediated cytotoxicity by halothane and nitrous oxide. *Anesthesiology* 1976;44:386.

127. Bruce D L. Halothane action on lymphocytes does not involve cyclic AMP. *Anesthesiology* 1976;44:151–154.

128. Moller-Larsen F, Moller-Larsen A, Haahr S. The influence of general anesthesia and surgery on cell-mediated cytotoxicity and interferon production. *J Clin Lab Immunol* 1983;12:69–75.

129. Duncan P G, Cullen B F, Ray-Keil L. Thiopental inhibition of tumor immunity. *Anesthesiology* 1977;46:97–101.

130. Woods G M, Griffith D M. Reversible inhibition of natural killer cell activity by volatile anaesthetic agents *in vitro*. *Br J Anaesth* 1986;58:535–539.

131. Griffith C D M, Kamath M B. Effect of halothane and nitrous oxide anaesthesia on natural killer lymphocytes from patients with benign and malignant breast disease. *Br J Anaesth* 1986;58:540–543.

132. Whelan P, Morris P J. Immunological responsiveness after transurethral resection of the prostate: general versus spinal anesthetic. *Clin Exp Immunol* 1982;48:611–618.

133. Salo M, Eskola J, Nikoskelainen J. T- and B-lymphocyte function in anesthetics. *Acta Anaesth Scand* 1984;28:292–295.

134. Salo M. Effect of anaesthesia and open-heart surgery on lymphocyte responses to phytohaemagglutinin and concanavalin A. *Acta Anaesth Scand* 1978;22:471–479.

135. Puri P, Brazil J, Reen D J. Immunosuppressive effects of anesthesia and surgery in the newborn: 1. Short-term effects. *J Pediatr Surg* 1984;19:823–828.

136. Mollitt D L, Marmer D J, Steele R W. Age-dependent variation of lymphocyte function in the postoperative child. *J Pediatr Surg* 1986;21:633–635.

137. Park S K, Brody J I, Wallace H A, Blakemore W S. Immunosuppressive effect of surgery. *Lancet* 1971;i:53–55.

138. Watkins J, Salo M. *Trauma, stress and immunity in anaesthesia and surgery.* London: Butterworth & Co., 1982:218.

139. Doenicke A, Grote B, Suttmann H, et al. Effects of halothane on the immunological system in healthy volunteers. *Clin Res Rev* 1981;1:23.

140. Salo M. The effect of anaesthesia and total hip replacement on the phytohaemagglutinin and concanavalin A responses of lymphocytes. *Ann Chir Gynaecol* 1977;66:299–303.

141. Moudgil G C, Singal D P, Gordon J. Comparative effects of halothane and isoflurane anesthesia on perioperative lymphocyte function. *Anesthesiology* 1992;77:A354.

142. Ryhanen P, Jouppila R, Lanning M, Jouppila P, Hollmen A, Kouvalaninen K. Natural killer cell activity after elective cesarean section under general and epidural anesthesia in healthy parturients and their newborns. *Gynecol Obstet Invest* 1985;19:139–142.

143. Hole A, Unsgaard G, Breivik H. Monocyte functions are depressed during and after surgery under general anesthesia but not under epidural anesthesia. *Acta Anaesth Scand* 1982;26:301–307.

144. Fong Y, Moildawer L L, Shires T, Lowry S F. The biologic characteristics of cytokines and their implication in surgical injury. *Surg Gynecol Obstet* 1990;170:363–378.

145. Whitcer J T, Evans S W. Cytokines in disease. *Clin Chem* 1990;36:1269–1281.

146. Darling G, Goldstein D S, Stull R, Gorschboth C M, Norton J A. Tumor necrosis factor: immune endocrine interaction. *Surgery* 1989;106:1155–1160.

147. Kaplan E, Dinarello C A, Gelfand J A. Interleukin 1 and the response to injury. *Immunol Res* 1989;8:118–129.

148. Grzelak I, Olszewski W L, Rowinski W. Blood mononuclear cell production of IL-1 and IL-2 following moderate surgical trauma. *Eur Surg Res* 1989;21:114–122.

149. Duncan J J, Moldawer L L, Bistrian B R,

Blackburn G L. *In vitro* leukocyte and endogenous mediator production is not impaired following surgical stress in moderately malnourished patients. *JPEN J Parenter Enteral Nutr* 1984;8:174–177.

150. Shenkin A, Fraser W D, Series J, et al. The serum interleukin 6 responses to elective surgery. *Lymphokine Res* 1989;8:123–127.

151. Pullicino E A, Carli F, Poole S, Rafferty B, Malik S T A, Elia M. The relationship between circulating concentrations of interleukin 6 (IL-6), tumor necrosis factor (TNF) and the acute phase response to elective surgery and accidental injury. *Lymphokine Res* 1990;9:231–238.

152. Akiyoshi T, Koba F, Arinaga S, Miyazaki S, Wada T, Tsuji H. Impaired production of interleukin 2 after surgery. *Clin Exp Immunol* 1985;59:45–49.

153. Faist E, Ertel W, Cohnert T, Huber P, Inthorn D, Heberer G. Immunoprotective effects of cyclooxygenase inhibition in patients with major surgical trauma. *J Trauma* 1990;30:8–18.

154. Faist E, Ertel W, Mewes A, Alkan S, Walz A, Strasser T. Trauma-induced alterations of the lymphokine cascade. In: Faist E, Ninnemann J, Green D, eds. *Immune consequences of trauma, shock, and sepsis.* Berlin: Springer-Verlag, 1989:79–94.

155. Teodorczyk-Injeyan J A, McRitchie D I, Peters W J, Lalani S, Girotti M J. Expression and secretion of Il-2 receptor in trauma patients. *Ann Surg* 1990;212:202–208.

156. Brivio F, Lissoni P, Mancini D, et al. Effect of antitumor surgery on soluble interleukin 2 receptor serum levels. *Am J Surg* 1991;161;466–469.

157. Abraham E, Freitas A A. Hemorrhage produces abnormalities in lymphocyte function and lymphokine generation. *J Immunol* 1989;142:899–906.

158. Michie H R, Wilmore D W. Sepsis, signals, and surgical sequelae (a hypothesis). *Arch Surg* 1990;125:531–536.

159. Faist E, Mewes A, Baker C C, et al. Prostaglandin E_2 (PGE$_2$)-dependent suppression of interleukin $_\alpha$ (IL-2) production in patients with major trauma. *J Trauma* 1987;27:837–848.

160. Zapata-Sirvent R, Hansbrough J F, Bartle E J. Prevention of posttraumatic alterations in lymphocyte subpopulations in mice by immunomodulating drugs. *Arch Surg* 1986;121:116–122.

161. Hansbrough J, Peterson V, Zapata-Sirvent R, Claman H N. Postburn immunosuppression in an animal model. II. Restoration of cell-mediated immunity by immunomodulating drugs. *Surgery* 1984;95:290–296.

162. Livingstone D H, Appel S H, Wellhausen S R, Sonnenfeld G, Polk H C Jr. Depressed interferon gamma production and monocyte HLA-DR expression after severe injury. *Arch Surg* 1988;123:1309–1312.

163. Markovic S N, Knight P R, Murasko D M. Inhibition of interferon stimulation of natural killer cell activity in mice anesthetized with halothane or isoflurane. *Anesthesiology* 1993;78:700–706.

164. Salo M, Nissilä M. Cell-mediated and humoral immune responses to total hip replacement under spinal or general anaesthesia. *Acta Anaesth Scand* 1990;34:241–248.

165. Eskola J, Salo M, Viljanen M K, Ruuskanen O. Impaired B lymphocyte function during open heart surgery. Effects of anaesthesia and surgery. *Br J Anaesth* 1984;56:333–338.

166. Cohnen G. Changes in immunoglobulin levels after surgical trauma. *J Trauma* 1972;12:249–254.

167. Rem J, Nielsen O S, Brandt M R, Kehlet H. Release mechanisms of postoperative changes in various acute phase proteins and immunoglobulins. *Acta Chir Scand* 1980;502:51–56.

168. Grob P, Holch M, Fierz W, Glinz W, Geroulanos S. Immunodeficiency after major trauma and selective surgery. *Pediatr Infect Dis J* 1988;7:S37–S42.

169. Stevenson G W, Hall S C, Miller P J, et al. The effect of anesthetics agents on human immune system function. I. Design of a system to deliver inhalational anesthetics agents to leukocyte cultures *in vitro*. *J Immunol Methods* 1986;88:277–283.

170. Kinnaert P, Mahieu A, van Geertruyden N. Stimulation of antibody synthesis induced by surgical trauma in rats. *Clin Exp Immunol* 1978;32:243–252.

171. Kinnaert P, Mahieu A, van Geertruyden N. Stimulation of antibody synthesis induced by surgical trauma in rats. Revised statistical analysis. *Clin Exp Immunol* 1979;37:174–175.

172. Kinnaert P, Mahieu A, van Geertruyden N. Effect of surgical procedures on the humoral responsiveness of rats. *Surg Gynecol Obstet* 1980;151:85–88.

173. Cooper A J, Irvine J M, Turnbull A R. Depression of immunological responses due to surgery. *Immunology* 1974;27:393–399.

174. Markley K, Smallman E, Evans G. Antibody production in mice after thermal and tourniquet trauma. *Surgery* 1967;61:896–903.

175. Ferrero E, Ferrero M D, Marni A, et al. *In vitro* effects of halothane on lymphocytes. *Eur J Anaesthesiol* 1986;3:321–330.

176. Hansbrough J F, Zapata-Sirvent R L, Bartle E J, et al. Alterations in splenic lymphocyte subpopulations and increased mortality from sepsis following anesthesia in mice. *Anesthesiology* 1985;63:267–273.

177. Tubaro E, Borelli G, Croce C, Cavallo G, Santiangeli C. Effect of morphine on resistance to infection. *J Infect Dis* 1983;148:656–666.

178. Knight P R, Bedows E, Narhrwold M L, Maassab H F, Smitka C W, Busch M T. Alterations in influenza virus pulmonary pathology induced by diethyl ether, halothane, enflurane, and pentobarbital anesthesia in mice. *Anesthesiology* 1983;58:209–215.

179. Tait A R, Du Boulay P M, Knight P R. Alterations in the course of and histopathologic response to influenza virus infections produced

by enflurane, halothane, and diethyl ether anesthesia in ferrets. *Anesth Analg* 1988;67: 671–676.

180. MacLean L D. Host resistance in surgical patients. *J Trauma* 1979;19:297–304.

181. Daly J M, Dudrick S J, Copeland E M III. Intravenous hyperalimentation. Effect on delayed cutaneous hypersensitivity in cancer patients. *Ann Surg* 1980;192:587–592.

182. Christou N V, Tellado J M. *In vitro* polymorphonuclear neutrophil function in surgical patients does not correlate with anergy but with "activating" processes such as sepsis or trauma. *Surgery* 1989;106:718–724.

183. O'Mahony J B, Palder S B, Wood J J, et al. Depression of cellular immunity after multiple trauma in the absence of sepsis. *J Trauma* 1984;24:869–875.

184. Heideman M, Saravis C, Clowes G H A. Effect of nonviable tissue and abscesses on complement depletion and the development of bacteremia. *J Trauma* 1982;22:527–532.

185. Meakins J L, Pietsch J B, Christou N V, MacLean L D. Predicting surgical infection before the operation. *World J Surg* 1980;4:439–450.

186. LaRaja R D, Rothenberg R E, Odom J W, Mueller S C. The incidence of intraabdominal surgery in acquired immunodeficiency syndrome: a statistical review of 904 patients. *Surgery* 1989;105:175–179.

187. Eykyn S J, Braimbridge M V. Open heart surgery complicated by postoperative malaria. *Lancet* 1977;ii:411–412.

188. Agostino D, Cliffton E E. Anaesthetic effect on pulmonary metastases in rats. *Arch Surg* 1964; 88:735.

189. Schatten W E, Kramer W M. An experimental study of postoperative tumor metastases. II: Effect of anesthesia, operation and cortisone administration on growth of pulmonary metastases. *Cancer* 1958;11:460.

190. Moudgil G C, Frame B, Blajchman M A, Singal D P. Effects of anaesthesia on tumour metastasis. *Can Anaesth Soc J* 1990;38:A127.

191. Vose B M, Moudgil G C. Effect of surgery on tumor-directed leucocyte responses. *Br Med J* 1975;1:56–58.

192. Kumar J, Taylor G. Effect of surgery on lymphocytotoxicity against tumor cells. *Lancet* 1974;i:1564.

193. Kemp A S, Berke G. Inhibition of lymphocyte-mediated cytolysis by the local anesthetics benzyl and salicyl alcohol. *Eur J Immunol* 1973;3:674–677.

194. Lee S K, Singh J, Taylor R B. Subclasses of T cells with different sensitivities to cytotoxic antibody in the presence of anesthetics. *Eur J Immunol* 1975;5:259.

195. Jewell W R, Romsdahl M M. Recurrent malignant disease in operative wounds not due to surgical implantation from the resected tumor. *Surgery* 1965;58:806–809.

196. Lange P H, Hekmat K, Bosl G, Kennedy B J, Fraley E E. Accelerated growth of testicular cancer after cytoreductive surgery. *Cancer* 1978;45:1498–1506.

197. Stevenson H C. Tumor immunology. In: Virella G, Goust J M, Fudenberg H H, Patrick C P, eds. *Introduction to medical immunology.* New York: Marcel Dekker, 1989.

198. Koenig A, Koenig U D, Heicappel R, Stoeckel H. Differences in lymphocyte mitogenic stimulation pattern depending on anaesthesia and operative trauma: I. Halothane-nitrous oxide anaesthesia. *Eur J Anaesth* 1987;4:17–24.

199. Cullen B F, van Belle G. Lymphocyte transformation and changes in leukocyte count: effects of anesthesia and operation. *Anesthesiology* 1975;43:563–569.

200. Abraham E, Regan R F. The effects of hemorrhage and trauma on interleukin 2 production. *Arch Surg* 1985;120:1341–1344.

201. Cruickshank A M, Jennings G, Fearon K H, Elia M, Shenkin A. Serum interleukin 6 (IL-6)—effect of surgery and undernutrition. *Cli Nutr* 1991;10(suppl):65–69.

202. Kinnaert P, Mahieu A, Mahieu M, et al. Effect of surgical trauma on delayed type hypersensitivity. *J Surg Res* 1983;34:227–230.

203. Abraham E, Chang Y-H. Effects of hemorrhage on the inflammatory response. *Arch Surg* 1984; 119:1154–1157.

204. Bjornson A B, Bjornson H S, Altemeier W A. Serum-mediated inhibition of polymorphonuclear leukocyte function following burn injury. *Ann Surg* 1981;194:568–575.

205. Abraham E, Lee R J, Chang Y-H. The role of interleukin 2 in hemorrhage-induced abnormalities of lymphocyte proliferation. *Circ Shock* 1986;18:205–213.

206. Rodrick M L, Wood J J, Grbic J T, et al. Defective IL-2 production in patients with severe burn and sepsis. *Lymphokine Res* 1986;5: S75–80.

207. Brody J I, Pickering N J, Fink G B, Behr E D. Altered lymphocyte subsets during cardiopulmonary bypass. *Am J Clin Pathol* 1987;87:626–628.

208. Pollock R, Ames F, Rubio P, et al. Protracted severe immune dysregulation induced by cardiopulmonary bypass: a predisposing etiologic factor in blood transfusion-related AIDS? *J Clin Lab Immunol* 1987;22:1–5.

209. Finlayson D C, Zaidan J R, Hunter R L, Check I, Levy J H. Serum protein changes during cardiopulmonary bypass: implications for host defence. *Perfusion* 1990;5:101–106.

210. Knudsen F, Andersen L W. Immunological aspects of cardiopulmonary bypass. *J Cardiothorac Anesth* 1990;4:245–258.

211. Abraham E, Freitas A A. Hemorrhage in mice induces alterations in immunoglobulin-secreting B cells. *Crit Care Med* 1989;17: 1015–1019.

212. Abraham E, Chang Y-H. Hemorrhage in mice produces alterations in intestinal B cell repertoires. *Cell Immunol* 1990;128:165–174.

213. Abraham E. Physiological stress and cellular ischemia: relationship to immunosuppression

and susceptibility to sepsis. *Crit Care Med* 1991;19:613–618.

214. Deitch E A. Gut failure: its role in the multiple organ failure syndrome. In: Deitch E A, ed. *Multiple organ failure*. New York: Thieme Verlag, 1990:40–59.

215. Chaudry I H, Stephan R N, Harkema J M, Dean R E. Immunological alterations following simple hemorrhage. In: Faist E, Ninnemann J, Green D, eds. *Immune consequences of trauma, shock, and sepsis*. Berlin: Springer-Verlag, 1989:363–373.

216. Salo M. Immunosuppressive effects of blood transfusion in anaesthesia and surgery. *Acta Anaesth Scand* 1988;32(suppl 89):26–34.

217. Opelz G. Current relevance of the transfusion effect in renal transplantation. *Transplant Proc* 1985;17:1015–1022.

218. Dawes L G, Aprahamian C, Condon R E, Malangoni M A. The risk of infection after colon injury. *Surgery* 1986;100:796–803.

219. Tartter P I, Driefuss R M, Malon A M, Heimann T M, Aufses A H. Relationship of postoperative septic complications and blood transfusion in patients with Crohn's disease. *Am J Surg* 1988;155:43–48.

220. Maetani S, Nishikawa T, Hirakawa A, Tobe T. Role of blood transfusion in organ system failure following major abdominal surgery. *Ann Surg* 1986;203:275–281.

221. Shelby J, Hisatake G. Effect of ibuprofen and interleukin 2 on transfusion-induced suppression of cell-mediated immunity. *Arch Surg* 1988;123:1397–1399.

222. Nielsen H J, Hammer J H, Moesgaard F, Kehlet H. Ranitidine prevents postoperative transfusion-induced depression of delayed hypersensitivity. *Surgery* 1989;105:711–717.

223. Waymack J P, Miskell P, Gonce S. Alterations in host defense associated with inhalation anesthesia and blood transfusion. *Anesth Analg* 1989;69:163–168.

224. Galandiuk S, George C D, Pietsch J D, Byck D C, DeWeese R C, Polk H C Jr. An experimental assessment of the effect of blood transfusion on susceptibility to bacterial infection. *Surgery* 1990;108:567–571.

225. Waymack J P, Fernandes G, Cappelli P J, et al. Alterations in host defense associated with anesthesia and blood transfusions. II. Effect on response to endotoxin. *Arch Surg* 1991;126:59–62.

226. Yones R N, Rogatko A, Vydelingum N A, Brennan M F. Effects of hypovolemia and transfusion on tumor growth in MCA-tumor-bearing rats. *Surgery* 1991;109:307–312.

227. Parrott N R, Lennard T W J, Taylor R M R, Proud G, Shenton B K, Johnston I D A. Effect of perioperative blood transfusion on recurrence of colorectal cancer. *Br J Surg* 1986;73:970–973.

228. Kampschöer G H M, Maruyama K J, Sasako M, Kinoshita T, van de Velde C J H. The effects of blood transfusion on the prognosis of patients with gastric cancer. *World J Surg* 1989;13:637–643.

229. Wobbes Th, Bemelmans B L H, Kuypers J H C, Beerthuizen G I J M, Theeuwes A G M. Risk of postoperative septic complications after abdominal surgical treatment in relation to perioperative blood transfusion. *Surg Gynecol Obstet* 1990;171:59–62.

230. Hauser W E Jr, Remington J S. Effect of antibiotics on the immune response. *Am J Med* 1982;72:711–716.

231. Miller T E, North D K. Clinical infections, antibiotics and immunosuppression: a puzzling relationship. *Am J Med* 1981;71:334–336.

232. Prete P, Levin E R, Pedram A. The *in vitro* effects of endogenous opiates on natural killer cells, antigen-specific cytolytic T cells, and T-cell subsets. *Exp Neurol* 1986;92:349–359.

233. Shavit Y, Lewis J W, Terman G W, Gale R P, Liebeskind J C. Opioid peptides mediate the suppressive effects of stress on natural killer cell cytotoxicity. *Science* 1984;223:188–190.

234. Bryant H U, Bernton E W, Holaday J W. Morphine pellet-induced immunomodulation in mice: temporal relationships. *J Pharmacol Exp Ther* 1988;245:913–920.

235. Yahya D M, Watson R R. Minireview immunomodulation by morphine and marijuana. *Life Sci* 1987;41:2503–2510.

236. Mukwaya G. Immunosuppressive effects and infections associated with corticosteroid therapy. *Pediatr Infect Dis J* 1988;7:499–504.

237. Posey W C, Nelson H S, Branch B, Pearlman D S. The effects of acute corticosteroid therapy for asthma on serum immunoglobulin levels. *J Allergy Clin Immunol* 1978;62:340–348.

238. Bone R C, Fisher C J, Clemmer T P, et al. A controlled clinical trial of high-dose methylprednisolone in the treatment of severe sepsis and septic shock. *N Engl J Med* 1987;317:653–658.

239. Veterans Administration Systemic Sepsis Cooperative Study Group. Effect of high-dose glucocorticoid therapy on mortality in patients with clinical signs of systemic sepsis. *N Engl J Med* 1987;317:659–665.

240. Moudgil G C, Singal D P, Gordon J, Forrest J B. Effects of steroids and barbiturate therapy on the immune response *in vitro*. *Anesthesiology* 1984;61:A128.

241. Scordamaglia A, Ciprandi G, Ruffoni S, et al. Brief communications: theophylline and the immune response: *in vitro* and *in vivo* effects. *Clin Immunol Immunopathol* 1988;48:238–246.

242. Peura D A, Johnson L F. Cimetidine for prevention and treatment of gastroduodenal mucosal lesions in patients in an intensive care unit. *Ann Intern Med* 1985;103:173–177.

243. Lanza F L, Sibley C M. Role of antacids in the management of disorders of the upper gastrointestinal tract: review of clinical experience 1975–1985. *Am J Gastroenterol* 1987;82:1223–1241.

244. Ershler W B, Hacker M P, Burroughs B J, Moore A L, Myers C F. Cimetidine and the immune response. *Clin Immunol Immunopathol* 1983;26:10–17.

Anesthetic Toxicity, edited by
Susan A. Rice and Kevin J. Fish.
Raven Press, Ltd., New York © 1994.

14

Pulmonary Effects of Anesthesia

Brian P. Kavanagh and Ronald G. Pearl

*Department of Anesthesia, Stanford University School of Medicine,
Stanford, California 94305*

The pulmonary effects of anesthetics arise from the physiologic alterations in neural and muscular control, changes in pulmonary vascular and airway tone, and alterations in ciliary function and lung mechanics. The direct toxicology of anesthetics on the pulmonary system constitutes a minor area of research because of the clear absence of clinical pulmonary toxicity associated with modern anesthetic practice. With the exception of i.v. administration of liquid volatile anesthetics, pulmonary toxicity of anesthetics has been described only in animal models using obsolete agents, frequently in high doses, and with pharmacologic manipulation designed to maximize the production of toxic metabolites. This chapter, therefore, focuses on the adverse pulmonary physiologic and pathophysiologic changes associated with anesthesia with regard to pulmonary mechanics, the pulmonary vasculature, airway caliber, direct anesthetic pulmonary toxicity, airway irritation, ciliary function, and oxygen toxicity.

PULMONARY MECHANICS

General anesthesia involves the use of i.v. and inhaled agents, frequently in conjunction with muscle paralysis. This section concentrates on the effects of general anesthetics on lung mechanics. The effects of anesthesia on central nervous system (CNS) control of respiration and on the tone of the upper airway have been the subject of excellent reviews (1,2).

Induction of anesthesia is associated consistently with a reduction in the functional residual capacity (FRC) of approximately 18% (3). This decrease in FRC is not altered by neuromuscular blockade, and further reduction in FRC at time periods after the induction of anesthesia is minimal. The use of high fractional inspired concentrations of O_2 (FIO_2) does not accentuate the reduction in FRC. The reduction in FRC associated with induction of anesthesia is not observed in semi-recumbent patients (4). The etiology of the reduction of FRC is unclear, but several mechanisms have been proposed, including altered thoracic cage recoil, cephalad displacement of the diaphragm, altered recoil of the pulmonary parenchyma, and redistribution of the intrathoracic blood volume (5,6). The measurement of many of these variables was not consistent between studies and may have resulted in bias in the interpretation of results.

Reduction of chest wall recoil is suggested by two findings: partial paralysis by itself in the absence of anesthesia results in reduced FRC, and induction of anesthesia is associated with a loss of tone in several inspiratory muscle groups (7). Although cephalad displacement of the diaphragm has been documented following induction of anesthesia (8), this effect does not appear to be a consistent finding (9). Nonetheless, cephalad diaphragmatic displacement does appear to occur as a direct effect of induction of anesthesia, as opposed to a secondary effect of alteration in the recoil properties of either the thoracic cage or the abdomen. The possibility that the reduced FRC is due to increased lung recoil of the pulmonary parenchyma is thought to be unlikely because chest wall tension rather than lung parenchymal tension is altered by anesthesia (10). Thus, increased pulmonary recoil may occur as a result of losses in FRC rather than being the actual cause of the reduction in FRC. Increased expiratory muscle tone may occur during anesthesia from elevations in abdominal muscle activity. However, the use of muscular paralysis does not reduce the diminution in FRC, which would be anticipated if increased expiratory muscle tone was responsible. An altered distribution of central blood volume has been proposed as a potential mechanism to explain reductions in the FRC. Studies using radiolabeled erythrocytes suggest, however, that there is no net redistribution of central thoracic or abdominal blood volumes under halothane anesthesia (5).

The consequences of reduced FRC can be considered under two main topics: alterations of pulmonary gas exchange and alterations of pulmonary airflow resistance and compliance. Compression atelectasis, as diagnosed by serial computer-assisted tomographic examinations, occurs following i.v. or inhalational anesthesia, although not in patients with significant chronic obstructive lung disease (11) or in patients receiving i.v. ketamine for induction of anesthesia (12). With compression atelectasis, there are areas of increased density observed in the caudal portions of the lungs that contribute to increased intrapulmonary shunting (10). Although application of positive end-expiratory pressure (PEEP) reverses these areas of microatelectasis, it does not reliably improve the impairment in gas exchange. Reduction of FRC below the pulmonary closing volume results in lung airway closure, with resultant shunting of pulmonary blood through hypoventilated lung units. Maneuvers designed to increase the FRC, such as PEEP, produce little improvement in arterial oxygenation because the nonperfused areas are preferentially expanded. Much pulmonary tissue may not develop either airway closure or compression atelectasis but may, nevertheless, have extremely low ventilation to perfusion ($\dot{V}/\dot{Q}$) ratios on a regional basis, resulting in impairment in systemic oxygenation.

As FRC decreases, the airway pressure tends to increase. Increases in airway pressure may be further exacerbated by either increases in resistance due to the presence of an endotracheal tube or by the development of upper airway obstruction at the level of the pharynx or larynx. It appears, however, that these effects may be offset by the potent bronchodilator effects of the inhaled volatile agents used in anesthesia. This is the case during anesthesia for young healthy patients with normal body habitus, but patients with obesity or preexisting obstructive lung disease may develop significant net elevations in airway pressure.

In addition to the changes described, the decreased FRC caused by induction of anesthesia is associated with approximately a 20% reduction in pulmonary compliance. Factors contributing to this decreased compliance (representing pulmonary as opposed to thoracic cage alterations) may include alterations in surfactant activity. Decreased compliance is likely the result of a shift in the pulmonary pressure–volume relationships due to decreased FRC. The consequences of this reduction in pulmonary compliance include increased $\dot{V}/\dot{Q}$ mismatching because of regions of atelectasis and increased work of breathing. When intermittent positive pressure ventilation is used, the decreased compliance may be associated with increases in airway pressure. In contrast with the inhalational agents or other i.v. agents, i.v. ketamine does not alter pulmonary compliance (13).

Physiologic dead space increases with anesthesia primarily due to increases in alveolar dead space. This may result in the development of a higher proportion of zone 1 conditions (ventilated areas that are not being perfused) as a result of increased mean airway pressure or ventilation of areas with existing high $\dot{V}/\dot{Q}$ ratios.

ANESTHESIA AND THE PULMONARY VASCULATURE

Many reviews have focused on the effects of general anesthesia on the pulmonary vasculature (14,15). This section focuses on the vascular causes of impaired gas exchange during anesthesia and then briefly reviews the available data on the specific effects of anesthesia on the pulmonary vasculature.

The initial interest in the pulmonary vascular effects of anesthesia stemmed from the original observations by Marshall et al. (16) and Nunn (17) that breathing halothane (1% to 4%) resulted in an increase in venous admixture from a normal value of less than 5% to approximately 14%. These increases persisted in the postoperative period, and during this period, the resultant hypoxemia was due to a persistently increased level of venous admixture rather than to respiratory depression. Comparison of inhaled and i.v. anesthetics confirms that diminished oxygenation during general anesthesia is not fully accounted for by the observed alterations in pulmonary mechanics. Intravenous and inhalational anesthesia result in similar alterations in pulmonary mechanics, as outlined previously, but volatile agents result in greater degrees of hypoxemia compared with equipotent concentrations of i.v. anesthesia. There is, therefore, an additional effect of volatile anesthetic agents, which results in decreased oxygenation, but not on the basis of altered lung mechanics.

Research to date has focused on the effects of general anesthesia on hypoxic pulmonary vasoconstriction (HPV). HPV may be defined as local pulmonary vasoconstriction occurring in response to regional alveolar hypoxia. The reduced local perfusion results in diminished shunting of pulmonary blood flow through underventilated areas. Several important facts are known about the physiology of HPV. Marshall and Marshall (18) investigated the principal determinants of magnitude of HPV. They found that alterations in alveolar P_{O_2} (P_{AO_2}) were more important than changes in mixed venous P_{O_2} ($P\bar{v}_{O_2}$), although both influenced the degree of HPV response. These data indicated that the site of action of HPV was probably at the level of the small pulmonary arteries. Th exact mechanisms of HPV have not been fully elucidated, but the effect may in part be mediated by calcium-dependent channels located in the precapillary pulmonary arterioles. These mechanisms have been reviewed recently by Pearl (15).

HPV may be considered as comprising three separate systems: on O_2 sensor, a transducer, and an effector system. Reduced nicotinamide adenine dinucleotide phosphate (NADPH) oxidase may represent the O_2 sensor system in the lung, just as it is known to do in the carotid body. Potassium channels may be involved in the transduction and effector systems, as hypoxia can inhibit calcium-sensitive potassium channels in canine pulmonary artery cells (19). Stimulation of these cells results in reduced potassium conductance and depolarization, with subsequent calcium entry and vascular smooth muscle contraction.

The role of mechanical factors in the autoregulatory response to lobar atelectasis has been investigated (20). In pulmonary atelectasis, the major cause of flow diversion is active HPV, not compression secondary to reductions in the lobar volume.

The extent of the hypoxic area also is important in determining the extent of the HPV response (21). As the area of alveolar hypoxemia is increased, the extent of the HPV, as inferred by flow diversion and by increases in measured pulmonary artery pressure, also increases. Maximum HPV responses occur at P_{AO_2} values of approximately 30 mm Hg. HPV is unimportant when either very small or very large areas of lung tissue are rendered hypoxic (22). The major clinical importance of HPV is in cases where moderate amounts of lung tissue are hypoxic, as in cases of single-lung ventilation.

The specific effects of anesthesia can now be considered. Assessment of the effects of individual anesthetic agents on the pulmonary vasculature has been complicated by the myriad of different models used. A modification of the proposed classification (22) of the models used in the investigation of HPV is as follows: human, *in vitro*, and *in vivo*, with the latter subdivided into intact (closed-chest) and nonintact (open-chest) versions.

Although there are confounding factors, such as the effects of anesthetic agents on cardiac output and mixed venous hemoglobin saturation ($S\bar{v}_{O_2}$), the human studies of HPV are likely to be the most relevant to the clinical situation. An uncontrolled case series examined the effects of i.v. ketamine anesthesia on oxygenation with double-lung followed by single-lung ventilation (23). No patients developed Pa_{O_2} of less than 70 mm Hg, and the mean Pa_{O_2} was 130 mm Hg during one-lung ventilation with 100% O_2. The results were considered by the authors to indicate that i.v. ketamine infusion was an acceptable alternative to volatile agents for the anesthetic management of single-lung anesthesia. Contrary evidence was provided by a study that compared i.v. ketamine with a control group who received inhaled enflurane for single-lung anesthesia (24). Rees and Gaines measured shunt fraction (Q_s/Q_t) in addition to Pa_{O_2} and reported no significant differences between these variables in the two study groups during single-lung ventilation (24).

The pulmonary effects of the addition of halothane or isoflurane to an i.v. anesthetic regimen consisting of either ketamine or methohexital was studied by Rogers and Benumof in a series of patients undergoing thoracic surgery (25). The authors concluded that there was no difference between the i.v. and inhaled agents in terms of arterial oxygenation. Another group determined that the addition of either isoflurane (26) or enflurane (27) in low concentrations did not significantly affect the reduction in pulmonary blood flow observed in response to unilateral ventilation with a hypoxic gas mixture. Discontinuation of halothane and conversion to an i.v. regimen consisting of thiopental, fentanyl, and diazepam resulted in significant improvements in arterial oxygenation and reductions in Q_s/Q_t (28). Similar directional, but not statistically significant, changes were observed when isoflurane rather than the i.v. regimen was substituted for halothane. The magnitude of the observed effects led the authors to suggest that the inhibition of HPV by volatile agents was modest. Controversy in terms of the correct interpretation of the data, possibly caused by the small sample sizes and minor observed effects, resulted from this work.

Overall, there appears to be a general consensus that commonly used i.v. anesthetic agents do not significantly impair HPV, although some of the newer i.v. agents have not been studied. Furthermore, it appears that the effects of volatile agents are minimal if used in low concentrations. Significant difficulty in interpretation of the diverse data has resulted from failure to control for alterations in cardiac output and changes in $P\bar{v}_{O_2}$. Two studies using *in vivo* intact models have added to the controversy (29,30). Domino et al. examined the effects of increasing concentrations of inhaled isoflurane on HPV in a closed-chest canine model and controlled fluctuations in the cardiac output by altering the amount of blood flow through an artificial arteriovenous fistula (29). They found that the percentage depression of HPV was linearly related to the alveolar concentration of isoflurane. These data did not confirm the findings of Sykes et al. who found that low concentrations of inhaled halothane had no significant effect on HPV (30).

Studies from multiple centers using a range of models have resulted in confusion about the effects of volatile agents on HPV. Studies have suggested that volatile agents either inhibit, have no effects on, or actually potentiate HPV (22). These inconsistencies between these studies may be related to possible inherent differences in the actual agents used, intraspecies variations, differences in the models used, failure to control for altered physiologic variables, and methodologic differences in measurement of blood flow, cardiac output, and venous admixture.

Because of the assumed critical importance of HPV in patients under general anesthesia and the assumption that the commonly used volatile anesthetic agents may inhibit HPV to some extent, various drugs have been used in an attempt to potentiate HPV. High-dose almitrine bimesylate, a carotid body stimulant, has been assessed in canine models (31). High-dose almitrine was associated with potent pulmonary vasoconstriction, but this vasoconstriction was most marked in areas of low pulmonary vascular tone. The net effects of almitrine, at these doses and in this model, were to increase the overall pulmonary vascular resistance but worsen the matching of ventilation and perfusion. A study in nonanesthetized patients with chronic obstructive pulmonary disease (COPD) has demonstrated that almitrine may improve arterial oxygenation, even in the absence of demonstrable effects on respiratory drive or minute ventilation (32). Other authors have examined the effects of prostacyclin (PGI_2) and leukotrienes in the modulation of HPV under anesthesia (33,34). No clear consensus has emerged on the roles of these mediators in HPV, but this again may be due to methodologic or species differences or both. A lack of HPV responsiveness to nitrous oxide (N_2O) was restored following administration of acetylsalicylic acid (ASA), suggesting a role for cyclooxygenase products in the development of HPV (35). A consensus on the role of leukotrienes suggests that they appear not to be mediators of HPV but rather play a role in modulating the magnitude of the response in a species- and model-dependent manner (36,37).

AIRWAY CALIBER

Understanding the factors regulating airway caliber during anesthesia is important. Reduction of airway caliber, sometimes referred to as bronchospasm, may occur during anesthesia and surgery, especially following instrumentation of the larynx and trachea in a patient with asthma or chronic bronchitis. If the airway constriction is significant, it may become difficult or impossible to ventilate the lungs, thereby endangering the patient's life. Knowledge of the mechanisms involved in bronchospasm is necessary for the effective prevention and reversal of this potentially life-threatening condition.

Airway caliber is modulated by three basic factors: intraluminal, mural, and extramural components. Extramural compression is usually the result of a compressive mass and is generally of acute significance only when a large proximal airway is compromised. The intraluminal component consists of secretions and occasional debris, and the mural component consists of the airway smooth muscle tone and the degree of mucosal edema. Most research in recent years has focused on the mechanisms of airway smooth muscle constriction.

The cellular basis for many of these events has been outlined by Hirshman and Bergman (38). The biochemical events underlying airway smooth muscle tone are complex. Signal transduction following receptor activation is now known to involve activation of several post-receptor signaling systems, many of which are interdependent. These include G-proteins, cyclic nucleotides (cAMP, cGMP), protein kinase A, inositol phosphate compounds, and ionized calcium. This myriad of second messenger systems allows interaction between the products of beta-adrenergic receptor and muscarinic cholinergic receptor stimulation. This is thought to result in bronchomotor tone being modulated by alterations in the cytosolic level of ionized calcium.

The extracellular mechanisms that regulate these intracellular processes are equally complex and have been reviewed in detail (39). The effects of the CNS on airway caliber are complex and result from regulation of vagal (parasympathetic) tone via reflex mechanisms. Vagal efferent fibers release acetylcholine, which results in bronchoconstriction. Although there is no direct sympathetic innervation of the bronchial tree, CNS-mediated alterations in the levels of circulating catecholamines (epinephrine rather than norepinephrine) counterbalance the parasympathetic vagal effects. Recently, novel neuropeptides have been described that mediate these effects via noncholinergic, nonadrenergic mechanisms. Vasoactive intestinal polypeptide (VIP), substance P, and a range of tachykinins form a heterogeneous group and have varied effects on bronchomotor tone. VIP results in bronchodilation, and its control is not yet fully understood. Substance P and tachykinins result in bronchoconstriction and may further exacerbate reductions in airway caliber through mediation of acute inflammatory responses resulting in mucosal edema. Furthermore, tachykinins are cleared by endopeptidase enzymes, and thus mucosal disruption or damage may increase the bronchoconstrictive effects (40). Finally, mucosal edema, reflecting acute airway inflammatory changes, has a potent effect on narrowing the airway lumen.

The inhalational agents halothane, enflurane, and isoflurane were considered to have comparable bronchodilating effects with similar mechanisms of action (41,42).

Recent work has cast doubt on these assumptions. Brown et al. (43) used high-resolution computer-assisted tomography to compare the bronchodilator effects of halothane and isoflurane. Halothane and isoflurane dilated histamine-constricted airways in a dose-dependent manner, but halothane was a more potent bronchodilator. Many sites of action are possible for these agents. Korenaga et al. reported that neural release of acetylcholine was reduced with halothane, resulting in a reduced intensity of muscular contraction (44). Others reported that equipotent concentrations of halothane and isoflurane had minimal direct effects on airway tone (45). Further data from a canine model suggested that halothane was equivalent to atropine in the prevention of histamine-induced bronchoconstriction and that there was no synergism demonstrable between the two agents. This suggested that halothane may mediate bronchodilation by inhibition of vagal reflexes. A study using isolated second and third order canine bronchial rings, which had been preconstricted with acetylcholine, serotonin, or electrical field stimulation, elegantly demonstrated that halothane-induced bronchodilation is not dependent on the presence of airway epithelium (46).

Halothane has not been shown previously to alter the basal beta-adrenergic tone (38), and the only evidence for a direct effect of halothane on basal smooth muscle tone was in the context of excessively high levels of halothane. High-resolution computed tomography, which is devoid of the direct irritant effects inherent in the traditionally used tantalum bronchography, has shed more light on these mechanisms (47). Brown et al., using this novel technique, demonstrated that halothane regulates canine airway caliber by blockade of basal vagal tone (47). The prevailing consensus appears to be that at clinically relevant concentrations, all volatile agents have potent bronchodilating effects. A single study reporting that isoflurane may actually increase baseline bronchomotor tone (48) may have been interpreted falsely because of several confounding issues, including the effects of reduction of FRC with induction of anesthesia and the irritating effects of an endotracheal tube (38).

The mechanisms of action of ketamine-induced bronchodilation are not limited to inhibition of neural reflexes but also include vagal inhibition, direct relaxation of airway smooth muscle, and increases in the levels of circulating catecholamines, resulting in heightened beta-adrenergic effect (38). Ketamine has been shown to prevent induced bronchospasm in a greyhound model (49). That study demonstrated that the prevention of bronchospasm was mediated through a beta-adrenergic mechanism.

Barbiturates in large doses can prevent endotracheal tube-induced reflex broncho-constriction (38). Light anesthesia in conjunction with thiobarbiturates maintains airway reflexes (50). It is likely that clinically used doses of thiobarbiturates may result in direct bronchoconstriction but that higher doses result in bronchodilation (38). Bronchoconstriction is not observed with the use of the non-thiobarbiturates.

Nondepolarizing neuromuscular blocking drugs are muscarinic agonists, two of which (D-tubocurarine, atracurium) are clinically associated with histamine release. D-Tubocurarine is associated with increases in airway resistance when compared with pancuronium (51). However, as Hirshman and Bergman have discussed, histamine levels were not reported in that study, and the effects of histamine antagonists were not assessed (38). Anticholinergics, which are used to reverse the effects of nondepolarizing muscle blockade, result in an increase in the local concentration of acetylcholine. This increased acetylcholine concentration may increase bronchomotor tone through parasympathomimetic effects. The greater understanding of the complexity of muscarinic cholinergic receptor subtypes and the availability of specific agonists and antagonists may assist in the elucidation of mechanisms and the development of a new gen-

eration of therapies. Overall, the effects of nondepolarizing relaxants on bronchomotor tone are minimal, and histamine release can be minimized by the use of slow infusion rates for these agents.

PULMONARY TOXICITY OF GENERAL ANESTHETICS

Compared with the extensive literature describing hepatic or renal toxicity associated with anesthesia, the pulmonary toxicity of general anesthetic agents has received little attention. Instead, interest has focused on the physiologic and functional pulmonary changes associated with anesthesia. This has occurred because direct pulmonary toxicity in the absence of other causes does not seem to occur as a consequence of administration of the modern inhaled anesthetics.

The pulmonary toxicity of the volatile agents was described initially with the observation of fluroxene (2,2,2-trifluroethyl-vinyl ether) toxicity. Because of the association of human fluroxene toxicity with the use of microsomal enzyme-inducing drugs, Murson et al. examined the effects of phenobarbiturate pretreatment on the development of toxicity secondary to fluroxene or its metabolites in Rhesus monkeys (52). The animals were exposed to inhaled flourxene at an estimated alveolar concentration of 5.5%. Biochemical and histologic data from all of the major organ systems, including the lungs, were recorded. There was no evidence of pulmonary toxicity. When the animals were pretreated with phenobarbital, subsequent fluroxene exposure was associated with fatal lung toxicity in all the animals. These pretreated animals developed profound dyspnea, hypoxia and florid pulmonary edema and died of respiratory failure. At necroscopy, the lungs were hemorrhagic and edematous, with areas of atelectasis. Histologic examination revealed alveolar and interstitial edema, in addition to intraalveolar hemorrhage. There were no consistent changes to indicate that the histologic appearance was the result of an inflammatory process. Whereas the concentration of inspired fluroxene was equal for all animals, the pretreated group had significantly higher levels of fluroxene metabolites. These included higher expired concentrations of trifluroethylene, higher blood and serum concentrations of nonvolatile organic fluoride, and greater urinary concentrations of both trifluroethylene and nonvolatile organic fluoride. The Rhesus monkey can survive fluroxene exposure without any evidence of pulmonary toxicity and is similar to humans in this regard. However, pretreatment with barbiturates, and perhaps other inducers of microsomal drug metabolism, also results in evidence of accelerated biotransformation, with the production of toxic metabolites (52).

Intraperitoneal administration of trichloroethylene (TCE) has been associated with pulmonary toxicity in murine models (53). Mortality was dose related, and histologic examination showed morphologic damage that varied with the doses administered. A dose of 2000 mg/kg of TCE was associated with clara cell vacuolization, which was most marked in the terminal bronchioles. Larger doses resulted in exfoliation of the clara cells and necrotic changes in the terminal bronchioles, with associated parenchymal changes consisting of reduced lamellar bodies in the type II cells and microvillus disruption. There was no alveolar edema nor any detected alteration in the intracellular calcium levels.

In an effort to determine the effects of anesthetic agents on the bronchoalveolar lavage (BAL) fluid content, Henderson and Lowrey tested the effects of four different anesthetic regimens (54). The four regimens [inhaled halothane 3.5%, i.v. sodium pentobarbitone, 100% CO_2, and no intervention (controls)] were administered to groups of rats and hamsters before cervical dislocation. When the subsequent BAL samples were analyzed using enzymatic assessment and cellular counts, the BAL samples from the halothane-exposed animals most closely resembled the control group, indicating that of these regimens, halothane may be the most innocuous. The clinical significance of these findings, however, is difficult to predict.

The i.v. administration of halothane, either accidentally or as a mode of suicide, is usually fatal in humans (55). Sandison et al. studied the effects of i.v. administration in dogs (56). The initial response following administration to spontaneously breathing dogs was apnea, cyanosis, and coma, followed by spontaneous recovery. Invasive monitoring revealed that the left atrial pressure decreased and the pulmonary artery pressure, which became elevated quickly, did not return completely to baseline. Lung histology revealed alveolar hemorrhage and edema, the extent of which appeared to be dose related. The histologic results were interpreted as demonstrating signficant perivascular injury at the level of the pulmonary arterioles and capillaries. The exact mechanism of this pulmonary toxicity is unknown, but the authors suggested two possible explanations. First, halothane reaches the pulmonary vasculature as an insoluble i.v. bolus and exerts its effects through its primary irritant properties. An alternative explanation is that the halothane disperses into multiple i.v. emboli, resulting in acute pulmonary vascular obstruction. Left ventricular failure was not observed in this study, suggesting that the pulmonary arterial hypertension had its basis in pulmonary vascular occlusion.

The possibility that acute left ventricular failure may occur following passage of i.v. halothane through the pulmonary circulation and emerging into the coronary circulation was investigated in a canine model (57). This study confirmed that pulmonary vascular disruption with concomitant pulmonary artery hypertension, rather than left ventricular failure, was responsible for the development of the alveolar edema (57). The study also documented marked elevations in the levels of circulating thromboxane B_2, indicating increased production of the parent active pulmonary vasoconstrictor thomboxane A_2 (TXA$_2$). Although TXA$_2$ usually is derived from platelets, the authors noted that it may be synthesized in pulmonary vascular endothelium following local thrombus formation and suggested that this may be the case following i.v. halothane. Regardless of its source, TXA$_2$ is a potent pulmonary vasoconstrictor and may be responsible for much of the pulmonary pathology observed following i.v. halothane. Several other reports have documented the effects of i.v. halothane in humans (58–60). Dwyer and Coppel measured the pulmonary vascular pressures in a patient following i.v. halothane and confirmed the pulmonary artery hypertension found in the animal studies (55). Neither the exact cause of death nor the optimal therapeutic approach has been determined for patients following i.v. halothane administration (61).

Xylazine, an alpha$_2$-agonist, is a commonly used anesthetic in veterinary anesthesia because of its potent sedative, analgesic, and muscle relaxant properties (62). Rats treated parenterally with high doses of xylazine develop extensive pulmonary edema, which is rich in cellular debris and protein (63). Reduction of the pulmonary edema by pretreatment with allopurinol led the authors of this study to suggest that the pulmonary toxicity may be mediated, in part, by superoxide radicals (63). The increased use of systemic and regional alpha$_2$-agonists in modern anesthetic practice, however, has not been associated with any reports of direct pulmonary toxicity.

AIRWAY IRRITATION BY VOLATILE ANESTHETICS

Airway irritation is especially important when performing inhalational induction of anesthesia because of the increased incidence of coughing, breathholding, prolongation of induction, and laryngospasm. The rank order of irritation by volatile agents has been determined in healthy volunteers in the following ascending order of magnitude: sevoflurane < halothane < enflurane < isoflurane, with 1 MAC of agent, and sevoflurane = halothane < enflurane < isoflurane, with 2 MAC of agent (64). (The MAC of a volatile anesthetic agent is the inspired concentration required to prevent any movement in response to surgical stimulation in 50% of patients.) This study was limitations, however, as the exposures were extremely brief (15 seconds), there were brief intervals between exposure to the different agents, the subjects were volunteers and not patients, dry air was used to deliver the agents, and the maximum dose of agent used was 2 MAC, which is lower than commonly used for inhalational induction of anesthesia.

Nishimo et al. examined the effects of nasal insufflation of volatile agents on pulmonary, laryngeal, and tracheal reflexes (65). They found that nasal application of 5% halothane, enflurane, or isoflurane to orally intubated patients produced pulmonary effects manifested as prolongation of the expiratory time. Halothane was the least irritant, and enflurane was the most irritant. There were no changes detected in laryngeal or tracheal smooth muscle tone.

In children, studies have confirmed that isoflurane is associated with a more complicated inhalational induction than halothane, as indicated by increased incidences of salivation, coughing, breathholding, and laryngospasm (66,67). Significant problems have been recorded in pediatric anesthesia with the use of desflurane (68). The high incidence of complications related to the irritant properties of the agent led the authors to suggest that desflurane is not a suitable agent for inhalational induction in children (68).

CILIARY FUNCTION AND MUCOCILIARY CLEARANCE

The significance of impaired mucociliary clearance after general anesthesia lies in the association of endobronchial mucous retention and obstruction, with the resultant development of postoperative atelectasis (69).

Forbes and Gamsu compared the effects of i.v. thiopental (25 mg/kg), inhaled halothane (1.2 MAC for either 2 or 6 hours), and inhaled diethylether (1.2 MAC for 2 hours) in dogs (69). Using tantalum bronchography and serial chest roentgenographs, they found that whereas thiopental had no effect on the rate of mucociliary clearance, both halothane and ether significantly decreased the clearance rate. These data supported findings from a previous study in female patients undergoing halothane endotracheal anesthesia for gynecologic procedures (70). Using a fiberoptic method of assessing the velocity of endobronchially placed Teflon discs, the investigators reported that the mucous velocity was significantly reduced over time with the halothane anesthesia. There were, however, no control patients in this study. Another method, using radioactive isotope droplets, has been studied in dogs (71). These authors documented no changes in mucous velocity with thiopental but approximate 50% reductions in velocity with 1.2 to 1.8 MAC of inhaled enflurane.

The clinical significance of these studies relates to the development of bronchial obstruction and postoperative atelectasis. Gamsu et al. (72) documented that although complete clearance of radiopaque tantalum occurred in less than 48 hours in their patients undergoing peripheral lower limb procedures, abdominal surgery under general endotracheal anesthesia was associated with delays in clearance of up to 6 days. These delays were associated with the subsequent development of pulmonary atelectasis. The authors did not provide any information about the type of anesthetic agents used, the mode of ventilation, concomitant use of regional anesthetic techniques, or the efficacy or method of postoperative analgesia.

The underlying mechanism of this inhibition of clearance may be inhibition of cellular ciliary function, as documented by Nunn et al. (73). These authors studied the effects of a range of formerly commonly used inhalational anesthetics on the swim-

ming velocity of the flagellate *Tetrahymena pyriformis*. Depression of ciliary activity by 50% occurred at the same concentrations of the agents, with the exception of cyclopropane, required to prevent movement in response to surgical incision in 50% of patients. This depression of motility was not associated with any ultrastructural changes identifiable by electron microscopy. Furthermore, large increases in the concentration of the agents resulted in deciliation, or loss of the cilia, distal to the level of the axosome and in mitochondrial swelling.

PULMONARY OXYGEN TOXICITY

The use of high concentrations of inspired O_2 (30% to 100%) is an integral component of general anesthetic practice. The issues involved in hyperoxic pulmonary toxicity have been reviewed extensively (74–77). The question of hyperoxic lung toxicity is always present, sometimes to a trivial extent, when greater than 35% O_2 is used. Anesthesiologists, therefore, always attempt to use the minimum safe level of inspired O_2. Guidelines exist concerning the safe maximum level of O_2 in terms of concentration and duration of exposure, but these guidelines may be misleading because of their reliance on changes in vital capacity as indicators of pulmonary toxicity (74). Furthermore, the duration of exposure during general anesthesia is almost uniformly brief, suggesting that pulmonary hyperoxic toxicity is unlikely to be a significant issue for general anesthesia in most cases.

Studies of the minimum duration of exposure required to cause the earliest detectable manifestations of O_2 toxicity are difficult to interpret. Pentane, a product of free radical-induced alveolar lipid peroxidation, is detectable in the expired gas in humans after only 30 minutes of ventilation with 100% O_2 (78). A significant alveolar–capillary leakage can be detected in BAL fluid to albumin and transferrin following ventilation with 95% O_2 for 17 hours (79) and to albumin following ventilation with 30% O_2 for 45 hours (80). Many studies that have examined ways of detecting early and reversible signs of hyperoxic toxicity are described in reviews of the topic (74,75). The clinical relevance of these methods of detection of early pulmonary toxicity remains to be determined.

The pathogenesis of O_2 toxicity has been reviewed extensively (74). The histologic changes involve pericapillary fluid accumulation in the earlier stages, followed by infiltration with platelets, pulmonary macrophages, and polymorphonuclear cells (81). There are interspecies differences in the subacute responses to continued hyperoxic exposure. In humans, continued exposure results in destruction of type I alveolar epithelial cells with resultant hyperplasia of the type II cells, which proliferate and replace the whole alveolar epithelial layer (82). More chronic changes are associated with further proliferation of the type II cells, proliferation of pulmonary fibroblasts, and pulmonary vascular remodeling. The last is responsible for the pulmonary vascular obliterative changes that result in pulmonary hypertension.

The biochemical basis for pulmonary O_2 toxicity has been reviewed in detail by Klein (74). Cellular O_2 produces reactive O_2 species (free radicals) as part of the normal metabolic processes, and the concentrations of these radicals are increased greatly in the hyperoxic states. Further increases may be mediated by the activity of pulmonary endothelial xanthine oxidase (83). Superoxide anions are transformed to hydroxyl free radicals and singlet O_2 radicals, both of which are highly reactive and capable of lipid peroxidation and other toxic actions.

Reactive O_2 species activate the arachidonic acid metabolic pathway, and eicosanoids are released (84). Although lipoxygenase and cyclooxygenase pathways are stimulated, it appears that the lipoxygenase metabolites (i.e., the leukotrienes) are capable of enhancing the pulmonary toxicity.

Hyperbaric oxygen is associated with reduction in pulmonary compliance, which is thought to represent a diminution in the quantity of pulmonary surfactant. It is not clear if this represents a direct destructive effect of O_2 radicals on the formed surfactant or an inhibitory effect on surfactant production.

Many xenobiotics, including such commonly used agents as bleomycin, methotrexate, busulphan, and cyclophosphamide, or their metabolites are sources of free radicals. There are no similar data available, however, concerning the effects of general anesthetic agents on the pathogenesis of hyperoxic lung toxicity (74). Toxicity associated with the use of high concentrations of O_2 during anesthesia in patients receiving bleomycin (85–87) and mitomycin (88) has been described. In patients receiving bleomycin therapy, the incidence of postoperative pulmonary toxicity has been most closely correlated with the peak inspired concentration of O_2. Although the nature of the studies does not permit exact prediction of the safe levels of F_{IO_2}, no deaths were reported in one study of patients receiving general anesthesia following bleomycin therapy when the F_{IO_2} was less than 0.26, and no survivors were reported when the F_{IO_2} exceeded 0.34 (85). Patients undergoing mitomycin treatment in addition to thoracic radiotherapy also developed postoperative pulmonary toxicity that was directly related to the magnitude of the inspired O_2 concentration (88). In this study, patients developed pulmonary toxicity when the F_{IO_2} exceeded 0.50, and none developed pulmonary toxicity when the F_{IO_2} was less than 0.30. These cytotoxic drugs produce high levels of superoxide radicals, and the interaction between the O_2 and the drugs almost certainly involves an accentuation of the superoxide radicals due to the high ambient O_2 concentrations (89). The clinical implication of these effects is that the minimum possible F_{IO_2} should be used as determined by careful and continuous monitoring of systemic oxygenation.

CONCLUSIONS

Anesthetic agents exert effects on the pulmonary system at multiple levels. Traditionally, the physiologic alterations of the pulmonary volumes and pulmonary circulation were the targets for anesthetic research, and the issues of pulmonary toxicity involved only anesthetic agents that are no longer used clinically. However, knowledge of these effects and mechanisms provides clinicians and scientists with the underlying principles with which to investigate the pathophysiologic and potential toxicologic effects of newer i.v. and inhaled anesthetic agents.

REFERENCES

1. Nunn J F. Effects of anaesthesia on respiration. *Br J Anaesth* 1990;65:54–62.
2. Lumb A B. The respiratory muscles. *Curr Opinion Anesth* 1991;4:845–847.
3. Laws A K. Effects of induction of anaesthesia and muscle paralysis on functional residual capacity of the lungs. *Can Anaesth Soc J* 1968; 15:325–331.
4. Shah J, Jones J G, Galvin J, Tomlin P J. Pulmonary gas exchange during induction of anaesthesia with nitrous oxide in seated subjects. *Br J Anaesth* 1971;43:1013–1021.
5. Drummond G B, Pye D W, Annan F J, Tothill P. Changes in blood volume distribution associated with general anaesthesia. *Br J Anaesth* 1988; 60:12–21.
6. Marsh H M, Southorn P A, Rehder K. Anesthesia, sedation and the chest wall. In: Jones *Effects of anesthesia and surgery on pulmonary mechanisms and gas exchange*. J G, ed. Boston: Little, Brown & Co, 1984:1–12.
7. Muller N L, Bryan A C. Chest wall mechanics and respiratory muscles in infants. *Pediatr Clin North Am* 1979;26:503–516.
8. Froese A B, Bryan A C. Effects of anesthesia and paralysis on diaphragmatic mechanics in man. *Anesthesiology* 1974;41:242–255.
9. Krayer S, Rehder K, Vetterman J, Didier E P, Hoffman E A. Position and motion of the diaphragm during anesthesia-paraylsis. *Anesthesiology* 1987;70:891–898.
10. Wahba R W M. Perioperative functional residual capacity. *Can J Anaesth* 1991;38:384–400.
11. Gunnarsson L, Strandberg A, Brismar B, Tokics L, Lundquist H, Hedenstierna G. Atelectasis and gas exchange impairment during enflurane/nitrous oxide anaesthesia. *Acta Anaesthesiol Scand* 1989;33:629–637.
12. Tokics L, Hedenstierna G, Strandberg A, Brismar B, Lundquist H. Lung collapse and gas exchange during general anesthesia: effects of spontaneous breathing, muscle paralysis and positive end-expiratory pressure. *Anesthesiology* 1987;66:157–167.
13. Shulman D, Beardsmore C S, Aronson H B, Godfrey S. The effect of ketamine on the functional residual capacity in young children. *Anesthesiology* 1985;62:551–556.
14. Eisenkraft J B. Effects of anaesthetics on the pulmonary circulation. *Br J Anaesth* 1990;65: 63–78.
15. Pearl R G. The pulmonary circulation. *Curr Opinion Anaesthesiol* 1992;5:848–854.
16. Marshall B E, Cohen P J, Klingenmaier C H, Aukberg S. Pulmonary venous admixture before, during and after halothane: oxygen anesthesia in man. *J Appl Physiol* 1969;27:653–657.
17. Nunn J F. Factors influencing the arterial oxygen tension during halothane anaesthesia with spontaneous respiration. *Br J Anaesth* 1964;36: 327–341.
18. Marshall C, Marshall B E. Site and sensitivity for stimulation of hypoxic pulmonary vasoconstriction. *J Appl Physiol* 1983;55:711–716.
19. Post J M, Hume J R, Archer S L, Weir E K. Direct role for potassium channel inhibiton in hypoxic pulmonary vasoconstriction. *Am J Physiol* 1992;262:C883–C890.
20. Domino K B, Wetstein L, Glasser S A, et al. Influence of mixed venous oxygen tension on blood flow to atelectatic lung. *Anesthesiology* 1983;59:428–434.
21. Marshall B E, Marshall C, Benumof J L, Saidman L J. Hypoxic pulmonary vasoconstriction in dogs: effects of lung segment size and oxygen tension. *J Appl Physiol* 1981;51:1543–1551.
22. Benumof J L. One-lung ventilation and hypoxic pulmonary vasoconstriction: implications for anesthetic management. *Anesth Analg* 1985;64: 821–833.
23. Weinreich A I, Silvay G, Lumb P D. Continuous ketamine infusion for one-lung anaesthesia. *Can Anaesth Soc J* 1980;27:485–490.
24. Rees D I, Gaines G Y. One-lung anesthesia—a comparison of pulmonary gas exchange during anesthesia with ketamine or enflurane. *Anesth Analg* 1984;63:521–525.
25. Rogers S N, Benumof J L. Halothane and isoflurane do not decrease Pao₂ during one-lung ventilation in intravenously anesthetized patients. *Anesth Analg* 1985;64:946–954.
26. Carlsson A J, Bindslev L, Hedenstierna G. Hypoxia-induced pulmonary vasoconstriction in the human lung. The effect of isoflurane anaesthesia. *Acta Anaesthesiol Scand* 1987;66: 312–316.
27. Carlsson A J, Hedenstierna G, Bindslev L. Hypoxia-induced pulmonary vasoconstriction in human lung exposed to enflurane anaesthesia. *Acta Anaesthesiol Scand* 1987;31:57–62.
28. Benumof J L, Augustine S D, Gibbons J A. Halothane and isoflurane only slightly impair ar-

terial oxygenation during one-lung ventilation in patients undergoing thoracotomy. *Anesthesiology* 1987;67:910–915.

29. Domino K B, Borowec L, Alexander C M, et al. Influence of isoflurane on hypoxic pulmonary vasoconstriction in dogs. *Anesthesiology* 1986; 64:423–429.

30. Sykes M K, Gibbs J M, Loh L, Obdrzalek L, Arnot R N. Preservation of the pulmonary vasoconstrictor response to alveolar hypoxia during administration of halothane to dogs. *Br J Anaesth* 1978;50:1185–1196.

31. Chen L, Miller F L, Malmkvist G, Clerque F X, Marshall C, Marshall B E. High-dose almitrine bimesylate inhibits hypoxic pulmonary vasoconstriction in closed-chest dogs. *Anesthesiology* 1987;67:534–542.

32. Bardsley P A, Howard P, Tang O, et al. Sequential treatment with low-dose almitrine bimesylate in hypoxemic chronic obstructive airways disease. *Eur Respir J* 1992;5:1054–1061.

33. Gottlieb J E, McGeady M, Adkinson N F, Sylvester J T. Effects of cyclo-and lipoxygenase inhibitors on hypoxic pulmonary vasoconstriction in isolated ferret lungs. *J Appl Physiol* 1988;64:936–943.

34. Marshall C, Kim S D, Marshall B E. The actions of halothane, ibuprofen and BW755C on hypoxic pulmonary vasoconstriction. *Anesthesiology* 1987;66:537–542.

35. Lejune P, Deloof T, Leeman M, Melot C, Naeije R. Multipoint pulmonary vascular pressure/flow relationships in hypoxic and in normoxic dogs: Effects of nitrous oxide with and without cycloxygenase inhibition. *Anesthesiology* 1988;68: 92–99.

36. Pearl R G. Cromolyn sodium does not inhibit hypoxic pulmonary vasoconstriction in sheep. *Anesth Analg* 1990;71:183–187.

37. Pearl R G, Prielipp R C. Leukotriene synthesis inhibition and receptor blockade does not inhibit hypoxic pulmonary vasoconstriction in sheep. *Anesth Analg* 1991;72:169–176.

38. Hirshman C A, Bergman N A. Factors influencing intrapulmonary airway calibre during anaesthesia. *Br J Anaesth* 1990;65:30–42.

39. Freed A N, Hirshman C A. Airflow-induced bronchoconstriction: a model of airway reactivity in humans. *Anesthesiology* 1988;69:923–932.

40. Borson D B, Brokaw J J, Sekizawa K, McDonald D M, Nadel J A. Neutral endopeptidase and neurogenic inflammation in rats with respiratory infections. *J Appl Physiol* 1989;66: 2653–2658.

41. Alexander C M, Chen L, Ray R, Marshall B E. The influence of halothane and isoflurane on pulmonary collateral ventilation. *Anesthesiology* 1985;62:135–140.

42. Vettermann J, Beck K C, Lindahl S H E, Brichant J F, Rehder K. Actions of enflurane, isoflurane, vecuronium, atracurium and pancuronium on pulmonary resistance in dogs. *Anesthesiology* 1988;69:688–695.

43. Brown R H, Zerhouni E A, Hirshman C A. Comparison of low concentrations of halothane and isoflurane as bronchodilators. *Anesthesiology* 1993;78:1097–1011.

44. Korenaga S, Takeda K, Ito Y. Differential effects of halothane on airway nerves and muscles. *Anesthesiology* 1984;60:309–318.

45. Shah M V, Hirshman C A. Mode of action of halothane on histamine-induced airway constriction in dogs with reactive airways. *Anesthesiology* 1986;65:170–174.

46. Sayinen A, Lorenz R R, Warner D O, Rehder K. Bronchodilation by halothane is not modulated by airway epithelium. *Anesthesiology* 1991;75: 75–81.

47. Brown R H, Mitzner W, Zerhouni E, Hirshman C A. Direct *in vivo* visualization of bronchodilation induced by inhalational anesthesia using high-resolution computed tomography. *Anesthesiology* 1993;78:295–300.

48. Rehder K, Mallow J E, Fibuch E E, Krabill D R, Sessler A D. Effects of isoflurane anesthesia and muscle paralysis on respiratory mechanics in normal man. *Anesthesiology* 1974;41: 477–485.

49. Hirshman C A, Downes H, Farbood A, Bergman N A. Ketamine block of bronchospasm in experimental canine asthma. *Br J Anaesth* 1979; 51:713–718.

50. Jackson D M, Richards I M. The effects of pentobarbitone and chloralose anaesthesia on the vagal component of bronchoconstriction produced by histamine aerosol in the anaesthetized dog. *Br J Pharmacol* 1977;61:251–256.

51. Crago R R, Bryan A C, Laws A K, Winestock A E. Respiratory flow resistance after curare and pancuronium measured by forced oscillations. *Can Anaesth Soc J* 1972;19:604–614.

52. Munson E S, Malagodi M H, Shields R P, et al. Fluroxene toxicity induced by phenobarbital. *Clin Pharmacol Ther* 1975;687–699.

53. Forkert P G, Sylvestre P L, Poland J S. Lung injury induced by trichloroethylene. *Toxicology* 1985;35:143–160.

54. Henderson R F, Lowrey J S. Effect of anesthetic agents on lavage fluid parameters used as indicators of pulmonary injury. *Lab Anim Sci* 1983;33:60–62.

55. Dwyer R, Coppel D L. Intravenous injection of liquid halothane. *Anesth Analg* 1989;69: 250–255.

56. Sandison J W, Sivapragasam S, Hayes J A, Woo-Ming M O. An experimental study of pulmonary damage associated with intravenous injection of halothane in dogs. *Br J Anaesth* 1970;42:419.

57. Kawamoto M, Suzuki N, Takasaki M. Acute pulmonary edema after intravenous liquid halothane in dogs. *Anesth Analg* 1992;74:747–752.

58. Berman P, Tattersall M. Self-poisoning with intravenous halothane. *Lancet* 1982;ii:340.

59. Sutton J, Harrison G A, Hickie J B. Accidental intravenous injection of halothane. *Br J Anaesth* 1971;43:513–520.

60. Wig J, Chakravarty S, Krishnamurthy K, Mehta

D. Coma following ingestion of halothane. *Anaesthesia* 1983;38:552–555.

61. Stemp L I. Intravenous injection of liquid halothane [Letter]. *Anesth Analg* 1990;70:568.

62. Greene S A, Thurmon J C. Xylazine—a review of its pharmacology and use in veterinary medicine. *J Vet Pharmacol Ther* 1988;11:295–313.

63. Amouzadeh H R, Sangiah S, Qualls C W J, Cowel R L, Mauromoustakos A. Xylazine-induced pulmonary edema in rats. *Toxicol Appl Pharmacol* 1991;108:417–427.

64. Doi M, Ikeda K. Airway irritation produced by volatile anaesthetics during brief inhalation: comparison of halothane, enflurane, isoflurane and sevoflurane. *Can J Anaesth* 1993;40:122–126.

65. Nishino T, Tanaka A, Ishikawa T, Hiraga K. Respiratory, laryngeal, and tracheal responses to nasal insufflation of volatile anesthetics in anesthetized humans. *Anesthesiology* 1991;75:441–444.

66. Phillips A J, Brimacombe J R, Simpson D L. Anaesthetic induction with isoflurane or halothane in unpremedicated children. *Anesthesia* 1988;43:927–929.

67. Pandit U A, Steude G M, Leach A B. Induction and recovery characteristics of isoflurane and halothane anesthesia for short outpatient operations in children. *Anaesthesia* 1985;40:1226–1230.

68. Taylor R H, Lerman J. Induction, maintenance and recovery characteristics of desflurane in infants and children. *Can J Anaesth* 1992;39:6–13.

69. Forbes A R, Gamsu G. Mucociliary clearance in the canine lung during and after general anesthesia. *Anesthesiology* 1979;50:26–29.

70. Lichtiger M, Landa J E, Hirsh J A. Velocity of tracheal mucus in anesthetized women undergoing gynecologic surgery. *Anesthesiology* 1975;42:753–756.

71. Forbes A R, Horrigan R W. Mucociliary flow in the trachea during anesthesia with enflurane, ether, nitrous oxide, and morphine. *Anesthesiology* 1977;46:319–321.

72. Gamsu G, Singer M M, Vincent H H, et al. Postoperative impairment of mucous transport in the lung. *Am Rev Respir Dis* 1976;114:673–679.

73. Nunn J F, Sturrock M E, Wills E J, et al. The effect of inhalational anaesthetics on the swimming velocity of *Tetrahymena pyriformis*. *J Cell Sci* 1974;15:537–554.

74. Klein J. Normobaric pulmonary oxygen toxicity. *Anesth Analg* 1990;70:195–207.

75. Deneke S M, Franburg B L. Normobaric oxygen toxicity of the lung. *N Engl J Med* 1980;303:76–86.

76. Deneke S M, Franbrug B L. Oxygen toxicity of the lung: an update. *Br J Anaesth* 1982;54:737–749.

77. Frank L, Massaro D. Oxygen toxicity. *Am J Med* 1980;69:117–126.

78. Morita S, Snider M T, Inada Y. Increased N-pentane excretion in humans: a consequence of pulmonary oxygen exposure. *Anesthesiology* 1986;64:730–733.

79. Davis W B, Rennard S I, Bitterman P B, Crystal R G. Pulmonary oxygen toxicity. Early reversible changes in human alveolar structure induced by hyperoxia. *N Engl J Med* 1983;309:878–883.

80. Griffith D E, Holden W E, Morris J F, Min L K, Krishnamurthy G T. Effects of common therapeutic concentrations of oxygen on lung clearance of ^{99m}Tc-DPTA and bronchoalveolar lavage albumin concentration. *Am Rev Respir Dis* 1986;134:233–237.

81. Crapo J D. Morphologic changes in pulmonary oxygen toxicity. *Annu Rev Physiol* 1986;48:721–731.

82. De los Santos R, Seidenfeld J J, Anzueto A, et al. One hundred percent oxygen lung injury in adult baboons. *Am Rev Respir Dis* 1987;136:657–661.

83. Rodell T C, Cheronis J C, Ohnemus C L, Piermattei D J, Repine J E. Xanthine oxidase mediates elastase-induced injury to isolated lungs and endothelium. *J Appl Physiol* 1987;63:2159–2163.

84. Sporn H S, Peters-Golden M, Simon R H. Hydrogen peroxide-induced arachidonic acid metabolism in rat alveolar macrophage. *Am Rev Respir Dis* 1988;137:49–56.

85. Goldiner P L, Carlon G C, Cvitkovic E, Schweizer O, Howland W S. Factors influencing postoperative morbidity and mortality in patients treated with bleomycin. *Br Med J* 1978;1:1664–1667.

86. Toledo C H, Ross W E, Hood C L, Block E R. Prevention of bleomycin toxicity by oxygen. *Cancer Treat Rep* 1982;66:359–362.

87. Tryka A F, Godleski J J, Skornik W A, Brain J D. Bleomycin and 70% oxygen exposure, early and late effects. *Am Rev Respir Dis* 1982;125:92.

88. Franklin R, Buroker T R, Vaishampayan G V, Vaitkevicious V K. Combined therapies in esophageal squamous cell cancer. *Proc Am Assoc Cancer Res* 1979;20:223.

89. Klein D S, Wilds P R. Pulmonary toxicity of antineoplastic agents: anaesthetic and postoperative implications. *Can Anaesth Soc J* 1983;30:399–405.

Anesthetic Toxicity, edited by
Susan A. Rice and Kevin J. Fish.
Raven Press, Ltd., New York © 1994.

15

Biomarkers of Anesthetic Toxicity

C. Murray Ardies

*Center for Exercise Science and Cardiovascular Research, Northeastern Illinois University,
Chicago, Illinois 60625*

The use of markers to indicate that a specific biologic response has occurred is well established in medicine and anesthesiology. For example, eyelash reflex, respiratory rate, heart rate, blood pressure, and electrocardiogram patterns are all common physiologic markers that may be used to indicate the depth of anesthesia (1). These physiologic-based markers are monitored without removing biologic samples from the patient, and they provide timely and valuable information regarding the physiologic state of the patient.

Biomarkers, like physiologic markers, also have been used in medicine for many years to assess specific aspects of a patient's status. The term "biomarker" also refers to markers that are used to indicate that a biologic event has occurred. Unlike physiologic markers, biomarkers are measured in biologic fluids or tissues (e.g., blood and urine) taken from the patient or subject. As defined by the Committee on Biological Markers of the National Research Council (2), a biomarker is simply any indicator of events within a biologic system. Depending on the specific makeup of the biomarker, it may be used to indicate prior exposure, toxic (or injurious) outcome, or risk of future reaction (2–5).

This chapter discusses biomarkers and the application of biomarkers to the study and identification of anesthetic toxicity. The potential use of biomarkers in clinical and research arenas is discussed, and the biochemical rationale for specific anesthetic biomarkers is presented briefly. Finally, new developments in immunochemical detection of anesthetic-related biomarkers are discussed because they represent some of the most exciting technologic developments for enhancing anesthetic safety.

BIOMARKERS

Biomarkers of Exposure, Effect, and Susceptibility

When the original chemical or its metabolite can be measured in a biologic sample, e.g., serum, hair, skin, or saliva, this substance is, by definition, a biomarker. Biologic molecules that indicate a biologic, biochemical, or molecular response following chemical exposure also qualify as biomarkers. Three classes of biomarkers were proposed by the Committee on Biological Markers: biomarkers of exposure, effect, and susceptibility (2).

A biomarker of exposure indicates that a specific compound entered the body via some route and was absorbed. This class of biomarkers includes the agent itself and its distinctive metabolites. The metabolites may either be free or bound to a biomolecule.

A biomarker of effect indicates that a biologic response has occurred as a result of a specific exposure. This class of biomarkers includes compounds that are biologically produced as a direct result of the exposure.

A biomarker of susceptibility indicates that a particular individual may be more susceptible to a specific biologic outcome than another.

In the context of this chapter, the main biologic outcome under consideration is toxicity. Therefore, the biomarkers of effect that we will deal with are biomarkers of toxicity. Elevated blood urea nitrogen (BUN) concentrations or serum transaminase activities are examples of biomarkers of toxicity. Some biologic responses are not a direct result of toxicity but may lead to other events that are. Any biologically produced compound that results from exposure and leads to toxicity, such as a toxic metabolite, can be termed a "biomarker of risk" (for developing a toxic reaction). A nontoxic metabolite that is produced from the parent compound concurrently with the toxic metabolite or as a direct result of the toxic metabolite also could qualify as a biomarker of risk.

Any biologic marker that indicates an individual has much greater than normal cytochrome P450-2E1 activity is a biomarker of susceptibility for cytochrome P450-2E1-mediated toxic reactions. For example, the production of toxic intermediates from acetaminophen (6) and enflurane (7), N-acetyl-benzoquinoneimine and fluoride, respectively, are clinically relevant reactions that are catalyzed by cytochrome P450-2E1.

Several books and reviews on biomarkers (2–5) suggest that the term and its use originated in the field of environmental toxicology. There was a need in environmental toxicology for tools to link a measured environmental burden of a specific chemical to the toxic responses in humans. The mere presence of a chemical in the environment does not necessarily mean that a toxic reaction will follow. Before toxicity will be manifest, a three-step process generally occurs. First, the chemical is absorbed; the route of exposure and the subsequent ab-

sorption are directly linked to the environmental source. Second, a chemical-specific biologic response that can lead to toxicity occurs. Third, the response must be sufficiently above the threshold to produce toxicity (injury). When these criteria are met, the presence of a chemical can be linked to a specific toxic reaction. Evidence for each of these conditions may be obtained, in part, by the use of appropriate biomarkers of exposure and effect. A detailed knowledge of the etiology of the chemically induced toxic reaction is necessary before appropriate biologic markers of exposure, effect (toxicity), or susceptibility can be selected and then used.

Measuring appropriate biomarkers of anesthetic exposure, toxicity, and risk in an individual is appropriate for highly susceptible individuals as well as for normally susceptible individuals because the same etiology of toxicity should exist. In general, individuals who are more susceptible to toxicity merely suffer a toxic reaction at a lower dose. There are exceptions, however, and for that reason, the following discussion is limited to biomarkers of exposure, toxicity (effect), and risk for developing a toxic reaction. The exceptions generally are identified by differences in pharmacogenetics (see chapter by Wood).

BIOMARKERS OF ANESTHETIC EXPOSURE, TOXICITY, AND RISK

Although clinically significant toxic reactions to anesthetics are relatively rare, the development of biomarkers of anesthetic toxicity may result in timely medical intervention to prevent or attenuate toxicity and any attendant suffering. Thus, the rationale for using biomarkers in anesthesia is to predict injury or other adverse outcome following anesthetic exposure. As previously mentioned, a sound understanding of the various mechanisms that contribute to the toxic process is necessary to determine if a potential biomarker is predictive of toxicity. Figure 1 illustrates a flow chart of the production of three generic types of biomarkers subsequent to anesthetic exposure.

If the biomarker is produced as a consequence of cell damage or cell death, it is a biomarker of toxicity. Biomarkers of anesthetic toxicity, by the simplest definition, include any indicator of cell damage or cell death that occurs as a direct or indirect result of anesthetic exposure. Biomarkers of toxicity might include elevated concentrations of serum creatinine or urea nitrogen in the case of kidney damage or elevated serum transaminases (aspartate aminotransferase, AST, and alanine aminotransferase, ALT) in the case of liver damage. Such biomarkers are not specific and result from many different toxic reactions. In order to link these biomarkers of toxicity to a specific anesthetic, a biomarker of a specific anesthetic exposure must also be used.

A biomarker of exposure indicates only that the anesthetic was absorbed. Using enflurane as an example, biomarkers of exposure include enflurane and its immediate metabolites, difluoromethoxydifluoroacetic acid and inorganic fluoride (F^-). Because there may be sources of F^- other than enflurane, F^- would not necessarily be a good biomarker of enflurane exposure. In the case of surgical patients, a biomarker of anesthetic exposure is not of practical use because a sedated or anesthetized patient has obviously been exposed to a known agent. A biomarker of exposure would be useful, however, for operating room personnel who by virtue of their presence in the operating theater may inadvertently be exposed to volatile anesthetic agents.

To be a biomarker of risk the marker must be directly involved in the toxic reaction or directly attributable to the toxic reaction. For example, a biomarker of risk for developing kidney damage is an elevated serum concentration of F^- because F^- is intimately involved in the toxic process. The nontoxic, defluorinated metabolite, difluoromethoxydifluoroacetic acid, also may constitute a biomarker of risk because its presence indicates an equimolar production of F^-. Because of the nonspecific nature of F^-, its use as a biomarker of risk necessitates the use of a biomarker of exposure. Inorganic fluoride is a biomarker of risk for kidney damage, but linkage with an anesthetic exposure is necessary before F^- can be a biomarker of anesthetic-associated kidney damage.

In rare circumstances, certain compounds may be produced or modified as a result of exposure in addition to being intimately involved in causing the toxic reaction. Thus, a single biomarker may provide not only evidence of prior exposure or risk of toxicity on subsequent exposures but also evidence of an ongoing toxic reaction.

Research Applications

Once appropriate biologic markers of exposure, toxicity, and risk have been selected, they can be employed in research and tested for their use in the clinical arena. An association between exposure to anesthetics and various negative health outcomes has been observed in several studies (8–12). With the development and use of appropriate biomarkers of anesthetic toxicity, a proof of causal relationship between exposure and toxicity may be possible. One of the major research applications of biomarkers is for the epidemiologic assessment of adverse health effects following exposure to anesthetics. Many published studies of anesthetic exposure and negative pregnancy outcomes are based on retrospective analyses of exposure (based on questionnaires or patient records or both) in patient populations or in operating room personnel (8–12) (see chapter by Ebi and Rice). Some reports documented a positive association between anesthetic exposure and adverse outcomes (8–10), whereas others observed no association (11,12). Small differences in methodologies and end point criteria may explain some of the qualitative differences in results. However, a sensitive and objec-

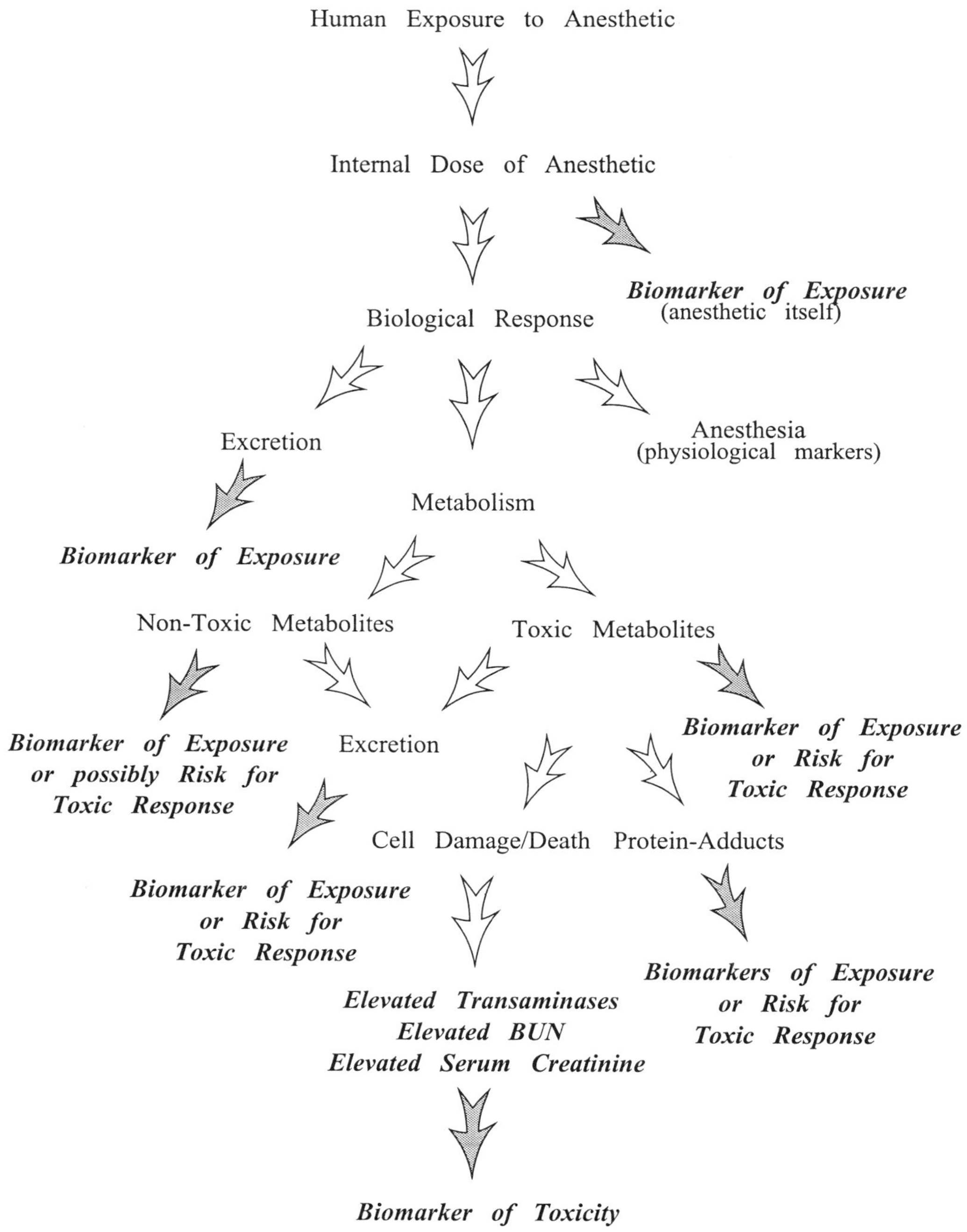

FIG. 1. Production of biomarkers following exposure to anesthetics.

tive biomarker of exposure is necessary to provide measurements of exposure that are more accurate than are responses to a questionnaire. Certainly, such use of biomarkers would enable researchers to eliminate a large source of uncertainty in determining which subjects were truly exposed to biologically relevant amounts of anesthetics. An example from environmental epidemiology illustrates this point. Answers from a questionnaire designed to determine which women in a Yugoslav community had exposure to lead from a local smelter were poor predictors of exposure when compared to the actual serum concentrations of lead (13).

Selecting appropriate biomarkers of anesthetic exposure, risk, and toxicity for further research and ultimately documenting the clinical applications of biomarkers would provide information that could vastly decrease the incidence and degree of complications associated with anesthetic use. A sound understanding of the various mechanisms that contribute to the toxic response(s) caused by an anesthetic is necessary to determine which biomarkers are potentially useful. The rest of this chapter focuses on several of the well-studied anesthetic agents and discusses the known and the potential biomarkers of a number of these agents. The inhalational anesthetics are discussed first, followed by the i.v. and local anesthetics. Finally, the technologic development of immunochemical methods for detecting biomarkers of anesthetic exposure, toxicity, and risk is discussed.

INHALATIONAL ANESTHETICS

Nitrous Oxide (N$_2$O)

Nitrous oxide (N$_2$O) is eliminated very rapidly in the expired gas, and detection methods are too insensitive to determine just how much is metabolized or even if biotransformation occurs at all. Because there

is as yet no evidence that N$_2$O actually is metabolized by mammalian systems, there is little potential to develop a marker for exposure based on metabolites. The best marker of exposure is the anesthetic itself. For occupational exposures, this means continuous measurement of N$_2$O in the ambient air. This approach, however, is not completely satisfactory for obvious reasons.

In part because N$_2$O is eliminated so rapidly and is not metabolized, there are no real toxicologic alterations resulting from the direct effects of N$_2$O on cellular function due to an acute exposure. On the other hand, N$_2$O can directly oxidize the cobalt atom of vitamin B$_{12}$, and long-term exposure to low concentrations of N$_2$O may decrease the amount of functional vitamin B$_{12}$. Subsequently, the activity of biologic functions dependent on vitamin B$_{12}$ may decrease (14,15). In both experimental animals and humans, a neuropathy and a form of megaloblastic anemia have been observed following chronic exposure to relatively high concentrations of N$_2$O (16–19) (see chapter by Koblin). These changes appear to be a result of the inactivation of methionine synthase (a vitamin B$_{12}$-dependent enzyme) and the subsequent decrease in DNA synthesis. The neuropathy also has been observed in some dentists, who regularly used N$_2$O as an anesthetic in an unscavenged dental operatory. Based on the target organ of N$_2$O-induced toxicity, a potential biomarker of N$_2$O toxicity is diminished white blood cell and red blood cell counts. Of course, the decreased blood cell counts must be coupled with a history of prolonged or repeated N$_2$O exposure for them to constitute a biomarker of N$_2$O toxicity. Because changes in blood cells occur subsequent to altered vitamin B$_{12}$ status, decreased vitamin B$_{12}$ or methionine synthase activity coupled with a history of prolonged or frequent exposure to N$_2$O may constitute a biomarker of risk for the development of megaloblastic anemia and neuropathy.

The duration of surgical procedures on healthy patients generally is too short to result in any toxic effect as a result of interaction with vitamin B_{12} and inhibition of methionine synthase (see chapters by Koblin and by Rice). The toxic effects of N_2O generally are confined to those who are exposed repeatedly to high concentrations of N_2O. This exposure can occur either intentionally, as with abuse, or when the anesthetic is administered under conditions where less than adequate N_2O scavenging occurs.

In summary, because of the very rapid elimination of N_2O, the anesthetic itself is the only available biomarker of exposure. Reduced red and white blood cell counts coupled with a history of N_2O exposure (or N_2O availability in the case of suspected abuse) may constitute a biomarker of N_2O toxicity, whereas a reduced vitamin B_{12} status in the same person may be a biomarker of risk.

Fluorinated Inhalational Anesthetics

The use of the fluorinated inhalational anesthetics occasionally is associated with clinically significant toxic reactions. Malignant hyperthermia has been observed in rare instances following use of some of these anesthetics (20) (see chapter by Larach). Briefly, malignant hyperthermia may be caused by a defect in the uptake of calcium by the sarcoplasmic reticulum of skeletal muscle in those individuals who are genetically susceptible. If recognized early enough, hyperthermia is effectively stopped by removing the anesthetic and administering dantrolene, which directly decreases the ability of the sarcoplasmic reticulum to release calcium. The best means to avoid problems associated with malignant hyperthermia is to closely monitor the appropriate physiologic marker, body temperature.

Halothane is associated with the highest incidence of hepatotoxicity. Hepatotoxicity resulting from other anesthetics is compared to the forms produced by halothane (see chapter by Baker and Van Dyke). Briefly, halothane is associated with two forms of hepatotoxicity. One is a mild transient form, and the other is a rare form of severe hepatitis (halothane hepatitis), which has been observed in approximately 1:35,000 anesthetic administrations (21). With this latter form of hepatitis, a fever usually develops 2 to 5 days after exposure, and analysis of the blood reveals elevated serum hepatic transaminases typical of hepatocellular damage or death. This condition often progresses to complete hepatic failure and death.

Understanding the metabolic fate of halothane can lead to the development of biomarkers of risk for halothane hepatitis. Although halothane hepatitis is almost unheard of in the United States because halothane is seldom used, there are other countries, such as South Africa, where the drug is still used extensively. An elevated concentration of liver enzymes in serum following exposure to halothane constitutes biomarkers for both forms of halothane hepatotoxicity. However, considering the consequences of halothane hepatitis, a marker of risk for this form might prove more valuable. A biomarker of risk for developing halothane hepatitis would help the clinician to decide if an anesthetic agent other than halothane should be used by identifying those individuals who are at high risk for developing halothane hepatitis. Additionally, a biomarker of risk along with an early appearance of a biomarker of toxicity would provide timely information indicating the need for prompt clinical intervention in those patients who are administered halothane.

Approximately 60% to 80% of the absorbed halothane is eliminated unchanged in the exhaled gas within the first 24 hours. Because halothane has a relatively high oil/gas partition coefficient, a few days are necessary for its complete elimination as it slowly diffuses from fat depots. Of the remaining amount, approximately half is metabolized by cytochrome P450-dependent mixed-function oxidases to yield trifluoroacetate (TFA) and free bromide (22). Most of the rest is exhaled, but a small amount is metabolically reduced to yield F^-, 2-chloro-1,1-difluoroethylene, and 2-chloro-1,1,1-trifluoroethane (23) (see chapter by Waskell). Any unmetabolized halothane is primarily exhaled. With repeated exposure to some drugs, such as isoniazid, specific cytochrome P450s that are capable of metabolizing halothane are induced. Bromide and TFA production are increased following halothane exposure after such treatment (24,25).

From the results of animal studies, TFA production apparently is associated most closely with developing the rare, fulminant form of hepatic necrosis. TFA is produced by cytochrome P450-mediated oxidation of halothane via a highly reactive intermediate, trifluoroacetyl chloride. This activated species can react with and subsequently bind to the free amino groups of proteins (26,27), as well as phospholipids that have an amino group such as phosphatidyl-ethanolamine (28,29), to yield the corresponding amide. This creates a TFA adduct of the protein or phospholipid. Any endogenous protein that has been modified chemically in this manner may be recognized by the immune system as a foreign protein, and this recognition initiates an immune response.

The TFA-modified proteins are responsible for initiating the production of antibodies and are termed "neoantigens." Antibodies are produced in response to these TFA neoantigens as a result of the first exposure to halothane. Presumably, these antibodies will then react with any future TFA adducts formed on the hepatocyte surface in response to a subsequent halothane exposure. Antibody-dependent events that may lead to cell necrosis are then initiated. There is considerable evidence that antibodies that recognize TFA adducts are involved in an immune-mediated, delayed,

fulminant form of hepatic necrosis caused by halothane (30–36). Both TFA-modified liver proteins (31,32,34) and TFA-specific antibodies (30,33,35) have been observed in patients following exposure to halothane or enflurane. Thus, an elevated serum conentration of antibodies that recognize TFA-modified proteins (anti-TFA antibodies) would be a useful biomarker of exposure to halothane. Antibody concentrations in serum usually are expressed as a titer. A high titer of anti-TFA antibodies also may be a biomarker of risk for developing the delayed, fulminant form of halothane-induced hepatic necrosis.

The production of TFA adducts (and presumably anti-TFA antibodies) following exposure to halothane apparently is not related to the development of the transient, nonfulminant form of halothane hepatitis (see chapter by Baker and Van Dyke). Alterations in calcium homeostasis and halothane-mediated hepatic hypoxia may be more relevant mechanisms for the production of this form of hepatotoxicity, although these mechanisms are not well understood. Because this form of halothane hepatotoxicity may be caused by a poorly understood direct effect of halothane on cellular physiology, a biomarker of risk is difficult to identify. Elevated concentrations of AST and ALT in serum are well-established biomarkers that indicate liver damage. When these biomarkers are elevated following halothane exposure, they provide evidence of halothane-induced hepatotoxicity. If these biomarkers are elevated in conjunction with a high titer of antibodies that recognize TFA adducts, the patient may be in the process of developing, or at least be at high risk for developing, halothane hepatitis. If a patient has a high titer of anti-TFA antibodies before scheduled surgery, the use of halothane as the anesthetic of choice may be contraindicated because of the implied risk for developing the delayed, fulminant form of halothane hepatitis. Although longitudinal studies have yet to be performed to provide conclusive evidence in support of the implied risk associated with a high titer of anti-TFA antibodies, an anesthesiologist with this knowledge would be wise to choose an anesthetic other than halothane. Measurement of anti-TFA antibodies, however, is only a theoretical possibility except for those few institutions pursuing research in this area.

The incidence of hepatotoxicity associated with other anesthetics is much less than that with halothane. Severe hepatic necrosis following repeated administrations of enflurane is even more rare than that observed for halothane. In those cases where it does occur, the patient usually has a history of halothane exposure (36). The mechanism for the rare severe form of hepatotoxicity with enflurane is most likely similar to that discussed for halothane (36), although few data exist to support or refute this hypothesis. Substantiated isoflurane-mediated hepatotoxicity has not been reported.

From a metabolic standpoint, toxic reactions to enflurane and isoflurane should be very rare, and the incidence of toxic reactions following the use of these anesthetics is much less than that associated with halothane. In addition to being relatively resistant to metabolism, both isoflurane and enflurane are eliminated in the expired gas much more quickly than halothane, leaving less time for metabolism to occur. Over 90% of these absorbed anesthetics are expired unchanged; 2% to 5% of enflurane and less than 1% of isoflurane are metabolized to difluoromethoxydifluoroacetic acid and F^- and to TFA and F^-, respectively (37–40).

The main toxic metabolite of enflurane and isoflurane is F^-, a nephrotoxin. Serum concentrations of F^-, however, seldom increase above 20 μM, whereas the normal threshold for clinical signs of kidney toxicity is greater than 50 μM. For this reason, renal toxicity in patients exposed to enflurane or isoflurane is very rare. As previously mentioned, under hypoxic conditions, reductive metabolism of halothane also releases F^- (23), but the amount is of little clinical relevance. Metabolism of methoxyflurane (also producing F^-) is extensive (41). Serum concentrations of F^- following administration of methoxyflurane can easily exceed 50 μM (42). When serum concentrations of F^- increase beyond the toxic threshold, serum concentrations of urea nitrogen and creatinine increase, indicating kidney damage. Serum urea nitrogen and creatinine and their clearances have been used extensively as biomarkers of toxicity and of risk for renal failure (see chapter by Fish).

Sevoflurane (clinical studies are in progress in the United States) and desflurane (recently released for clinical use) are relatively new fluorinated anesthetics that also deserve mention. Although both F^- and TFA are metabolites (F^- from both agents and TFA from desflurane) and could be used as biomarkers of exposure, F^- is too nonspecific to be a biomarker for sevoflurane, and too little TFA (next to none) is produced from desflurane to be of any practical value (43–45). The lack of reported toxic reactions to these agents (46) may be due to the fact that these anesthetics have been in clinical use for a relatively short time.

In summary, biomarkers of exposure for all of the fluorinated anesthetics include the individual anesthetics and their various metabolites. An elevated serum concentration of F^- is a direct biomarker of immediate risk for kidney toxicity. Antibodies that recognize TFA adducts may qualify as a biomarker of exposure to halothane and as a biomarker of risk for developing halothane hepatitis. Biomarkers of hepatotoxicity include elevated serum concentrations of AST and ALT, and nephrotoxicity would be indicated by elevated serum urea nitrogen or creatinine levels.

Any of the biomarkers for exposure, toxicity, and risk discussed above also would be beneficial in research for correlating long-term exposure to health outcomes. The various biomarkers of exposure would be useful to establish that exposure had occurred in occupational or recreational (abuse) settings. The biomarkers of toxicity and risk would be useful in relating the degree of biologic response to the degree of exposure.

Anesthetics and their metabolites, however, may not be too useful as biomarkers of exposure or risk if determinations are made several days or weeks after the exposures are terminated. The half-life of these compounds is much too short to make them of practical value other than for the period soon after exposure. When the time span between exposure and testing is more than a week, a different biomarker of exposure is necessary. Detection of antibodies directed against modified proteins would provide a much less time-sensitive biomarker. For instance, if anti-TFA antibodies are detected in serum, it is possible that an exposure to either halothane, isoflurane, or desflurane has occurred. In addition, because these antibodies may be directly involved in halothane hepatitis, these antibodies also constitute biomarkers of risk.

An additional type of biomarker not previously discussed that also may have some use in research on toxic exposures to anesthetics is a nonspecific biomarker of stress. Such a biomarker might be useful in screening operating room personnel because of the potential for exposure to anesthetics throughout the work week. A single marker that indicates a biologic response to anesthetic exposure would save both the time and the expense of testing everyone for the individual biomarkers associated with all the various anesthetics used during the week. Only those subjects with evidence of a stress response need to be tested further.

One such nonspecific biomarker of stress is a heat-shock protein (HSP-72). HSP-72 increases following halothane exposure under conditions that produce hepatotoxicity (47). Heat-shock proteins are considered stress proteins because they are synthesized in response to a variety of endogenous and environmental stressors (48,49). Because this protein is synthesized in re-

sponse to conditions associated with the production of hepatocellular damage following halothane exposure, it also may be a nonspecific indicator of a potentially toxic exposure to other anesthetics. This hypothesis has not been tested.

Local and Intravenous Anesthetics

The main toxicologic considerations with regard to these classes of anesthetics are seizures and cardiac arrhythmias produced by an apparent overdose of local anesthetics (see chapter by Feldman) and anaphylactoid reactions associated with some i.v. anesthetics (50,51). It is difficult to determine which i.v. anesthetics are involved in precipitating the anaphylactoid reaction because of the nature of the report from the anesthetic reactions advisory service at Royal Hallamshire Hospital, Sheffield, England (50). It appears, however, that thiopentone is most often associated with anaphylactoid reactions following exposure, and antibodies that recognize thiopentone have been observed in 30% of anesthetic reactors (50). As was the case with halothane, anesthetic-specific antibodies appear, in part, to be involved in mediating the toxic response. Assays for the presence of these antibodies would prove useful as a biomarker of risk for those persons who may be prone to immune-mediated toxic responses. A hypersensitivity response to propofol may have been responsible for the prostanoid reaction observed in one patient (51), and results of a drug-sensitivity test may, therefore, constitute a biomarker of risk for such a reaction to occur following administration of an anesthetic of this type.

Toxic reactions to these classes of anesthetics are either physiologically based (seizures/arrhythmias) or anaphylactic in nature. Therefore, biomarkers of toxicity may not be useful. Monitoring the appropriate physiologic indices may provide a much more timely indication that a toxic reaction is underway than testing biologic fluids or tissues. However, because anaphylactic responses may be mediated by the immune system, results of tests for drug sensitivity or for antibodies that recognize thiopentone or other agents may constitute viable biomarkers of risk.

TECHNOLOGIC CONSIDERATIONS

The purpose of this section is to discuss methodologies involved in measuring the proposed biomarkers. The development of tests for detecting antibodies is the main focus because such techniques are the result of some of the most exciting research in anesthetic toxicology. The type of technology used in this research has the potential to revolutionize clinical anesthesiology practice by vastly increasing anesthetic safety.

Methods for measuring some biomarkers can be very complex and time consuming, whereas for others, results can be obtained in a relatively short time. A biomarker of risk, such as F^-, is easily determined because ion-specific electrodes are available. A serum sample need only be diluted into a specific buffer, and the concentration of F^- can then be determined by immersing the electrode in the solution. Because this assay can be accomplished within an hour of obtaining serum, timely information can be obtained regarding impending nephrotoxicity. A high concentration of F^- can be detected before concentrations of serum creatinine or urea nitrogen are elevated.

Inhalational anesthetics and their volatile metabolites also can be determined quickly. Gas chromatographic and mass spectrographic techniques exist for most, and samples of expired gas or serum or both can be tested relatively easily. Thus, these biomarkers of exposure can be measured in a timely manner. From a clinical standpoint, however, biomarkers of risk generally provide more valuable information.

Because the immune system may be involved in many adverse reactions to an-

esthetics, methodologies that can detect anesthetic-specific or metabolite-specific antibodies that are biomarkers of risk may provide valuable tools for identifying individuals who are prone to toxic reactions. Once such individuals are identified, appropriate (alternative) anesthetics can be chosen to minimize risk. The extensive research on halothane hepatitis provides good examples of this type of technology.

Enzyme-linked immunosorbant assays (ELISA) are useful for detecting anti-TFA antibodies (52) that may be biomarkers of risk for developing halothane hepatitis. A typical ELISA procedure for detecting these antibodies has been described (53). Briefly, a solution containing TFA-modified protein is incubated in the wells of a 96-well, microtiter plate for several hours to adsorb the proteins to the plastic. The plates are washed to remove any unbound TFA-modified protein and incubated with another protein solution to bind any remaining unbound protein-binding sites on the plates. The sample to be tested for the presence of antibody (serum from patients, for example) is serially diluted, and samples at each dilution are incubated at room temperature in the microtiter plate for 1 to 3 hours. This is usually sufficient time for any anti-TFA antibody that may be in the diluted samples of serum to react with the TFA-modified proteins. The wells are washed with a buffered casein solution to remove the serum. Next, they are incubated for 3 hours at room temperature with a solution of peroxidase-conjugated antibody that recognizes human IgG. The perioxidase-conjugated anti-human IgG will bind only to those wells in which anti-TFA antibodies are present. When a color-producing substrate for the peroxidase is incubated in the wells, the amount of color produced in each well is directly dependent on the amount of antibody that recognized the adsorbed TFA-protein. In this manner, not only can the presence of anti-TFA antibody be confirmed, but the titer of antibody can be determined as well. The lowest detectable dilution, expressed as the inverse of the dilution, is the titer. The higher the titer, the greater the initial concentration of antibody.

As with any test of this nature, one must have access to proteins that have been modified by trifluoroacetyl chloride. One possible method for obtaining TFA-modified proteins for this assay has been described (53). Rabbits were anesthetized with 1% halothane in 99% oxygen for 45 minutes, and 18 hours later, the animals were killed and the livers were removed. The livers were homogenized, and a microsomal fraction was obtained by differential centrifugation. (Microsomes are composed of revesicularized fragments of endoplasmic reticulum that precipitate during centrifugation at 100,000 g.) The microsomal fraction is a good source of TFA-modified proteins (31,33,34) because the cytochrome P450 enzymes that metabolize halothane to TFA are located in the endoplasmic reticulum. This source of TFA-modified proteins has the theoretical advantage of supplying as a test antigen those TFA neoantigens that were produced by the rabbit *in vivo* (other animals possibly could be used). As mentioned previously, TFA neoantigens are proteins that are modified by TFA *in vivo,* which then stimulate the immune system to produce anti-TFA antibodies. In theory, the neoantigens produced in a rabbit (and located in the endoplasmic reticulum) following exposure to halothane are similar to those neoantigens produced in a human because cytochrome P450 enzymes in both species metabolize halothane to TFA.

In an ELISA procedure such as that described, antibody reactions against TFA-modified proteins have to be compared to a reaction against non-TFA-modified proteins to subtract out any background or non-TFA-specific antibody reactions. In the example given, microsomes obtained from rabbits that were not treated with halothane are used as the source of nonmodified proteins to coat the nonreactive wells.

A major drawback to this source of TFA-

modified/non-modified proteins is the great amount of reactivity toward unmodified microsomal proteins from liver of non-anesthetized rabbits. This makes it difficult to determine a positive reaction when sera from patients will react with unmodified proteins. To attenuate this problem, sera can be mixed with microsomes from control rabbits before the ELISA procedure to neutralize nonanti-TFA antibodies that interfere with the test.

Strong background reactions occur with this source of TFA-modified proteins because evidently some regions of the TFA neoantigen that do not contain the TFA adduct, as well as those that do, are antigenic. Those neoantigens in humans are very likely similar to those in rabbits. Therefore, following halothane exposure in humans, antibodies are produced that recognize both nonmodified and TFA-modified portions of neoantigens from rabbits. In addition, some antibodies may react with proteins that were not TFA-modified and are not capable of TFA modification. These proteins simply may have a region with structural similarities to the antigenic portion of the TFA neoantigen(s). Figure 2 illustrates the production of antibodies from TFA neoantigens.

An alternative source of TFA-modified proteins can diminish, although not eliminate, the propensity of human sera to react with nonmodified proteins from other species. For example, a single purified protein, such as rabbit serum albumin (RSA), can be acetylated with ethylthiotrifluoroacetate (ethylthio-TFA). Most procedures used to produce TFA-RSA are similar to the one described by others (54). Ethylthio-TFA is added to RSA and incubated. Extensive dialysis against a neutral buffer to remove the nonreacted chemical yields a preparation of RSA in which approximately 85% of the lysine residues are modified by TFA (54). During the reaction, the ethylthio group leaves as the TFA binds to an exposed lysine. The TFA-RSA can then be used, instead of the liver microsomes from halo-

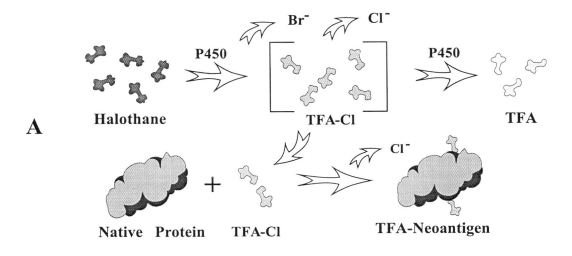

A

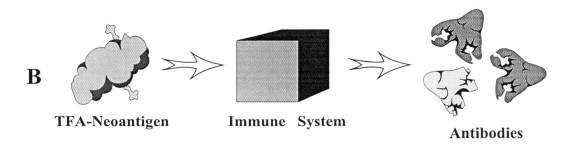

B

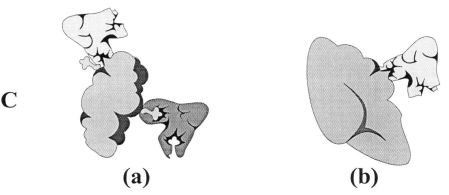

C

(a) **(b)**

FIG. 2. Production of antibodies following exposure to halothane. **A.** Halothane metabolism by cytochrome P450 produces TFA (via TFA-Cl). Some of the TFA-Cl may react with protein to produce TFA neoantigens. **B.** TFA neoantigen is presented to the immune system, and antibodies are produced against this protein. **C. (a)** Antibodies reacting against the TFA-modified portion of the TFA neoantigen. **(b)** Some antibodies may also crossreact with regions of other proteins that have structural similarities to a portion of the TFA neoantigen.

thane-treated rabbits, to coat the microtiter plates.

This substitution with RSA greatly reduces the amount of reaction that patient sera will have against the unreacted rabbit protein because the neoantigens in humans most likely do not have many antigenic portions that are similar to RSA. In addition, producing the test antigen in this manner is far faster and much less expensive than preparing cell fractions from tissue obtained from halothane-treated animals.

Using TFA-RSA does not completely eliminate the reaction of antibodies from patients' sera against unmodified RSA (33). In addition, because a single protein is being used as the TFA antigen, some of the antibodies that would recognize a TFA-modified protein (other than TFA-RSA) will not be detected, thus diminishing the sensitivity of the screening test.

Identifying those TFA conjugates that are likely to be involved in immune reactions producing halothane hepatitis would lead to the development of an ELISA test to predict risk more accurately. If the original neoantigens can be identified, ELISA tests that incorporate only these TFA-modified proteins rather than heterogeneous mixtures of modified and nonmodified proteins (microsomes) can be developed. Such screening tests should provide a much greater degree of sensitivity and accuracy compared to the tests currently in use.

To identify the TFA neoantigens, one must first have a mechanism to identify the non-TFA-modified protein. Antibodies that recognize both the TFA group and nonmodified portions of the TFA neoantigen are produced following exposure to halothane (Fig. 2). One can take advantage of this to identify the nonmodified neoantigen (55).

When liver microsomes from halothane-treated rats are subjected to polyacrylamide electrophoresis and the proteins are electrophoretically transferred onto nitrocellulose paper in a Western Blot procedure, anti-TFA antibodies from rabbits and sera from humans previously exposed to halo-

thane recognize the same proteins (55,56). Of the proteins recognized, the major one (a 59 kDa protein) is also recognized by the anti-TFA antibodies and sera even if the microsomes were obtained from nonhalothane-treated rats. Because sera obtained from patients with halothane hepatitis recognized the same protein from liver microsomes of halothane-treated and nonexposed rats (56), this rat protein might be the same or very similar to one of the neoantigens that produced initial sensitization to the TFA adduct. The amino acid sequence of this 59 kDa protein was determined, and the protein was identified as a serine-type carboxylesterase (55). Because this protein may represent one of the neoantigens that are modified by TFA, the use of this single protein as test antigen (when chemically modified by ethylthio-TFA) and as a control (nonmodified) in an ELISA procedure may produce a more sensitive test for anti-TFA antibodies.

Targets other than TFA-modified proteins also may be involved in the production of halothane hepatitis. Recently, TFA adducts of phospholipids were identified as a potential target for anti-TFA antibodies (54,57). Because a subset of anti-TFA antibodies apparently crossreacts with TFA-phospholipid adducts, the development of ELISA tests in the future that incorporate both TFA-protein and TFA-phospholipid adducts may provide information that predicts risk for hepatic damage even more accurately.

Through the continued efforts in immunotoxicologic research, the actual mechanisms of antibody-mediated cell damage in halothane hepatitis may one day be elucidated. Once the neoantigens and cell surface recognition sites are identified and their respective roles in the etiology of liver failure are determined, highly sensitive and accurate tests for determining risk for the development of such conditions can be produced, and strategies for the prevention of such conditions can be developed.

Similar immune mechanisms may be

involved in the production of toxic reactions to anesthetics other than halothane. Therefore, detection of anesthetic-specific (or metabolite-specific) antibodies based on similar techniques should provide a means to measure the appropriate biomarkers of risk for other anesthetics as well.

SUMMARY

The continuing development of tests for biomarkers of toxicity and risk, such as those described, will provide clinicians with the appropriate tools to select anesthetic agents that are least likely to precipitate a toxic reaction or recognize a toxic reaction in a timely manner so appropriate intervention can be initiated. With judicious use of the appropriate tests as they are developed, the apparent risks associated with anesthetic use may be greatly reduced.

ACKNOWLEDGMENT

I would like to thank Dale A. Chrystof, M.S., for her expert technical assistance in the preparation of this manuscript.

REFERENCES

1. Marshall B E, Longnecker D E. General anesthetics. In: Gilman A G, Rall T W, Nies A S, Tayler P, eds. *Goodman and Gilman's the pharmacological basis of therapeutics, 8th ed.* Elmsford, NY: Pergamon Press, 1990:285–310.
2. Committee on Biological Markers of the National Research Council. Biological markers in environmental health research. *Environ Health Persp* 1987;74:3–9.
3. Hulka B. Using biomarkers: views from an epidemiologist. *Health Environ* 1991;7:1–7.
4. Subcommittee on Immunotoxicology, Committee on Biologic Markers, of the National Research Council. *Biologic markers in immunotoxicology.* Washington, DC: National Academy Press, 1992.
5. Huggett R J, Kimerle, R A, Mehrle P M Jr, Bergman H L eds. *Biomarkers: biochemical, physiological, and histological markers of anthropogenic stress.* Chelsa, MI: Lewis Publishers, 1992.
6. Morgan E T, Koop D R, Coon M J. Comparison of six rabbit liver cytochrome P450 isozymes in formation of a reactive metabolite of acetaminophen. *Biochem Biophys Res Commun* 1983;112:8–13.
7. Tsutsumi R, Leo M A, Kim C-I, et al. Interaction of ethanol with enflurane metabolism and toxicity: role of P450-IIE1. *Alcohol Clin Exp Res* 1990;14:174–179.
8. Guirguis S S, Pelmear P L, Roy M L, Wong L. Health effects associated with exposure to anesthetic gases in Ontario hospital personnel. *Br J Ind Med* 1990;47:490–497.
9. Cohen E N, Bellvile J W, Brown, B W. Anesthesia, pregnancy and miscarriage—a study of operating room nurses and anesthetists. *Anesthesiology* 1971;35:343–347.
10. Knill-Jones R P, Moir D D, Rodrigues L V, Spence A A. Anaesthetic practice and pregnancy controlled survey of women anaesthetists in the United Kingdom. *Lancet* 1972;i:1326–1328.
11. Knill-Jones R P, Newman B J, Spence A A. Anesthetic practice and pregnancy-controlled survey of male anaesthetists in the United Kingdom. *Lancet* 1975;ii:807–809.
12. Pharoah P O D, Alberman E, Doyle P. Outcome of pregnancy among women in anesthetic practice. *Lancet* 1977;i:34–36.
13. Hague, C J R, Brewster M A. The potential of exposure markers in epidemiological studies of reproductive health. *Environ Health Persp* 1991;90:261–269.
14. Chanarin I. The effects of nitrous oxide on cobalamine, folates, and on related events. *CRC Crit Rev Toxicol* 1982;10:179–213.
15. Nunn J F. Clinical aspects of the interaction between nitrous oxide and vitamin B_{12}. *Br J Anaesth* 1987;59:3–13.
16. Kripke B J, Talarico L, Shah N K, Kelman A D. Hematologic reaction to prolonged exposure to nitrous oxide. *Anesthesiology* 1977;47:342–348.
17. Suzuki K S, Konno M, Kirikae T, et al. Effects of prolonged nitrous oxide exposure on hematopoietic stem cells in splenectomized mice. *Anesth Analg* 1990;1:389–393.
18. Chanarin I, Deacon R, Lumb M, Muir M, Perry J. Cobalamin-folate interrelationships: a critical review. *Blood* 1985;66:479–489.
19. O'Sullivan H, Jennings F, Ward K, et al. Human bone marrow biochemical function and megaloblastic hematopoiesis after nitrous oxide anesthesia. *Anesthesiology* 1981;55:645–649.
20. Gronert G A. Malignant hyperthermia. *Anesthesiology* 1980;53:294–312.
21. Bunker J P, Forrest W H, Mosteller F, et al. A study of the possible association between halothane anesthesia and postoperative hepatic necrosis In: *National halothane study.* Washington, DC: US Government Printing Office, 1969.
22. Rehder K, Forbes J, Alter H, Hessler O, Stier A. Halothane biotransformation in man: a quantitative study. *Anesthesiology* 1967;28:711–715.
23. Goldblum A, Loew G H. Quantum chemical

studies of anaerobic reductive metabolism of halothane by cytochrome P450. *Chem Biol Interact* 1980;32:83–99.

24. Rice S A, Sbordone L, Mazze R I. Metabolism by rat hepatic microsomes of fluorinated ether anesthetics following isoniazid administration. *Anesthesiology* 1980;53:489–493.

25. Jenner M A, Plummer J L, Cousins M J. Influence of isoniazid, phenabarbital, phenytoin, pregnenolone 16-α-Carbonitrile, and β-napthoflavone on halothane metabolism and hepatotoxicity. *Drug Metab Disp* 1990;18:819–822.

26. Van Dyke R A, Gandolfi A J. Studies on the irreversible binding of radioactivity from [¹⁴C]-halothane to rat hepatic microsomal lipids and protein. *Drug Metab Disp* 1974;2:469–476.

27. Edmunds H N, Trudell J R, Cohen E N. Low-level binding of halothane metabolites to rat liver histones *in vivo*. *Anesthesiology* 1981; 54:298–304.

28. Cohen E N, Trudell J R, Edmunds H N, Watson E. Urinary metabolites of halothane in man. *Anesthesiology* 1975;43:392–401.

29. Muller R, Stier A. Modifications of liver microsomal lipids by halothane metabolites: a multinuclear NMR spectroscopic study. *Naunyn-Schmiedeberg Arch Pharmacol* 1982;321:234–237.

30. Pohl L R, Satoh H, Christ D D, Kenna J G. The immunological and metabolic basis of drug hypersensitivities. *Annu Rev Pharmacol* 1988;28:367–368.

31. Kenna J G, Neuberger J, Williams R. Identification by immunoblotting of three halothane-induced liver microsomal polypeptide antigens recognized by antibodies in sera from patients with halothane-associated hepatis. *J Pharmacol Exp Ther* 1987;242:733–740.

32. Satoh H, Fukuda Y, Anderson D K, Ferrans V J, Gillette J R, Pohl L R. Immunological studies on the mechanism of halothane-induced hepatotoxicity: Immunohistochemical evidence of trifluoroacetylated hepatocytes. *J Pharmacol Exp Ther* 1985;233:857–862.

33. Hubbard A K, Roth T P, Gandolfi A J, Brown B R Jr, Webster N R, Nunn J F. Halothane hepatitis patients generate an antibody response toward a covalently bound metabolite of halothane. *Anesthesiology* 1988;68:791–796.

34. Pohl L R, Kenna J G, Satoh H, Christ D, Martin J L. Neoantigens associated with halothane hepatitis. *Drug Metab Rev* 1989;20:203–217.

35. Callis A H, Brooks S D, Roth T P, Gandolfi A J. Characterization of a halothane-induced humoral immune response in rabbits. *Clin Exp Immunol* 1987;67:343–351.

36. Christ D D, Kenna J G, Kammerer W, Satoh H, Pohl L R. Enflurane metabolism produces covalently bound liver adducts recognized by antibodies from patients with halothane hepatitis. *Anesthesiology* 1988;69:833–838.

37. Mazze R I, Calverly R K, Smith N T. Inorganic fluoride nephrotoxicity: prolonged enflurane and halothane anesthesia in volunteers. *Anesthesiology* 1977;46:265–271.

38. Dooley J R, Mazze R I, Rice S A, Borel J D. Is enflurane defluorination inducible in man? *Anesthesiology* 1979;50:213–217.

39. Greenstein L R, Hitt B A, Mazze R I. Metabolism *in vitro* of enflurane, isoflurane, and methoxyflurane. *Anesthesiology* 1975;42:420–424.

40. Blitt C D, Gandolfi A J, Soltis J J, Brown B R Jr. Extrahepatic biotransformation of halothane and enflurane. *Anesth Analg* 1981;60:129–132.

41. Sakai T, Takaori M. Biodegradation of halothane, enflurane, and methoxyflurane. *Br J Anaesth* 1978;50:785–791.

42. Cousins M J, Mazze R I. Methoxyflurane nephrotoxicity: a study of dose–response in man. *JAMA* 1973;216:1611–1612.

43. Holaday D A, Smith F R. Clinical characteristics and biotransformation of sevoflurane in healthy volunteers. *Anesthesiology* 1981;54:100–106.

44. Frink E J, Ghantous H, Malan T P, et al. Plasma inorganic fluoride with sevoflurane anesthesia: correlation with indices of hepatic and renal function. *Anesth Analg* 1992;74:231–235.

45. Koblin D D. Characteristics and implications of desflurane metabolism and toxicity. *Anesth Analg* 1992;75:S10–S16.

46. Weiskopf R B, Eger E I II, Ionescu P, et al. Desflurane does not produce hepatic or renal injury in human volunteers. *Anesth Analg* 1992;74:570–574.

47. Van Dyke R A, Mostafapour S, Marsh H M, Li Y, Chopp M. Immunocytochemical detection of the 72-kilodalton heat shock protein in halothane-induced hepatotoxicity in rats. *Life Sci* 1991;50:PL41–PL45.

48. Lindquist S. The heat-shock response. *Annu Rev Biochem* 1986;55:1151–1191.

49. Lindquist S, Craig E A. The heat-shock proteins. *Annu Rev Genet* 1988;22:631–677.

50. Watkins J W. Second report from an anesthetic reactions advisory service. *Anesthesia* 1989;44:157–159.

51. Dold M, Konarzewski W H. Delayed allergic response to propofol. *Anesthesia* 1989;44:533.

52. Martin B M, Kenna J G, Satoh H, Pohl L R. Assays for the detection of antibodies directed against halothane-induced liver neoantigens in the sera of patients with halothane hepatitis. *Anesthesiology* 1988;69:A439.

53. Kenna J G, Neuberger J, Williams R. An enzyme-linked immunosorbant assay for detection of antibodies against halothane-altered hepatocyte antigens. *J Immunol Methods* 1984;75:3–14.

54. Trudell J R, Ardies C M, Anderson W R. Antibodies raised against trifluoroacetyl-protein adducts bind to N-trifluoroacetyl-phosphatidylethanolamine in hexagonal phase phospholipid micelles. *J Pharmacol Exp Ther* 1991;257:657–662.

55. Satoh L, Martin B M, Schulick A H, Christ D D, Kenna J G, Pohl L R. Human anti-endoplasmic reticulum antibodies in sera of patients with halothane-induced hepatitis are directed

against a trifluoroacetylated carboxylesterase. *Proc Natl Acad Sci USA* 1989;86:322–326.

56. Kenna J G, Satoh H, Christ D D, Pohl L R. Metabolic basis for a drug hypersensitivity: antibodies in sera from patients with halothane hepatitis recognize liver neoantigens that con-

tain the trifluoroacetyl group derived from halothane. *J Pharmacol Exp Ther* 254:1103–1109.

57. Trudell J R, Ardies C M, Anderson W R. The effect of alcohol and anesthetic metabolites on cell membranes: a possible direct immune mechanism. *Ann NY Acad Sci* 1991;625,806–817.

Subject Index

Aspartate aminotransferase, AST (*contd.*)
  in halothane treated rats, 75
  in hepatotoxicity, 74,287,288

B
Barbiturates, in animal anesthesia, 24–25
Biologic response modifiers, BRM
  activities of, 243,253–254
  anesthesia effects on, 253–254
  nonspecific immune response and, 242–243
Biomarkers of toxicity
  ALT as,74, 283,287,288
  antibodies as, 287–288,290–294
  AST as, 74,75,283,287,288
  causal relationship proof and, 283,285
  defined, 281,283
  ELISA use in, 290,291
  exposure, 281
  fluoride as, 283,290
  of fluorinated anesthetics, 286–289
  generic types of, 283,284
  of intravenous anesthetics, 289–290
  of local anesthetics, 289–290
  measurement methods, 290–294
  of nitrous oxide, 285–286
  physiological markers and, 281
  of risk, 283
  stress proteins as, 289
  of susceptability, 282
β-Blockers, local anesthetic toxicity and, 118
Body temperature, *see also* Malignant hyperthermia
  regulation, 10
Bronchospasm, *see* Airway caliber
Bupivacaine
  cardiac arrest by, 109
  chemical structure,111
  as CVS depressant, 120,121–122,123–124
  development of, 108,109
  physiochemical properties, 111
  toxicity, 109,115,116,117,121,121,122
Butyrylcholinesterase, BChE
  dibucaine inhibition, 212
  genetic variants of, 199,200, 212–213
  liver synthesis, 212
  succinylcholine hydrolysis and, 199,200, 211–212

C
Calcium
  channels in MH, 210,220–221
  hepatotoxicity and, 79–80
  homeostasis, 79
  ryanodine receptor and, 220–221
  skeletal muscle contraction and, 220
Carbon dioxide, animal anesthesia and, 26

Carcinogenicity
  immune response and, 255–256,257
  isoflurane and, 61
  of volatile anesthetics, 6
Cardiovascular system, CVS
  arrhythmias and, 121–122
  cardiac output and, 120
  intracardiac conduction and, 121
  local anesthetic suppression, 120–124
  local anesthetic toxicity, 109–110,112,116, 117,119–124
  toxicity treatment, 124–125
Central nervous system, CNS
  arrhythmias and, 122–123,125
  convulsions and, 111–112,114,119
  depression, 118–119
  EEG monitoring, 119
  local anesthetic toxicity, 109,111–112,117, 118–119,122–123
  signs/symptoms of toxicity, 118–119
  toxicity treatment, 124–125
Chemotherapy, nitrous oxide enhancement, 149
Children
  airway irritation in, 275
  halothane toxicity in, 74–75
  isoflurane use in, 275
  local anesthetic toxicity in, 116–117
  sevoflurane use in, 101
Chloral hydrate, in animal anesthesia, 25
2-Chloro-1,1-difluorethane, CDE, as halothane metabolite, 75,76
Chloroprocaine
  physicochemical properties, 111
  toxicity,114
Cholinesterase, *see* Butyrylcholinesterase
Chronic obstructive pulmonary disease, COPD, HPV potentiation in, 271
Cimetidine
  immune response and, 259
  local anasthetic toxicity and, 118
  in prevention of anesthetic toxicity, 78
Cocaine
  addiction, 108
  historical aspects, 107–108
  as local anasthetic, 107, 108
  in spinal anesthesia, 108
  toxicity, 108
Codeine
  analgesic response to, 210
  metabolism, 210
Congenital abnormalities
  anesthetic exposure and, 45–46,176,177, 178–179,180,181,182–195
  gender differences in, 192
Continous spinal anesthesia, CSA
  microbore catheter use in, 126–127
  neurotoxicity of anesthetics in, 126–127
Cyclosporine, anesthetic toxicity and, 100

of isoflurane, 163,166
in vitro test systems, 160–161,170
in vivo test systems, 161–171
of local anesthetics, 170
methionine synthase and, 168,169
of methoxyflurane, 160,163,166
models of, 158–160
of nitrous oxide, 146,148,160–161,166–169
Reproduction and developmental toxicity, humans
abortion rate and, 182–189
conception rate and, 186
congenital abnormalities and, 45–46,176,
177,178–179,180,181,182–186,187
general anesthesia and, 176
local anesthetics and, 176
malformations and, 176
maternal/paternal exposure, 188–192
meta-analysis of, 195–196
nitrous oxide and, 160–161,163,166–169,
176,177–180,186
in nonobstetric surgery anesthesia,
176–181
in occupational anesthesia exposure, 5–6,
145–146,177,181–195
perinatal studies, 175–176
sex ratio and, 182–185
spinal anesthesia and, 176,179
stillbirths and, 181,182–185
Ropivacaine
CVS effects, 122
physiochemical properties, 111,115
toxicity, 115,116,120
Ryanodine receptor
genetics, 210–211,220
MH and, 210–211,220–221

S

Sendai virus infection, in research animals,
13–15,18
Sevoflurane
advantages/disadvantages, 101–102
chemical structure, 93
children and, 101
hepatotoxicity, 84
metabolism, 65–66,84,101–102
metabolism in obese, 54,55
nephrotoxicity, 101–102,104,288
safety of, 288
Smoking, enflurane metabolism and, 95
Spinal anesthesia
neutrophil migration in, 247
reproduction and development toxicity,
176,179
Stress proteins
halothane induced, 83
TFA proteins and, 83,289

Succinylcholine
BChE variant and, 199,200,212–213
MH induction, 210,220,228
pharmacogenetics, 211–213
Sudden infant death syndrome, SIDS, MH
association, 228
Superoxide
bactericidal activity and, 251–252
cytochrome P450 generation, 51
oxygen toxicity and, 277

T

Temperature regulation, anesthesia and, 221
Teratogenicity
of barbiturates, 169–170
factors influencing, 158
mechanisms, 158–159
methionine synthase inactivation and,
168,169
of nitrous oxide, 166–169
Tetracaine
local neurotoxicity of, 126
physiochemical properties, 111
toxicity, 115
Tetracycline
methoxyflurane use and, 100
renal fluoride and, 100
Therapeutic index, defined, 2
Toxicity
acid-base balance and, 113
acute, 2
age and, 116
chronic, 2
determinants, 1,4–5
dose-response curves, 2–3
epidemiology, 35–47,175–197
of fluoride, 89–104
lipid solubility and, 112
mechanisms, 3–4
metabolic disposition and, 10
neural, 125–127
preexisting conditions and, 98–100,116–117
prevention, 78
quantification, 1–2
reversibility, 4,157
species differences in, 10
threshold dose for, 3
treatment, 124–125
Tranquilizers
anesthesia potentiation by, 23–24
in animal anesthesia, 23–24
Tribromoethanol, in animal anesthesia, 25
Trifluoroacetate, TFA
antibodies, 81–82,287–288,290–294
as biomarker of toxicity, 287–288,289,
290–294
desflurane and, 65,101